Neuromodulation

Editors

SCOTT T. AARONSON
NOAH S. PHILIP

PSYCHIATRIC CLINICS OF NORTH AMERICA

www.psych.theclinics.com

Consulting Editor
HARSH K. TRIVEDI

September 2018 • Volume 41 • Number 3

ELSEVIER

1600 John F. Kennedy Boulevard • Suite 1800 • Philadelphia, Pennsylvania, 19103-2899

http://www.theclinics.com

PSYCHIATRIC CLINICS OF NORTH AMERICA Volume 41, Number 3
September 2018 ISSN 0193-953X, ISBN-13: 978-0-323-64132-6

Editor: Lauren Boyle
Developmental Editor: Kristen Helm

Psychiatric Clinics of North America (ISSN 0193-953X) is published quarterly by Elsevier Inc., 360 Park Avenue South, New York, NY 10010-1710. Months of issue are March, June, September, and December. Business and Editorial Offices: 1600 John F. Kennedy Blvd., Suite 1800, Philadelphia, PA 19103-2899. Periodicals postage paid at New York, NY and additional mailing offices. Subscription prices are $321.00 per year (US individuals), $666.00 per year (US institutions), $100.00 per year (US students/residents), $391.00 per year (Canadian individuals), $460.00 per year (international individuals), $838.00 per year (Canadian & international institutions), and $220.00 per year (Canadian & international students/residents). Foreign air speed delivery is included in all *Clinics*' subscription prices. All prices are subject to change without notice. **POSTMASTER:** Send address changes to *Psychiatric Clinics of North America*, Elsevier Health Sciences Division, Subscription Customer Service, 3251 Riverport Lane, Maryland Heights, MO 63043. **Customer Service: 1-800-654-2452 (US). From outside the United States, call 1-314-447-8871. Fax: 1-314-447-8029. E-mail: journalscustomerservice-usa@elsevier.com (for print support) and journalsonline support-usa@elsevier.com (for online support).**

Reprints. For copies of 100 or more, of articles in this publication, please contact the Commercial Reprints Department, Elsevier Inc., 360 Park Avenue South, New York, New York 10010-1710. Tel.: 212-633-3874, Fax: 212-633-3820, E-mail: reprints@elsevier.com.

Psychiatric Clinics of North America is covered in *MEDLINE/PubMed (Index Medicus)*, *Current Contents/Social and Behavioral Sciences, Social Science Citation Index, Embase/Excerpta Medica,* and PsycINFO.

Contributors

KEVIN A. CAULFIELD, MS
PhD Student, Brain Stimulation Laboratory, Medical University of South Carolina, Ralph H. Johnson VA Medical Center, Charleston, South Carolina, USA

CHARLES R. CONWAY, MD
Professor, Department of Psychiatry, Washington University School of Medicine, John Cochran VA Medical Center, St Louis, Missouri, USA

PAUL E. CROARKIN, DO, MS
Department of Psychiatry and Psychology, Mayo Clinic, Rochester, Minnesota, USA

DENIZ DORUK CAMSARI, MD
Department of Psychiatry and Psychology, Mayo Clinic, Rochester, Minnesota, USA

DARIN D. DOUGHERTY, MD, MMSc
Director, Division of Neurotherapeutics, Associate Professor, Department of Psychiatry, Massachusetts General Hospital, Harvard Medical School, Boston, Massachusetts, USA

SARAH L. GARNAAT, PhD
Assistant Professor (Research), Department of Psychiatry and Human Behavior, Warren Alpert Medical School of Brown University, Butler Hospital, Providence, Rhode Island, USA

MARK S. GEORGE, MD
Distinguished Professor of Psychiatry, Radiology, and Neuroscience, Layton McCurdy Endowed Chair, Director, Brain Stimulation Laboratory, Medical University of South Carolina, Ralph H. Johnson VA Medical Center, Charleston, South Carolina, USA

OLIVER M. GLASS, MD
Department of Psychiatry and Behavioral Sciences, Emory University School of Medicine, Atlanta, Georgia, USA

AISHWARYA K. GOSAI, BA
Department of Psychiatry, Massachusetts General Hospital, Harvard Medical School, Boston, Massachusetts, USA

BENJAMIN D. GREENBERG, MD, PhD
Butler Hospital, Brown University, VA RR&D Center for Neurorestoration and Neurotechnology, Providence VA Medical Center, Providence, Rhode Island, USA

ADRIANA P. HERMIDA, MD
Associate Professor, Geriatric Psychiatry Fellowship, Director, Department of Psychiatry and Behavioral Sciences, Emory University School of Medicine, Atlanta, Georgia, USA

MELISSA KIRKOVSKI, PhD
Deakin Child Study Centre, School of Psychology, Deakin University, Geelong, Australia

F. ANDREW KOZEL, MD, MSCR
HSR&D Center of Innovation on Disability and Rehabilitation Research (CINDRR), Mental Health and Behavioral Sciences, James A. Haley Veterans' Administration Hospital and Clinics, Department of Psychiatry and Behavioral Neurosciences, University of South Florida, Tampa, Florida, USA

COLLEEN K. LOO, MB BS, FRANZCP, MD
School of Psychiatry, University of New South Wales, Black Dog Institute, Prince of Wales Hospital, Sydney, New South Wales, Australia

WILLIAM V. McCALL, MD, MS
Professor, Department of Psychiatry and Health Behavior, Medical College of Georgia, Augusta University, Augusta, Georgia, USA

WILLIAM M. McDONALD, MD
Professor, JB Fuqua Chair for Late-Life Depression, Department of Psychiatry and Behavioral Sciences, Emory University School of Medicine, Atlanta, Georgia, USA

ALEXANDER McGIRR, MD, MSc, FRCPC
Department of Psychiatry, Hotchkiss Brain Institute, Mathison Centre for Mental Health Research and Education, University of Calgary, Calgary, Alberta, Canada

ADRIANO H. MOFFA, PsyD, Mphil
School of Psychiatry, University of New South Wales, Black Dog Institute, Prince of Wales Hospital, Sydney, New South Wales, Australia

STEVAN NIKOLIN, BSc, MCom
School of Psychiatry, University of New South Wales, Black Dog Institute, Prince of Wales Hospital, Sydney, New South Wales, Australia

NOAH S. PHILIP, MD
Associate Professor of Psychiatry and Human Behavior, Warren Alpert Medical School of Brown University, Director, Psychiatric Neuromodulation, Center for Neurorestoration and Neurotechnology, Providence VA Medical Center, Providence, Rhode Island, USA

PETER B. ROSENQUIST, MD
Professor, Department of Psychiatry and Health Behavior, Medical College of Georgia, Augusta University, Augusta, Georgia, USA

HADIA SHAFI, MD
Department of Psychiatry and Behavioral Sciences, Emory University School of Medicine, Atlanta, Georgia, USA

SANDARSH SURYA, MBBS
Assistant Professor, Department of Psychiatry and Health Behavior, Medical College of Georgia, Augusta University, Augusta, Georgia, USA

MUSTAFA TAHA BILGE, PhD
Department of Psychiatry, Massachusetts General Hospital, Harvard Medical School, Boston, Massachusetts, USA

HAIZHI WANG, MD, PhD
Resident Trainee, Department of Psychiatry and Human Behavior, Warren Alpert Medical School of Brown University, Providence, Rhode Island, USA

ALIK S. WIDGE, MD, PhD
Department of Psychiatry, Massachusetts General Hospital, Harvard Medical School, Boston, Massachusetts, USA; Picower Institute for Learning and Memory, Massachusetts Institute of Technology, Cambridge, Massachusetts, USA

WILLA XIONG, MD
PGY-4, Department of Psychiatry, Washington University School of Medicine in St. Louis, St Louis, Missouri, USA

NAGY A. YOUSSEF, MD
Associate Professor, Department of Psychiatry and Health Behavior, Medical College of Georgia, Augusta University, Augusta, Georgia, USA

SHIWEN YUAN, MD
Resident Trainee, Department of Psychiatry and Human Behavior, Warren Alpert Medical School of Brown University, Providence, Rhode Island, USA

Contents

The current practice of electroconvulsive therapy (ECT) has evolved over several decades with the implementation of safer equipment and advancement of techniques. In addition, modifications in the delivery of ECT, such as the utilization of brief and ultrabrief pulse widths and individualization of treatment parameters, have improved the safety of ECT without sacrificing efficacy. This article provides psychiatrists with a balanced, in-depth look into the recent advances in ECT technique as well as the evidence of ECT for managing depression in special populations and patients with comorbid medical problems.

The use of electroconvulsive therapy (ECT) for those suffering from major depressive disorder is well evidenced, time-honored, and recognized by most treatment guidelines. However, since its inception ECT has been used by practitioners for a broader range of neuropsychiatric conditions. This article reviews the highly variable evidence supporting the use of ECT in conditions other than depression, such as schizophrenia, bipolar manic states, catatonia, Parkinson disease, and posttraumatic stress disorder.

Deep brain stimulation has preliminary evidence of clinical efficacy but has been difficult to develop into a robust therapy, in part because its mechanisms are incompletely understood. The authors review evidence from movement and psychiatric disorder studies, with an emphasis on how deep brain stimulation changes brain networks. From this, they argue for a network-oriented approach to future deep brain stimulation studies. That network approach requires methods for identifying patients with specific circuit/network deficits. The authors describe how dimensional approaches to diagnoses may aid that identification. They discuss the use of network/circuit biomarkers to develop self-adjusting "closed loop" systems.

Deep brain stimulation has been used for decades in neurology to treat movement disorders. More recent work has focused on developing applications for deep brain stimulation in psychiatric illness. Initial studies have demonstrated positive results for treatment-refractory obsessive-compulsive disorder. Initial open-label studies of deep brain stimulation at targets for treatment-resistant depression have been encouraging. However, the only 2 published controlled trials that were conducted for potential US Food and Drug Administration approval for treatment-resistant depression were both negative. Future directions include potential use of alternate clinical trial designs, using tractography for more refined deep brain stimulation electrode targeting, and closed-loop deep brain stimulation approaches.

Stimulation of the left cervical vagus nerve, or vagus nerve stimulation (VNS), brings about an antidepressant response in a subset of patients with treatment-resistant depression (TRD). How this occurs is poorly understood; however, knowledge of the neuroanatomic vagal pathways, in conjunction with functional brain imaging studies, suggests several brain regions associated with mood regulation are critical: brainstem nuclei (locus coeruleus, dorsal raphe, and ventral tegmental area), thalamus, and insular and prefrontal cortex. Furthermore, animal studies suggest that VNS enhances neuroplasticity and changes in neuronal firing patterns. Continued study to better understand the mechanism of action of VNS in TRD is warranted.

Vagus nerve stimulation (VNS) has been studied for its effect on treatment-resistant depression. Open-label studies have shown a significant positive effect in an especially treatment-resistant depressive population. Insurance company support for VNS has been limited but may be reviewed given recent positive open-label data. Coming developments in novel external ways to stimulate the vagus nerve may revive interest in this area. This article reviews the clinical development of VNS starting with the first recognition of its potential for treating depression, parses the results of several large clinical trials, and suggests a future path for optimal clinical development and use.

Transcranial magnetic stimulation has emerged as a treatment option for treatment-resistant depression. Although existing data largely support efficacy of transcranial magnetic stimulation for major depressive disorder, ongoing research aims to optimize treatment parameters and identify biomarkers of treatment response. In this article, the authors describe data from controlled trials and ongoing efforts to enhance transcranial magnetic stimulation outcomes for major depressive disorder. Findings from preliminary research aimed at identifying neuroimaging and neurophysiologic biomarkers of transcranial magnetic stimulation effects are discussed.

Repetitive transcranial magnetic stimulation (rTMS) is being investigated
for psychiatric disorders, such as posttraumatic stress disorder (PTSD),
generalized anxiety disorder (GAD), and both phases of bipolar disorder.
Case series, open trials, and randomized controlled studies have demonstrated preliminary support for treating PTSD with rTMS alone as well as
with rTMS combined with psychotherapy. Similarly, there is some evidence that GAD can be treated with rTMS. The results for treating either
phase of bipolar disorder are mixed, with most of the current studies
showing lack of benefit over sham. Further study is required before
rTMS can be recommended for these disorders.

Transcranial direct current stimulation (tDCS) is a noninvasive brain stimulation technique that has been gaining favor as a viable tool in Psychiatry.
This review summarizes the evidence of tDCS as a treatment of disorders
such as depression, schizophrenia, and obsessive-compulsive disorder
(OCD). Current findings indicate that tDCS is probably effective in non-
treatment-resistant depressive patients. Regarding schizophrenia and
OCD, present evidence is not robust enough, although preliminary results
indicate that tDCS is a promising technique. Therefore, more trials are
needed before using tDCS in a clinical setting.

Recent advances and growing evidence supporting the safety and efficacy
of noninvasive neuromodulatory techniques in adults have facilitated the
study of neuromodulation applications in children and adolescents. Noninvasive brain stimulation methods such as transcranial direct current stimulation and transcranial magnetic stimulation have been considered in
children with depression, autism spectrum disorder, attention-deficit hyperactivity disorder, and other neuropsychiatric disorders. However, current clinical applications of neuromodulation techniques in children and
adolescents are nascent. There is a great need for developmentally
informed, large, double-blinded, randomized, controlled clinical trials to
demonstrate efficacy and safety of noninvasive brain stimulation in children and adolescents.

Although the application of noninvasive brain stimulation methods to
children and adolescents has been frequently studied in depression, autism
spectrum disorder, attention-deficit hyperactivity disorder, and other

PSYCHIATRIC CLINICS OF NORTH AMERICA

THE CLINICS ARE AVAILABLE ONLINE!
Access your subscription at:
www.theclinics.com

PSYCHIATRIC CLINICS OF
NORTH AMERICA

RELATED INTEREST

Preface

Neuromodulation

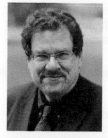 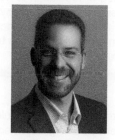

Scott T. Aaronson, MD   Noah S. Philip, MD
Editors

INTRODUCTION

Psychiatric neuromodulation is defined as any intervention intended to alter nervous system function using energy fields such as electricity, magnetism, or both, with the goal to improve psychiatric symptoms or related conditions. This concept is not new: neuromodulation, in one form or another, has been used to treat physical maladies for over a thousand years,[1] although its use for psychiatric disorders became popular in the past century. Since the 1930s,[2] electroconvulsive therapy (ECT) has been recognized as an effective treatment for severe depression, catatonia, and other severe mental health disorders. Over the following decades, newer technologies emerged, including vagus nerve stimulation (VNS), repetitive transcranial magnetic stimulation (rTMS), and deep brain stimulation (DBS); in the last decade, there has been renewed interest in other emerging technologies, including novel adaptations or approaches to rTMS (ie, those synchronized to brain rhythms; eg, Leuchter and colleagues[3]) or employing novel stimulation patterns (eg, Li and colleagues[4]), and low-intensity electrical stimulation.[5]

For a number of reasons, psychiatric neuromodulation has seen a recent surge of interest in clinical and research domains. Neuromodulation, at its core, targets electrical activity within brain networks, acting through different mechanisms than pharmacotherapy, offering the potential of treatment success, where medications have failed. Identifying and targeting specific neural circuitry or functional neural networks to reduce psychiatric symptoms may offer a level of mechanistic focality beyond that offered by ECT, pharmacotherapy, or most psychotherapies. Furthermore, despite decades of research, all currently available psychiatric pharmacology depends, in one form or another, on the manipulation of neurotransmitters related to the monoamine hypothesis.[6] While this approach was successful in bringing initial treatments to market, significant numbers of patients remain symptomatic despite the best evidence-based interventions.[7–9] Other systems, such as acetylcholine, seemed initially promising but ended in trial failure.[10,11] Furthermore, even the most promising new pharmacologic approach targeting the NMDA system with ketamine

Psychiatr Clin N Am 41 (2018) xiii–xvi
https://doi.org/10.1016/j.psc.2018.06.001
0193-953X/18/© 2018 Published by Elsevier Inc.

(eg, Murrough and colleagues[12]) has yet to translate into approved treatments, and early use indicates concern about safe long-term use.[13]

Another key driver in the application of clinical neuromodulation is its favorable side-effect profile. Clinicians, who are accustomed to managing and accepting a certain degree of side effects alongside clinical efficacy, may find the limited side effects of neuromodulation to be quite attractive. Neuromodulation is not associated with the risks of weight gain, diabetes, and sexual side effects shared by many pharmacologic interventions. Furthermore, outside of the risk of cognitive side effects of ECT, most adverse experiences with neuromodulation are constrained to treatment site discomfort and a very low risk of an isolated seizure event.[14]

DR PHILIP'S STORY

On a personal note, the story of how I started using neuromodulation was not straightforward. At the end of my psychiatry residency training, I worked under my mentor, Dr Linda Carpenter, on several different device-based clinical trials for depression at Butler Hospital. These included late-stage studies of VNS and DBS, and some of the early work in rTMS. This work continued into a neuromodulation fellowship, during which I more directly worked in rTMS while simultaneously managing an inpatient service at our local psychiatry hospital for about 3 years. During this time, I saw patients come and go, and despite my best efforts, many patients did not achieve meaningful improvement with my best-intentioned pharmacotherapy and psychotherapy. Yet, one observation was consistent: regardless of whether the medications worked, all my patients returned with a significant side-effect burden. A young man with first onset psychosis returned just as psychotic, and with diabetes and significant weight gain. A woman with severe depression returned with her depression, and now with no sexual drive and a feeling of emotional numbness. Another returned with crippling anxiety, now in addition to chronic gastrointestinal symptoms from their medication. Unfortunately, this is a partial list, and the memories go on. Some patients did quite well, but yet others did not, and not only did the medications not work, but also the patients were afflicted with side effects from my prescribing. As a physician, I took an oath to "do no harm," and I questioned whether I was doing the right thing. On the other hand, I was able to refer patients into this new area of neuromodulation, and particularly to our rTMS clinic. True, this didn't work for everyone, but when it didn't work, there were no crippling side effects with which to contend. After a few years, there was an opportunity for me to start my own neuromodulation service at the Providence VA, Rhode Island, and I took the opportunity as fast as I could. This is a field in its relative infancy, but the potential to reduce patients' symptoms is very real and reachable in the near term. While the greatest work to date remains in depression, I remain hopeful and optimistic that lessons learned from using neuromodulation in depression can be applied more broadly in the near term, to yield an entirely different way to care for patients suffering from these terrible diseases.

DR AARONSON'S STORY

I had never intended to become a "device guy." My career has been devoted to the recognition and treatment of severe, often treatment-refractory, mood disorders. After starting down a clinical/research path after residency, I grew frustrated with the limitations of clinical investigation and founded a large multidisciplinary outpatient practice with a focus on mood disorders, which, after 10 years, I further expanded to add a clinical trials component. This rekindled my research interests and led to my assuming the role of Director of the newly created Clinical Research Program at Sheppard Pratt Health System in

Baltimore, Maryland. Once established there doing phase 2 and 3 trials for the pharmaceutical industry in depression, I was asked to take over care for a cohort of VNS patients treated in the original double-blind trial and was also invited to be a rescue site for the original registration trial for the first TMS device. From there, my participation in device trials expanded exponentially to becoming the lead investigator for several VNS studies and a senior investigator in numerous TMS and tDCS trials as well as creating the new TMS service at my hospital, where we have treated over 300 patients over 9 years of operation.

At my core, my most fervent wish is that I do something to alleviate the suffering of people with severe mood disorders. I have been impressed by the science, the data, and the outcomes I've seen with my research and clinical work in neuromodulation.

SPECIAL ISSUE OF PSYCHIATRIC CLINICS OF NORTH AMERICA: NEUROMODULATION

With these thoughts in mind, this special issue of *Psychiatric Clinics of North America* is devoted to neuromodulation, to provide a concise, usable overview of current and future clinical brain stimulation. In editing this issue, we enlisted eminent thinkers who are both clinicians and researchers, to provide their thoughts on the dominant brain stimulation modalities. The issue is organized loosely by chronologic order, following the order in which the technologies were developed. It starts with the most ancient of technologies, convulsive therapy, and ends with reflections on future brain stimulation approaches. On the journey therein, we hope the reader will find a trove of valuable information and wisdom on transcranial magnetic and electrical stimulation. For those who already live and breathe neuromodulation, we hope our collection prompts you to think critically about your current practice and research, and for our newer colleagues and trainees, we hope this endeavor opens your eyes to one of the fastest-growing and most exciting areas in psychiatry.

Scott T. Aaronson, MD
Clinical Research Programs
Sheppard Pratt Health System
6501 North Charles Street
Baltimore, MD 21204, USA

Noah S. Philip, MD
Department of Psychiatry and Human Behavior
Alpert Medical School of Brown University
Psychiatric Neuromodulation
Center for Neurorestoration and Neurotechnology
Providence VA Medical Center
830 Chalkstone Avenue
Providence, RI 02908, USA

E-mail addresses:
SAaronson@sheppardpratt.org (S.T. Aaronson)
noah_philip@brown.edu (N.S. Philip)

REFERENCES

1. Heidland A, Fazeli G, Klassen A, et al. Neuromuscular electrostimulation techniques: historical aspects and current possibilities in treatment of pain and muscle wasting. Clin Nephrol 2013;79(suppl 1):S12–23.

2. Fink M. Meduna and the origins of convulsive therapy. Am J Psychiatry 1984; 141(9):1034–41.

3. Leuchter AF, Cook IA, Feifel D, et al. Efficacy and safety of low-field synchronized transcranial magnetic stimulation (sTMS) for treatment of major depression. Brain Stimul 2015;8(4):787–94.
4. Li CT, Chen MH, Juan CH, et al. Efficacy of prefrontal theta-burst stimulation in refractory depression: a randomized sham-controlled study. Brain 2014;137(7): 2088–98.
5. Philip NS, Nelson BG, Frohlich F, et al. Low-intensity transcranial current stimulation in psychiatry. Am J Psychiatry 2017;174(7):628–39.
6. Hillhouse TM, Porter JH. A brief history of the development of antidepressant drugs: from monoamines to glutamate. Exp Clin Psychopharmacol 2015;23(1):1–21.
7. Gaynes BN, Warden D, Trivedi MH, et al. What did STAR*D teach us? Results from a large-scale, practical, clinical trial for patients with depression. Psychiatr Serv 2009;60(11):1439–45.
8. Peters AT, Nierenberg AA. Stepping back to step forward: lessons from the Systematic Treatment Enhancement Program for Bipolar Disorder (STEP-BD). J Clin Psychiatry 2011;72(10):1429–31.
9. Swartz MS, Stroup S, McEvoy JP, et al. Special section on implications of CATIE: what CATIE found: results from schizophrenia trial. Psychiatr Serv 2008;59(5): 500–6.
10. Philip NS, Carpenter LL, Tyrka AR, et al. Nicotinic acetylcholine receptors and depression: a review of the preclinical and clinical literature. Psychopharmacology 2010;212(1):1–12.
11. Vieta E, Thase ME, Naber D, et al. Efficacy and tolerability of flexibly-dosed adjunct TC-5214 (dexmecamylamine) in patients with major depressive disorder and inadequate response to prior antidepressant. Eur Neuropsychopharmacol 2014;24(4):564–74.
12. Murrough JW, Iosifescu DV, Chang LC, et al. Antidepressant efficacy of ketamine in treatment-resistant major depression: a two-site randomized controlled trial. Am J Psychiatry 2013;170(10):1134–42.
13. Schak KM, Vande Voort JL, Johnson EK, et al. Potential risks of poorly monitored ketamine use in depression treatment. Am J Psychiatry 2016;173(3):215–8.
14. McClintock SM, Reti IM, Carpenter LL, et al. Consensus recommendations for the clinical application of repetitive transcranial magnetic stimulation (rTMS) in the treatment of depression. J Clin Psychiatry 2018;79(1). https://doi.org/10.4088/JCP.16cs10905.

Electroconvulsive Therapy in Depression

Current Practice and Future Direction

Adriana P. Hermida, MD*, Oliver M. Glass, MD, Hadia Shafi, MD,
William M. McDonald, MD

KEYWORDS

- Electroconvulsive therapy • Neuromodulation • Treatment-resistant depression
- Major depression • Review • Electrode placement • Cognitive side effects

KEY POINTS

- Electroconvulsive therapy (ECT) in conjunction with pharmacotherapy is superior to pharmacotherapy alone for management of treatment-resistant depression.
- Psychotic features and increased age are both positive predictive factors for a response to ECT. Acknowledging positive predictive factors can assist providers in deciding whether a patient would be a good candidate for ECT.
- Flexible treatment schedules after the acute course could improve remission rates and reduce unnecessary side effects.
- ECT tolerability and cognitive side effects can be improved by individualizing ECT treatment parameters.
- With refinements in the ECT technique for the treatment of special populations suffering from depression, complex medical conditions can be treated safely with ECT with fewer medical complications.

INTRODUCTION

It has been estimated that within the next 20 years depression will be the leading cause of disability in high-income nations.[1] Although pharmacotherapy may be effective for many with major depressive disorders (MDD), one-third of individuals will not

Disclosure Statement: No disclosures or conflict of interest (A.P. Hermida, O.M. Glass, and H. Shafi). Research support from the National Institute of Mental Health, National Institute of Neurological Disease and Stroke, Patient-Centered Outcomes Research Institute, Stanley Foundation, Soterix, Neuronetics, and Cervel Neurotherapeutics. Consultant on the Neurologic Devices Panel of the Medical Devices Advisory Committee, Center for Devices and Radiological Health, Food and Drug Administration, and member of an ad hoc member of several NIMH and NINDS study sections (W.M. McDonald).
Department of Psychiatry and Behavioral Sciences, Emory University School of Medicine, 12 Executive Park Drive Northeast, Atlanta, GA 30329, USA
* Corresponding author.
E-mail address: ahermid@emory.edu

Psychiatr Clin N Am 41 (2018) 341–353
https://doi.org/10.1016/j.psc.2018.04.001
0193-953X/18/© 2018 Elsevier Inc. All rights reserved.

respond to antidepressants.[2] As a result, a significant group of individuals with MDD will require alternative therapeutic modalities to address their depression. ECT has robust evidence to support its use in the treatment of MDD, particularly in patients with severe presentation of illness.

Unfortunately, electroconvulsive therapy (ECT) has historically suffered a damaging stigma that has limited its use. Much of the negative opinion can be traced back to the early years of ECT when it was administered without muscle relaxants and anesthesia. Memory loss remains a common primary concern among patients with ECT; however, the ECT electrode placement and parameters can now be modified to decrease the risk for that potential side effect. In addition, ECT machines used before the mid 1980s relied on a sinusoidal pulse wave that has been linked to significant cognitive deficits compared with the ultrabrief (UB) and brief (B) pulse waves that are used with modern technology.[3]

This article is intended to provide psychiatrists with a balanced, in-depth look at the recent advances in ECT technique as well as the evidence of ECT for managing depression including MDD in patients with comorbid medical problems.

THE MECHANISM OF ACTION

The mechanism of action of ECT remains poorly understood. Hypotheses range from ECT's involvement in targeting neurotransmitter and neuroendocrine dysregulation, GABAergic anticonvulsant effects, and involvement on the molecular level. Because ECT triggers a generalized seizure, there are biological changes that cannot be attributed to a singular mechanism of action.

ECT treatments are associated with normalization of hypothalamic–pituitary–adrenal axis in depressed patients, supporting a neuroendocrine mechanism.[4] The anticonvulsant theory,[5] the most widely accepted hypothesis, is based on the observation that ECT treatments result in an increase in the seizure threshold and a decrease in seizure duration over a course of ECT treatments. gamma-Aminobutyric acid (GABA) has been postulated as a key mediator of the ECT anticonvulsant effect.[5] The changes in GABA transmission secondary to ECT suggest that there may be an increase in tonic inhibition after repeated seizures.[6] The glutamate system is intrinsically related to GABA.[7] Seizures are accompanied by acute release of glutamate, which serves as the predominant mode of excitatory neurotransmission in the brain,[8] possibly causing the cognitive side effects.[9]

Imoto and colleagues[10] demonstrated that inducing seizures in animal models profoundly changed biochemical and physiologic features of mature granule cells in the hippocampal dentate gyrus (DG), more so than selective serotonin reuptake inhibitors treatments. The investigators of the same study suggested that "dematuration" of neurons in the DG could be a common cellular basis for antidepressant therapy.

Narp, an immediate early gene induced by electroconvulsive seizures (ECS), plays a key role in brain-derived neurotrophic factor (BDNF)–dependent synaptic modulation.[11] With repeated ECS, a rise in Narp protein can persist for nearly 24 hours, agglomerating in the hippocampus.[11] Chang and colleagues[11] concluded that Narp contributes to the antidepressant action of ECT and that ECS can induce dendritic arborization.

ECT has been shown to induce hippocampal neurogenesis[12] and neuroplasticity.[13] Schloesser and colleagues[14] reported that ECS leads to antidepressant effects with concurrent hippocampal neurogenesis. Neuroimaging studies[15] have revealed that ECT induces neuroplastic processes in the amygdala and hippocampus that are associated with improved clinical response in MDD. Although a complete understanding of how ECT works is not yet known, the ongoing advancement of technology and research is bringing it within our reach.

EFFICACY AND SAFETY

ECT is arguably the most efficacious treatment modality in psychiatry. ECT is superior to pharmacotherapy for unipolar major depression based on a UK meta-analysis published in the Lancet.[16] ECT has also been found to lower the number of readmissions to the hospital.[17] A retrospective longitudinal study by Cosculluela and colleagues[18] concluded that in a sample of 24 depressed patients, the hospital length of stay and number of hospitalizations over a period of 3 years became significantly reduced in patients receiving maintenance ECT (M-ECT). ECT is also associated with a decreased depression burden leading to improved quality of life.[19]

The adverse effects of ECT relate more to tolerability than safety. In fact, ECT is considered a safe treatment. Even though patients may fear death, the mortality rate is extremely low.[20] A recent systematic review[20] analyzed data from 766,180 ECT treatments across 32 countries yielding an ECT-related mortality rate of 2.1 per 100,000 treatments. Advances regarding anesthesia and improvements in the ECT technique over the years have not only decreased ECT-related complications but also improved cognitive outcomes and patient satisfaction.

WHEN TO CONSIDER ELECTROCONVULSIVE THERAPY IN THE TREATMENT OF DEPRESSION?

Unfortunately, the stigma revolving around ECT may limit its use. Some providers may still be under the impression that ECT should be left as a last resort for treating depression, even though the literature indicates the benefit of ECT is higher in those who have had fewer medications trials.[21] In the context of severe depression, ECT should be considered if the symptoms of depression are severely debilitating regardless of the number of medication trials attempted. Furthermore, ECT should also be considered as an early intervention in psychotic depression, where its efficacy is well-documented [22,23] and in emergency psychiatric cases (eg, suicidality, severe catatonia, neuroleptic malignant syndrome).[24–26] Perhaps most importantly, ECT has been shown to have a robust antisuicidal effect.[24] When patients are educated about the clinical efficacy of ECT, some may prefer to receive it earlier in the course of their depression than undergo several medication trials. Despite the wide range of benefits to ECT, the provider should carefully consider whether a patient is appropriate for ECT, by weighing the benefits versus risks.

CHOOSING ELECTRODE PLACEMENT AND TREATMENT PARAMETERS

Clinicians who use ECT should be familiarized with all modalities of electrode placement. There are 3 commonly used electrode placements in current ECT practice: right unilateral (RUL), bitemporal (BT), and bifrontal (BF), the last 2 of which are also referred to as bilateral (BL).

The decision on which electrode placement to use lies in the principle of maximizing efficacy while minimizing cognitive side effects. Advances in technology have led to improved efficacy with fewer cognitive side effects. The introduction of UB pulse width (eg, pulse width between 0.25 and 0.37 milliseconds) is one of the latest advances in ECT that has enhanced seizure efficiency with significantly fewer cognitive side effects. In a double-blind, randomized controlled trial[27] comparing UB-RUL-ECT (dosed at 8 times seizure threshold) to B-RUL-ECT (dosed at 5 times seizure threshold), the efficacy outcomes were not significantly different, but the UB group showed less cognitive impairment. A meta-analysis[28] comprising a total of 689 patients compared B with UB pulse RUL-ECT, and the results suggested that B-RUL-ECT has a small advantage in terms of efficacy, along with a higher remission rate. However, this slight increased efficacy in the B-RUL group came at the cost of significantly more cognitive side effects in all of the examined cognitive domains.

Current research supports initiating treatment with UB-RUL-ECT dosed at least 6 times the seizure threshold for major depression unless there are significant severity specifiers such as catatonia or previous failures to RUL treatments. If no response is achieved, then modification of the treatment can be implemented. Tew and colleagues[29] randomized 24 patients who failed to improve with moderate-charge RUL to either high-charge RUL or BL treatments. Patients in the BL group exhibited significantly greater cognitive impairment than those who received high-charge RUL-ECT. Clinical response in depressive symptom remission did not differ in the 2 groups. The investigators concluded that patients who fail to respond to moderate-charge RUL-ECT may benefit from a switch to high-charge RUL-ECT than to BL-ECT. In clinical practice, increasing the charge on UB-RUL seems an appropriate step. Some practitioners switch from UB-RUL to B-RUL after 4 to 6 treatments. However, the authors are currently unaware of any data that supports this strategy. Other clinicians may switch to BL if the patient fails to respond to RUL. The decision on whether to switch to BF or BT depends on cognitive function and the severity of symptoms. The authors are unaware of any systematic studies that compare these treatment approaches. More research is needed to establish an evidence-based step by step algorithm.

PREDICTORS OF RESPONSE

Several positive predictors of ECT response in MDD have been described in the literature. In a randomized clinical trial of 253 unipolar depressed individuals treated with ECT, Petrides and colleagues[30] found that those with psychotic depression had a significantly higher likelihood of obtaining remission compared with nonpsychotic depressed patients (83% vs 71%). Literature supports that older age and catatonic features are also positive predictors.[31,32]

The Consortium for Research in ECT[23] reported that an early response to ECT predicts long-term efficacy and greater severity of depression at baseline predicted a favorable response to ECT.

BDNF, the most widely distributed neurotrophin in the central nervous system with a central role in neurogenesis, has been suggested as a biomarker of response to ECT.[33] Higher serum levels of BDNF following ECT have been reported.[34] A recent meta-analysis[35] showed that higher levels of serum BDNF were associated with a successful course of ECT. BDNF serum elevation before an ECT course is associated with remission of depression, and a rise in BDNF after an ECT course has been shown to increase the likelihood for remission.[36] Although the sample size is small, functional MRI neuroimaging data suggest that a reduction in functional connectivity in the left dorsolateral prefrontal cortex post-ECT is associated with a therapeutic response in depressed patients.[37]

Some studies have supported the concept that MDD has hyperactive neuroinflammatory components that may be balanced by ECT.[38,39] Hestad and colleagues[40] described normalization of high pre-ECT serum tumor necrosis factor alpha levels, a cytokine involved in systemic inflammation, when patients responded favorably to an ECT course.

ADDRESSING RELAPSE

The relapse rate after an acute course of ECT has been reported to be between 50% and 84%[41,42] within 6 months. Several studies have shown that combining pharmacotherapy with M-ECT decreases relapse rates.[41,42] Literature has shown that when a patient is only provided with placebo after ECT, the risk of relapse can be as high as 84%.[42]

During the acute course of ECT, it is crucial for the clinician to consider changing the patient's failed antidepressant medications to a category that the patient has not failed or tried in the past.[43] Simply continuing the patient on their current unsuccessful antidepressant regimen may increase the chance of relapse.[43] Pharmacologically, tricyclic antidepressants have the largest evidence in relapse prevention after ECT.[41]

According to the Prolonging Remission in the Depressed Elderly (PRIDE) study, UB-RUL-ECT with venlafaxine is highly efficacious in the treatment of late life depression.[44] A recent meta-analysis[45] of 5 studies involving 436 patients, who entered remission after an acute course of ECT, showed that continuation ECT and M-ECT with pharmacotherapy was associated with significantly fewer relapses and recurrences within the first year when compared with pharmacotherapy alone.

Computer-assisted cognitive behavior therapy (CCBT) after an index course of ECT to prevent relapse has been reported.[46] The subjects in the study who achieved remission were treated in an open label study with CCBT and remained well at 6 months. Previous studies have reported that CBT in combination with antidepressants might be an effective continuation treatment to sustain response after successful ECT in patients with MDD.[47]

Traditionally, continuation ECT is administered at scheduled intervals in the 6 month after an acute ECT course. However, the PRIDE study[48] demonstrated effectiveness when rescue ECT was administered only when there was a worsening in depression, as measured by an increase in the HAM-D. Therefore, rather than stopping ECT, a slow taper with a flexible approach may be a reasonable strategy to minimize relapse.

MINIMIZING COGNITIVE SIDE EFFECTS

ECT may result in acute transient disorientation, immediately following treatment, and may also lead to anterograde and/or retrograde amnesia.[49] Although a small proportion of patients have reported permanent memory loss, most of the research studies have consistently demonstrated that memory impairment associated with ECT is transient and tends to resolve within a few months.[50]

Modern ECT mitigates cognitive side effects by individualizing the stimulus dosing, modifying the electrode placement, altering the pulse amplitude and width, and/or adjusting the administration frequency.

Individualizing Stimulus

Several strategies have been used to calculate the initial stimulus dosing. The "half-age method"[51] halves the patient's age, which then produces a number for the provider that can be used to set the initial percent charge. Although this method is used worldwide, providers do not take into consideration that in some parts of the world the output of the ECT is double the output of the machines used in the United States. Similarly, the age method, which would be double the half-age method, is still in use by some, but may use a charge that is substantially higher than the seizure threshold. Other stimulus dosing strategies include the fixed dose and calculated-dose paradigm, which refers to the use of preselected dosing tables provided by the machine manufacturer company.

However, neither the patient's age nor any other combination of demographic variables is a completely reliable means of estimating the seizure threshold[52] because concomitant medications may also affect the seizure threshold. In an attempt to individualize the stimulus relative to the individual seizure threshold, the seizure titration[53] method has been implemented. It provides a stepwise application of ECT stimuli at an initial level that is anticipated to be subthreshold and then at increasing levels until a seizure is elicited. The estimated seizure threshold is then used to guide dosing levels in subsequent sessions. Researchers have shown that patients who have been titrated have less cognitive side effects than those who have received a fixed dose.[52]

Electrode Placement

There is general consensus among psychiatry providers that RUL-ECT is associated with less cognitive side effects compared with BL-ECT. RUL-ECT at supra-seizure threshold (6×) has been demonstrated to be generally as effective as BT-ECT (1.5×) with significantly less severe and persistent cognitive effects.[54,55] BF-ECT,[56] which avoids direct stimulation of the temporal lobes, has been demonstrated to have equal antidepressant efficacy to BT-ECT but with fewer cognitive side effects.

Empirical data on the use of frontoparietal electrode placement[57] suggest efficacy with less cognitive side effects than RUL. Limited data from small double-blind and open trials relating to left anterior right temporal (LART) placement[58] have supported its efficacy and decreased cognitive side effects compared with BL-ECT.[59] More research is needed before adopting this approach in clinical practice.

Parameter Configuration

Theoretically, shortening the pulse width used can result in depolarizing neurons at lower energy and decreasing cognitive side effects while maintaining efficacy. UB pulse, where the pulse width is less than 0.5 milliseconds, has been shown to produce fewer cognitive side effects than B pulse (pulse width >0.5 milliseconds).[60] Robust research supports the fact that UB-RUL may be equivalent in efficacy to more intense forms of ECT, but with substantially less memory impairment.[61] Data looking at UB-RUL in the treatment of late life patients with severe depression demonstrated not only its efficacy but also an excellent safety and tolerability profile.[48]

Recent studies have explored the feasibility of low-amplitude ECT and have revealed that conventional amplitudes substantially exceed the neural activation threshold in most brain structures.[62] Low-amplitude stimulus can induce seizures effectively while producing fewer cognitive side effects.[63] In addition, researchers investigated the effect of creating more focal seizures (that may not generalize as readily to memory structures such as the hippocampus) using varying electrode placements[64] and high-energy magnetic stimulation pulses[65] to improve cognitive safety with ECT while maintaining efficacy.

Monitoring Electroconvulsive Therapy Memory Impairment

Early detection of the emergence of cognitive side effects during the ECT course is important because providers can then adjust the treatment approach. Bedside tools to monitor memory issues include the Montreal Cognitive Assessment (MOCA) and the Mini Mental Status Examination. These tools, however, were not developed to evaluate the cognitive deficits presented in the context of ECT. The ElectroConvulsive Cognitive Assessment (ECCA), a 30-question, easy to administer bedside test, has been designed to assess the specific cognitive domains that are affected in ECT, including retrograde autobiographical amnesia.[66] The ECCA has been shown to be more sensitive to ECT cognitive changes than the MOCA. Preliminary results show that the ECCA is a practical and sensitive tool during ECT clinical practice. The results of cognitive testing should be routinely reviewed during the course of treatment to influence appropriate clinical decision-making (eg, holding or ending treatment and/or changing ECT treatment parameters).

Memory loss is one of the most concerning side effects that may occur secondary to ECT. As outlined earlier, several aspects on the ECT technique can be modified to minimize this adverse effect. Furthermore, this particular risk is outweighed by the treatment's life-saving benefit. In fact, many patients may be willing to experience transient changes in memory function in exchange for the relief of suffering from their severe depression.

SPECIAL POPULATIONS

In this section, the authors review the available literature for individualizing ECT parameters for specific populations that may benefit from such treatment.

The Geriatric Population

Geriatric depression may respond to ECT more favorably than other ages.[67] Based on findings from the PRIDE study, patients receiving ~ 7 ECT treatments with UB-RUL, 3 times a week, at 6 times the seizure threshold along with venlafaxine, showed a response and remission rate of 70% and 61%, respectively.[44] An increase in stimulus dose by 50% midcourse for slow or no response seems to be beneficial.[44] In PRIDE Phase II, administration of four M-ECT treatments at a fixed interval along with rescue treatments with venlafaxine plus lithium resulted in lower depression severity at 24 weeks postinitial remission.[48] It should be noted that the prevalence of cognitive impairment post-ECT may be higher in geriatric patients.[2]

The Depressed Suicidal Patient

ECT seems to have rapid short-term beneficial effects in those with suicidality. Kellner and colleagues[68] showed that those with unipolar depression had rapid relief of suicidal intent after receiving BT-ECT. A nationwide retrospective cohort by Liang and colleagues[69] found that ECT treatment was associated with a 19.7% lower risk of suicide when compared with treatment with medication. Thus, ECT may be beneficial when considered earlier in the course of treatment when the patient is suicidal.

Parkinson Disease Depression

ECT is beneficial for treating the depressive symptoms secondary to Parkinson disease (PD), with improvement seen in up to 66% of affected patients. Patients with PD will likely see an improvement in motor symptoms, which is hypothesized to be secondary to ECT-mediated dopamine receptor responsiveness and transmission.[70]

M-ECT in patients with PD depression has been minimally studied, but cognitive complaints and delirium seem to be the most common reasons for discontinuing ECT.[71] Holding PD medication the morning of ECT, carefully monitoring cognition during the course of ECT, and treating with UB-RUL twice weekly[70] can mitigate the risks discussed earlier.

Poststroke Depression

Prevalence of poststroke depression (PSD) can be as high as 30%, and it is associated with poor recovery, greater cognitive impairment, and higher mortality rates.[72] Based on the authors' review of the literature, there are no controlled or comparison trials that demonstrate the effectiveness of ECT versus medication in the setting of

PSD. Guidelines are lacking in regard to the wait period between the occurrence of the stroke and initiation of ECT treatments, as well as regarding the safety of ECT in post-hemorrhagic stroke. Review of case reports for ECT in PSD showed that the time from stroke to first ECT treatment, when reported, usually ranges between 1 and 15 months. The patients with PSD receiving ECT were often older, had greater severity of depressive illness, or had a significant history of intolerance to antidepressants. There are reports of improvement in mood symptoms with both BL and RUL.[73,74] The role of M-ECT for PSD requires further study because relapse rates post-ECT have been shown to be high.[2] Although no worsening of cerebrovascular status has been reported in patients with PSD receiving ECT,[74] it is imperative to optimize cerebrovascular accident (CVA) risk factors, while weighing the risk versus benefits of ECT treatments before the administration of ECT. It is crucial for medical staff involved in the ECT treatments to be adequately trained in recognizing the early signs and symptoms of CVA.[75]

Depression in Pregnancy

Based on retrospective case reviews, both BL and RUL ECT are considered to be safe in all trimesters and no teratogenic or long-term deficit have been shown with intrauterine ECT exposure.[76,77] Transient fetal arrhythmia is the most commonly cited fetal adverse event, which is possibly because of fetal hypoxia, and can potentially be mitigated by pre-oxygenation, avoiding hyperventilation, and right hip tilt to relieve aorto-caval pressure.[77] Premature labor and uterine contractions seem to be the most commonly reported maternal adverse outcomes, the latter of which is due to a seizure-induced release of oxytocin. Furthermore, short-term use of tocolytics (labor suppressants), such as ritodrine or magnesium, have been found helpful in some cases of premature uterine contractions.[76,78] The efficacy of the abovementioned tocolytic agents have been found to be comparable, but magnesium has specific neuroprotective effects for preterm births that occur before 32 weeks.[79]

Psychotic depression in pregnancy usually responds well to ECT without significant adverse events.[77] Antipsychotic medications have teratogenic potential and lack safety data during pregnancy. This holds true especially during the first trimester, and so providers may prefer ECT as a treatment modality in this population group.[76,78]

Guidelines regarding maternal and fetal parameters are lacking. ECT treatment in itself does not seem to have a causal relationship with premature labor. Assessment of overall maternal risk by implementing collaboration between anesthesia, obstetrics, and psychiatry is crucial. A neonatal intensive care unit with an in-house obstetrician should be available as the pregnancy progresses.[76,78]

SUMMARY

ECT has evolved rapidly over the past decade with the implementation of safer equipment and advancement of techniques. Additionally, modifications in the delivery of ECT, such as modified anesthesia regimens have improved the safety of ECT. Adapting treatment plans to personalize the frequency of treatments needed to maintain remission, as supported by research outlined in the PRIDE study, encourages practitioners to consider less rigid treatment plans. Flexible treatment schedules after the acute course could improve remission rates and reduce unnecessary side effects. With refinements in the ECT technique for the treatment of special populations suffering from depression, complex medical conditions can be treated with fewer medical complications. Through a collaborative care model, different medical specialties should work together to elaborate comprehensive practice recommendations that focus on modifying the ECT technique according to each special population. Although ECT has been stigmatized historically, the current practice of ECT continues to improve through exciting state-of-the-art research. Looking retrospectively, some may marvel at the longitudinal resilience of the practice of ECT and understand that this signals its profound value. ECT continues to remain an important and highly effective treatment modality in the treatment of major depression.

REFERENCES

1. Gonzalez HM, Vega WA, Williams DR, et al. Depression care in the United States: too little for too few. Arch Gen Psychiatry 2010;67(1):37–46.
2. Riva-Posse P, Hermida AP, McDonald WM. The role of electroconvulsive and neuromodulation therapies in the treatment of geriatric depression. Psychiatr Clin North Am 2013;36(4):607–30.
3. Fujita A, Nakaaki S, Segawa K, et al. Memory, attention, and executive functions before and after sine and pulse wave electroconvulsive therapies for treatment-resistant major depression. J ECT 2006;22(2):107–12.
4. McKay MS, Zakzanis KK. The impact of treatment on HPA axis activity in unipolar major depression. J Psychiatr Res 2010;44(3):183–92.
5. Duthie AC, Perrin JS, Bennett DM, et al. Anticonvulsant mechanisms of electroconvulsive therapy and relation to therapeutic efficacy. J ECT 2015;31(3):173–8.
6. Farrant M, Nusser Z. Variations on an inhibitory theme: phasic and tonic activation of GABA(A) receptors. Nat Rev Neurosci 2005;6(3):215–29.
7. Petroff OA. GABA and glutamate in the human brain. Neuroscientist 2002;8(6): 562–73.
8. Cho CH. New mechanism for glutamate hypothesis in epilepsy. Front Cell Neurosci 2013;7:127.
9. Zhang J, Narr KL, Woods RP, et al. Glutamate normalization with ECT treatment response in major depression. Mol Psychiatry 2013;18(3):268–70.
10. Imoto Y, Segi-Nishida E, Suzuki H, et al. Rapid and stable changes in maturation-related phenotypes of the adult hippocampal neurons by electroconvulsive treatment. Mol Brain 2017;10(1):8.
11. Chang AD, Vaidya PV, Retzbach EP, et al. Narp mediates antidepressant-like effects of electroconvulsive seizures. Neuropsychopharmacology 2018;43(5): 1088–98.
12. Rotheneichner P, Lange S, O'Sullivan A, et al. Hippocampal neurogenesis and antidepressive therapy: shocking relations. Neural Plast 2014;2014:723915.
13. Abbott CC, Jones T, Lemke NT, et al. Hippocampal structural and functional changes associated with electroconvulsive therapy response. Transl Psychiatry 2014;4:e483.
14. Schloesser RJ, Orvoen S, Jimenez DV, et al. Antidepressant-like effects of electroconvulsive seizures require adult neurogenesis in a neuroendocrine model of depression. Brain Stimul 2015;8(5):862–7.
15. Joshi SH, Espinoza RT, Pirnia T, et al. Structural plasticity of the hippocampus and amygdala induced by electroconvulsive therapy in major depression. Biol Psychiatry 2016;79(4):282–92.
16. UK ECT Review Group. Efficacy and safety of electroconvulsive therapy in depressive disorders: a systematic review and meta-analysis. Lancet 2003; 361(9360):799–808.

17. Slade EP, Jahn DR, Regenold WT, et al. Association of electroconvulsive therapy with psychiatric readmissions in US hospitals. JAMA Psychiatry 2017;74(8): 798–804.
18. Cosculluela A, Cobo J, Martínez-Amorós E, et al. Effectivity and cost-effectivity of the maintenance electroconvulsive therapy: a mirror naturalistic analysis. Actas Esp Psiquiatr 2017;45(6):257–67.
19. McCall WV, Lisanby SH, Rosenquist PB, et al. Effects of continuation electroconvulsive therapy on quality of life in elderly depressed patients: a randomized clinical trial. J Psychiatr Res 2018;97:65–9.
20. Torring N, Sanghani SN, Petrides G, et al. The mortality rate of electroconvulsive therapy: a systematic review and pooled analysis. Acta Psychiatr Scand 2017; 135(5):388–97.
21. Prudic J, Sackeim HA, Devanand DP. Medication resistance and clinical response to electroconvulsive therapy. Psychiatry Res 1990;31(3):287–96.
22. Kellner CH, Knapp RG, Petrides G, et al. Continuation electroconvulsive therapy vs pharmacotherapy for relapse prevention in major depression: a multisite study from the consortium for research in electroconvulsive therapy (CORE). Arch Gen Psychiatry 2006;63(12):1337–44.
23. Husain MM, Rush AJ, Fink M, et al. Speed of response and remission in major depressive disorder with acute electroconvulsive therapy (ECT): a consortium for research in ECT (CORE) report. J Clin Psychiatry 2004;65(4):485–91.
24. Fink M, Kellner CH, McCall WV. The role of ECT in suicide prevention. J ECT 2014; 30(1):5–9.
25. Luchini F, Medda P, Mariani MG, et al. Electroconvulsive therapy in catatonic patients: efficacy and predictors of response. World J Psychiatry 2015;5(2):182–92.
26. Wittenauer Welsh J, Janjua AU, Garlow SJ, et al. Use of expert consultation in a complex case of neuroleptic malignant syndrome requiring electroconvulsive therapy. J Psychiatr Pract 2016;22(6):484–9.
27. Loo CK, Katalinic N, Smith DJ, et al. A randomized controlled trial of brief and ultrabrief pulse right unilateral electroconvulsive therapy. Int J Neuropsychopharmacol 2014;18(1) [pii:pyu045].
28. Tor PC, Bautovich A, Wang MJ, et al. A systematic review and meta-analysis of brief versus ultrabrief right unilateral electroconvulsive therapy for depression. J Clin Psychiatry 2015;76(9):e1092–8.
29. Tew JD Jr, Mulsant BH, Haskett RF, et al. A randomized comparison of high-charge right unilateral electroconvulsive therapy and bilateral electroconvulsive therapy in older depressed patients who failed to respond to 5 to 8 moderate-charge right unilateral treatments. J Clin Psychiatry 2002;63(12):1102–5.
30. Petrides G, Fink M, Husain MM, et al. ECT remission rates in psychotic versus nonpsychotic depressed patients: a report from CORE. J ECT 2001;17(4): 244–53.
31. Birkenhager TK, Pluijms EM, Ju MR, et al. Influence of age on the efficacy of electroconvulsive therapy in major depression: a retrospective study. J Affect Disord 2010;126(1–2):257–61.
32. Fink M, Kellner CH, McCall WV. Optimizing ECT technique in treating catatonia. J ECT 2016;32(3):149–50.
33. Fernandes B, Gama CS, Massuda R, et al. Serum brain-derived neurotrophic factor (BDNF) is not associated with response to electroconvulsive therapy (ECT): a pilot study in drug resistant depressed patients. Neurosci Lett 2009;453(3): 195–8.

34. Bocchio-Chiavetto L, Zanardini R, Bortolomasi M, et al. Electroconvulsive therapy (ECT) increases serum brain derived neurotrophic factor (BDNF) in drug resistant depressed patients. Eur Neuropsychopharmacol 2006;16(8):620–4.

35. Rocha RB, Dondossola ER, Grande AJ, et al. Increased BDNF levels after electroconvulsive therapy in patients with major depressive disorder: a meta-analysis study. J Psychiatr Res 2016;83:47–53.

36. Freire TF, Fleck MP, da Rocha NS. Remission of depression following electroconvulsive therapy (ECT) is associated with higher levels of brain-derived neurotrophic factor (BDNF). Brain Res Bull 2016;121:263–9.

37. Perrin JS, Merz S, Bennett DM, et al. Electroconvulsive therapy reduces frontal cortical connectivity in severe depressive disorder. Proc Natl Acad Sci U S A 2012;109(14):5464–8.

38. Hermida AP, McDonald WM, Steenland K, et al. The association between late-life depression, mild cognitive impairment and dementia: is inflammation the missing link? Expert Rev Neurother 2012;12(11):1339–50.

39. Brites D, Fernandes A. Neuroinflammation and depression: microglia activation, extracellular microvesicles and microRNA dysregulation. Front Cell Neurosci 2015;9:476.

40. Hestad KA, Tonseth S, Stoen CD, et al. Raised plasma levels of tumor necrosis factor alpha in patients with depression: normalization during electroconvulsive therapy. J ECT 2003;19(4):183–8.

41. Jelovac A, Kolshus E, McLoughlin DM. Relapse following successful electroconvulsive therapy for major depression: a meta-analysis. Neuropsychopharmacology 2013;38(12):2467–74.

42. Sackeim HA, Haskett RF, Mulsant BH, et al. Continuation pharmacotherapy in the prevention of relapse following electroconvulsive therapy: a randomized controlled trial. JAMA 2001;285(10):1299–307.

43. Sackeim HA. Continuation therapy following ECT: directions for future research. Psychopharmacol Bull 1994;30(3):501–21.

44. Kellner CH, Husain MM, Knapp RG, et al. Right unilateral ultrabrief pulse ECT in geriatric depression: phase 1 of the PRIDE study. Am J Psychiatry 2016;173(11):1101–9.

45. Elias A, Phutane VH, Clarke S, et al. Electroconvulsive therapy in the continuation and maintenance treatment of depression: systematic review and meta-analyses. Aust N Z J Psychiatry 2018;52(5):415–24.

46. Wilkinson ST, Ostroff RB, Sanacora G. Computer-assisted cognitive behavior therapy to prevent relapse following electroconvulsive therapy. J ECT 2017;33(1):52–7.

47. Brakemeier EL, Merkl A, Wilbertz G, et al. Cognitive-behavioral therapy as continuation treatment to sustain response after electroconvulsive therapy in depression: a randomized controlled trial. Biol Psychiatry 2014;76(3):194–202.

48. Kellner CH, Husain MM, Knapp RG, et al. A novel strategy for continuation ECT in geriatric depression: phase 2 of the PRIDE study. Am J Psychiatry 2016;173(11):1110–8.

49. Semkovska M, McLoughlin DM. Measuring retrograde autobiographical amnesia following electroconvulsive therapy: historical perspective and current issues. J ECT 2013;29(2):127–33.

50. Semkovska M, McLoughlin DM. Objective cognitive performance associated with electroconvulsive therapy for depression: a systematic review and meta-analysis. Biol Psychiatry 2010;68(6):568–77.

51. Petrides G, Fink M. The "half-age" stimulation strategy for ECT dosing. Convuls Ther 1996;12(3):138–46.

52. McCall WV, Reboussin DM, Weiner RD, et al. Titrated moderately suprathreshold vs fixed high-dose right unilateral electroconvulsive therapy: acute antidepressant and cognitive effects. Arch Gen Psychiatry 2000;57(5):438–44.

53. Petrides G, Braga RJ, Fink M, et al. Seizure threshold in a large sample: implications for stimulus dosing strategies in bilateral electroconvulsive therapy: a report from CORE. J ECT 2009;25(4):232–7.

54. Sackeim HA, Prudic J, Devanand DP, et al. A prospective, randomized, double-blind comparison of bilateral and right unilateral electroconvulsive therapy at different stimulus intensities. Arch Gen Psychiatry 2000;57(5):425–34.

55. Sackeim HA, Dillingham EM, Prudic J, et al. Effect of concomitant pharmacotherapy on electroconvulsive therapy outcomes: short-term efficacy and adverse effects. Arch Gen Psychiatry 2009;66(7):729–37.

56. Sienaert P, Vansteelandt K, Demyttenaere K, et al. Randomized comparison of ultra-brief bifrontal and unilateral electroconvulsive therapy for major depression: clinical efficacy. J Affect Disord 2009;116(1–2):106–12.

57. Loo CK, Bai S, Martin D, et al. Revisiting frontoparietal montage in electroconvulsive therapy: clinical observations and computer modeling: a future treatment option for unilateral electroconvulsive therapy. J ECT 2015;31(1):e7–13.

58. Swartz CM. Physiological response to ECT stimulus dose. Psychiatry Res 2000; 97(2–3):229–35.

59. Weiss AM, Hansen SM, Safranko I, et al. Effectiveness of left anterior right temporal electrode placement in electroconvulsive therapy: 3 case reports. J ECT 2015; 31(1):e1–3.

60. Sackeim HA, Prudic J, Nobler MS, et al. Effects of pulse width and electrode placement on the efficacy and cognitive effects of electroconvulsive therapy. Brain Stimul 2008;1(2):71–83.

61. Rasmussen KG. The PRIDE study and the conduct of electroconvulsive therapy: questions answered and unanswered. J ECT 2017;33(4):225–8.

62. Peterchev AV, Krystal AD, Rosa MA, et al. Individualized low-amplitude seizure therapy: minimizing current for electroconvulsive therapy and magnetic seizure therapy. Neuropsychopharmacology 2015;40(9):2076–84.

63. Youssef NA, Sidhom E. Feasibility, safety, and preliminary efficacy of low amplitude seizure therapy (LAP-ST): a proof of concept clinical trial in man. J Affect Disord 2017;222:1–6.

64. Borckardt JJ, Linder KJ, Ricci R, et al. Focal electrically administered therapy: device parameter effects on stimulus perception in humans. J ECT 2009;25(2): 91–8.

65. Cycowicz YM, Rowny SB, Luber B, et al. Differences in seizure expression between magnetic seizure therapy and electroconvulsive shock. J ECT 2017. https://doi.org/10.1097/YCT.0000000000000470.

66. Hermida AP, Henderson S, Tang Y, et al. Validation of a brief cognitive tool (ECA) designed specifically for use during and after electroconvulsive therapy ISEN abstracts. J ECT 2015;31(3):e32–9.

67. McDonald WM. Neuromodulation treatments for geriatric mood and cognitive disorders. Am J Geriatr Psychiatry 2016;24(12):1130–41.

68. Kellner CH, Fink M, Knapp R, et al. Relief of expressed suicidal intent by ECT: a consortium for research in ECT study. Am J Psychiatry 2005;162(5):977–82.

69. Liang CS, Chung CH, Ho PS, et al. Superior anti-suicidal effects of electroconvulsive therapy in unipolar disorder and bipolar depression. Bipolar Disord 2017. https://doi.org/10.1111/bdi.12589.
70. Kennedy R, Mittal D, O'Jile J. Electroconvulsive therapy in movement disorders: an update. J Neuropsychiatry Clin Neurosci 2003;15(4):407–21.
71. Kramer BA. A naturalistic review of maintenance ECT at a university setting. J ECT 1999;15(4):262–9.
72. Mitchell AJ, Sheth B, Gill J, et al. Prevalence and predictors of post-stroke mood disorders: a meta-analysis and meta-regression of depression, anxiety and adjustment disorder. Gen Hosp Psychiatry 2017;47:48–60.
73. Weintraub D, Lippmann SB. Electroconvulsive therapy in the acute poststroke period. J ECT 2000;16(4):415–8.
74. Murray GB, Shea V, Conn DK. Electroconvulsive therapy for poststroke depression. J Clin Psychiatry 1986;47(5):258–60.
75. Bruce BB, Henry ME, Greer DM. Ischemic stroke after electroconvulsive therapy. J ECT 2006;22(2):150–2.
76. Saatcioglu O, Tomruk NB. The use of electroconvulsive therapy in pregnancy: a review. Isr J Psychiatry Relat Sci 2011;48(1):6–11.
77. Anderson ELR, Reti IM. ECT in pregnancy: a review of the literature from 1941 to 2007. Psychosom Med 2009;71(2):235–42.
78. Leiknes KA, Cooke MJ, Jarosch-von Schweder L, et al. Electroconvulsive therapy during pregnancy: a systematic review of case studies. Arch Womens Ment Health 2015;18(1):1–39.
79. Kim MK, Lee SM, Oh JW, et al. Efficacy and side effect of ritodrine and magnesium sulfate in threatened preterm labor. Obstet Gynecol Sci 2018;61(1):63–70.

When All Else Fails
The Use of Electroconvulsive Therapy for Conditions Other than Major Depressive Episode

Peter B. Rosenquist, MD*, Nagy A. Youssef, MD,
Sandarsh Surya, MBBS, William V. McCall, MD, MS

KEYWORDS

- Electroconvulsive therapy • Indications • Schizophrenia • Bipolar disorder • Mania
- Post-traumatic stress disorder • Catatonia

KEY POINTS

- Draft guidance prepared by the FDA Office of Device Evaluation for the first time specifies a labeled indication for ECT, restricted to major depressive episode, but ECT practitioners may appropriately provide treatment of other "off-label" conditions.
- Limited evidence supports the inclusion of ECT in the treatment guidelines for treatment-resistant schizophrenia, bipolar mania, and mixed states and catatonia.
- Use of ECT in PTSD and Parkinson disease is encouraging; however, the overall body of evidence is insufficient to support use of ECT as a primary intervention in these conditions because of limited research, sample size, and design limitations. However, there is no rationale for foregoing ECT treatment of another primary indication if comorbid with these conditions, because anecdotal evidence suggests there may be symptomatic improvement and no clear evidence for harm.

INTRODUCTION

In 1938, the US Congress passed the Food, Drug and Cosmetic Act, which gave the Food and Drug Administration (FDA) the authority to oversee and ensure the safety of products meant for human consumption. That same year, the Italians, Ugo Cerletti and

Dr P.B. Rosenquist discloses current research funding from NIMH (R01MH09S776A1), American Foundation for Suicide Prevention, Lumosity Corporation (66324S-13), Merck (8S0073-9), ALS Association, GlaxoSmithKline, Harvard Stem Cell Institute, Neurologic Clinical Research Institute (701419-18), and MECTA Corporation (72200S-2). Dr N.A. Youssef discloses current research supported by American Foundation for Suicide Prevention (DIG-0-087-13), Merck, MECTA Corporation, ABR Corporation, and Veterans Administration. Dr S. Surya has no disclosures. Dr W. V. McCall discloses current research support from NIMH, American Foundation for Suicide Prevention, Merck, and MECTA Corporation.
Department of Psychiatry and Health Behavior, Medical College of Georgia at Augusta University, Augusta, GA, USA
* Corresponding author. 997 Street Sebastian Way, Augusta, GA 30912.
E-mail address: prosenquist@augusta.edu

Lucio Bini, collaborated to develop electroconvulsive therapy (ECT). In 1976, the Dalkon Shield intrauterine device injured at least 900,000 women in the United States, which aided passage of the Medical Device Regulation Act bringing medical devices under the purview of the FDA. Accordingly, ECT was afforded "grandfather" status and classified as a class III (highest risk) device until 2015 when the FDA Office of Device Management proposed new rules for the reclassification of ECT devices as class II (intermediate risk) in recognition of the large body of evidence with regard to its safety.[1] The draft guidance prepared by the FDA Office of Device Evaluation for the first time specified a labeled indication for ECT, restricted to major depressive episode associated with unipolar or bipolar disorder, and for those "patients 18 years of age and older who are treatment-resistant, or who require a rapid response due to the severity of their psychiatric or medical condition." The guidance identifies several populations for which there is "Lack of evidence for efficacy or safety", including, schizophrenia, schizophreniform disorder, schizoaffective disorder, and bipolar mania or mixed states."[2]

Although product labeling is an important mechanism for promoting safe and effective products, the FDA does not define scope of practice. It is therefore understood that physicians may prescribe treatments that are off-label in accordance with professional judgment. This practice is widespread and generally accepted. A recent survey indicated that in a group of commonly used medications in an office-based practice, 21% were for an off-label use, although of concern was the survey's judgment that 73% of those medications had poor or no scientific support for the stated indication.[3] Given the high frequency of treatment resistance across the full spectrum of mental disorders, it is likely that the judicious off-label use of ECT will continue. The impeccable clinician will consult the evidence, document the rationale, and communicate uncertainties as part of the informed consent process.

In this review, we examine certain conditions that are considered off-label indications for ECT under the proposed FDA reclassification, namely schizophrenia, bipolar mania, catatonia, Parkinson disease (PD), and post-traumatic stress disorder (PTSD). We weigh the published evidence to address two main questions: whether the evidence supports the use of ECT, and what recommendations may be offered as to how ECT should be used.

SCHIZOPHRENIA

Among the off-label indications for ECT, schizophrenia emerges as the most time-honored, has the largest empirical basis, and correspondingly greater inclusion in published treatment guidelines. However, there remain sufficient criticisms regarding the evidence base to give pause to clinicians and those who define the coverage policy for national health services and private insurance. The Schizophrenia Patient Outcomes Research Team: Updated Treatment Recommendations make no mention of ECT.[4] In the most recent versions of World Federation of Societies of Biological Psychiatry Guidelines, ECT achieved a low-ranking recommendation as a treatment option, reserved for treatment-resistant schizophrenia as an add-on to antipsychotic treatment and for schizophrenia with catatonic features.[5] The United Kingdom National Institute for Health and Care Excellence guideline on the use of ECT[6] concluded that there was insufficient evidence to endorse the general use of ECT in the management of schizophrenia but did allow that ECT might be effective in acute episodes of schizophrenia with catatonic features, might reduce the likelihood of relapses, and that the combination of ECT and pharmacotherapy might be more effective than pharmacotherapy alone.

Similar reserved endorsements emerged from a Cochrane review of randomized controlled trials (RCTs) of ECT for schizophrenia.[7] The authors note that most studies favor real ECT and suggest that ECT resulted in fewer relapses and a greater likelihood of being discharged from the hospital. In eight RCTs (n = 419 patients) that directly compared ECT with antipsychotic medications, the results favored medications, but importantly when ECT was added to antipsychotics the combination was superior to antipsychotics alone. ECT was considered an option when the treatment aim was rapid global improvement and symptomatic reduction, and for patients whose illnesses had shown only a limited response to medication alone.

A gold standard for clinical trials involving devices in the modern era includes a sham arm to compare with the active device. **Table 1** compares the sham-controlled published RCTs that reveal small sample sizes; heterogeneous approaches to patient selection, diagnosis, and outcome assessment; and ECT technique.[8–13] All studies included concurrent antipsychotic pharmacotherapy equally to all groups, so these studies are best characterized as ECT plus pharmacotherapy versus pharmacotherapy alone (sham ECT). Overall, ECT outperformed sham ECT in four of six trials, despite short treatment courses.

Several controlled trials have addressed the possible limitation of inadequate duration of ECT treatment, in the context of antipsychotic drug failure. Chanpattana and coworkers[14] studied a group of patients who had failed to respond during an acute exacerbation of psychosis to a minimum of two antipsychotics from at least two different classes, each equivalent to 750 mg chlorpromazine equivalents daily. Patients had a baseline Brief Psychiatric Rating Scale (BPRS) score of at least 35, and more than a 2-year duration of illness. In recognition of the chronic nature of the illness, the study used a two-phase design. The first phase was an open-label acute trial of ECT/antipsychotic medication in combination, followed by a 3-week stabilization period during which ECT was tapered. Responders who sustained improvement during the stabilization period were then randomized in a 6-month continuation phase to receive either treatment alone or in combination. In the acute phase 114 patients with schizophrenia were enrolled. The study also controlled antipsychotic doses, with all patients receiving flupenthixol, 12 mg/d, in the first week and increased as tolerated to 24 mg/d in the second week, while receiving bitemporal (BT) brief pulse ECT at threshold three times a week. ECT was continued until patients achieved the response criteria (defined a priori as a reduction in the BPRS to 25 or less) or received a maximum of 20 treatments at which time they were declared nonresponders. A total of 101 patients completed the study with 58 responders and 43 nonresponders. Baseline BPRS scores before/and after treatment were 49.1 ($\pm$ 9.6)/18.7 ($\pm$ 7.2) in responders and 51.4 ($\pm$ 9.4)/39.4 ($\pm$ 8.3) in nonresponders ($P<.001$). The average number of ECT treatments for responders was 13.9 ($\pm$ 4.8), and nonresponders received 20.4 ($\pm$ 0.8) treatments. In this study, and a subsequent larger study by the same authors (N = 293; 54.6% responders), responders were characterized as younger, with less extensive family history of schizophrenia, shorter durations of present episode and total illness, higher rates of psychiatric admission, more paranoid type, lower baseline negative symptoms, and higher baseline Global Assessment of Functioning score compared with nonresponders.[15]

In a randomized, single-blind study, Petrides and colleagues[16] focused on treatment-resistant patients with schizophrenia on a stable dose of clozapine for at least 8 weeks, with persistent psychotic symptoms ($\geq$12 in the BPRS psychosis subscale) and no current mood symptoms. Patients were subsequently randomized to receive 8 weeks of BT ECT (3 times a week for the first 4 weeks, then twice a week for 4 weeks) in addition to clozapine or to continue with clozapine treatment

Table 1
Randomized, controlled studies of ECT in schizophrenia

Study	Randomized Comparison	Sample	Diagnostic Criteria	ECT Technique	Outcome Measures	Main Results
Brandon et al,[8] 1984 "Leicester Trial"	BL ECT + antipsychotic (n = 9) vs sham ECT + antipsychotic (n = 8)	Inpatients with schizophrenia, referred for ECT No change in antipsychotic permitted during 4-wk study phase Chlorpromazine equivalents 273 mg in simulated ECT group, 317 mg in real ECT	Present State Examination	Sine wave ECT of unspecified dosage twice per week, for a total of 8 treatments	Blind ratings: MASS	Patients receiving real ECT had significantly greater improvement in MASS at 2 ($P = .02$) and 4 ($P = .05$) wk No difference between groups at extended 12- and 28-wk follow-up
Sarkar et al,[9] 1994	BL ECT + haloperidol (n = 15) vs sham ECT + haloperidol (n = 15)	Inpatients with schizophreniform disorder (illness <2 mo); confirmation of schizophrenia at 6 mo in 29/30 patients	DSM-III-R per Research Diagnostic Criteria	Sine wave fixed dosage BT ECT for a fixed course of 6 treatments	BPRS; clinician global rating weekly for 6 wk, and at 6 mo	Both groups improved over treatment course; no significant difference between groups at any time point
Ukpong et al,[10] 2002	BL (n = 9) + antipsychotic vs sham ECT + antipsychotic (n = 7)	ECT-naive patients with schizophrenia of <2 y duration, onset before 45 y (mostly inpatients) Chlorpromazine equivalent dose of 300 mg daily	ICD-10	Brief pulse fixed dosage BT ECT 3 d/wk, for a total of 6 treatments	Blinded (single rater) ratings BPRS; CGI-S and Scale for Assessment of Negative Symptoms at 2, 4, 6, 8, 12, 16, and 20 wk	Both groups improved in first 2 wk, with no significant difference between groups at any time point

Study	Design	Population	Diagnostic Criteria	ECT	Measures	Results
Masoudzadeh & Khalilian,[11] 2007	Sham ECT + clozapine vs ECT alone with sham clozapine vs ECT + clozapine (n = 6 each group)	Treatment-resistant schizophrenia (failure to respond to 2 adequate antipsychotic trials)	DSM-IV criteria confirmed by two psychiatrists	RUL ECT for 12 sessions given 3 times per week for 4 wk	PANSS	All groups improved; ECT + clozapine group significantly improved compared with other groups (see text for additional details)
Abraham & Kulhara,[12] 1987	ECT (n = 11) vs simulated ECT (n = 11) All patients received trifluoperazine, 20 mg daily	Inpatients or outpatients with schizophrenia; age of onset <40 y; ECT naive; illness not >2 y	Research Diagnostic Criteria	8 ECT twice weekly for 4 wk (electrode placement unspecified)	BPRS and CGIs administered q 2 wk for 26 wk	ECT superior to simulated ECT at all time points (CGI) and for first 12 wk (BPRS)
Goswami et al,[13] 2003	BT ECT (n = 15) vs sham ECT (n = 10)	Outpatients with schizophrenia, unresponsive to 3 courses of 2 different classes of neuroleptic (1000-mg chlorpromazine equivalents) in past 5 y, receiving neuroleptic at minimum of 500 CPZ equivalents for duration of study	DSM-IV	Brief pulse BT ECT at 50%–200% of seizure threshold, duration >25 s thrice-weekly; minimum of 6 tx, maximum and range unspecified	BPRS and CGI at baseline, weekly over 4 wk; rehospitalization rate	ECT superior to sham ECT after 2 wk No difference in CGI Rehospitalization rate 20% for ECT and 70% for sham group

Abbreviations: BPRS, Brief Psychiatric Rating Scale; BT, bitemporal; CGI, clinical global impression scale; CPZ, chlorpromazine; DSM-IV, Diagnostic and Statistical Manual-fourth edition; ICD, International Classification of Diseases; MASS, Montgomery Asberg Schizophrenia Scale; PANSS, Positive and Negative Syndrome Scale; RUL, right unilateral.

for 8 weeks. Patients in the pharmacotherapy-only arm who did not respond after 8 weeks were crossed over to the ECT arm and received the combination treatment for another 8 weeks in an open trial. The study used two levels of response: 20%, and 40% reduction in the psychosis items of BPRS. There were no responders in the pharmacotherapy group as defined by 20% reduction of the psychosis subscale, compared with 12 of 20 (60%; $P<.001$) in the ECT + clozapine group. There were 10 of 20 (50%; $P<.001$) responders in the ECT + clozapine group meeting the 40% reduction criterion. For those who did not respond to 16 weeks of clozapine treatment crossed over to the combination there were 11 of 15 (73.3%) responders when response was defined as 20% reduction and 6 of 15 (40%) when 40% was used.

Choice of Electrode Placement

Questions remain regarding optimal ECT technique particularly about electrode placements. An early randomized comparison of unilateral dominant (n = 18), unilateral nondominant (n = 17), and BT (n = 19) ECT for outpatients with schizophrenia showed no difference between groups in BPRS total scores or in the proportion of patients achieving 50% or greater reduction after a minimum of six ECT administered or at completion of treatment (average number of treatments, eight for unilateral and 9.4 for bilateral).[17] Phutane and colleagues[18] compared the speed of therapeutic response and cognitive adverse effects for patients randomized to receive bifrontal (BF) (n = 62) versus BT (n = 60) ECT administered at 1.5 times seizure threshold and with 1.5-ms pulse width setting, thrice-weekly with the total number of ECT treatments administered decided by the referring psychiatrist. Primary efficacy was determined by a response criterion of 40% reduction of total BPRS score. After six ECT sessions, 27/43 (63%) of BF met criteria as compared with 5/38 (13.2%) of patients administered BT ECT. By the end of the treatment course, 41/43 (95.3%) and 30/38 (78.9%) achieved response criteria for BF and BT ECT, respectively. Significant differences in favor of the BF group were found for recent memory, serial subtraction, digit span, and total controlled word association test. The authors conclude that BF offers significant advantages in speed and likelihood of clinical response and a more benign cognitive outcome.

Electroconvulsive Therapy for Maintenance

Two controlled trials have addressed the question of maintenance ECT (MECT) in schizophrenia. The earlier described study by Chanpattana and coworkers[14] used a second phase, during which continuation ECT was given weekly to patients who responded in the acute phase for 1 month (four treatments) and then biweekly for 5 months (10 treatments). Fifty-one patients were enrolled and 45 completed the second phase of the study. Among the completers, significantly more maintained remission after 6 months in the combined MECT + flupenthixol group (60%), whereas 93% relapsed in the MECT-alone and the flupenthixol-alone groups.

Yang and colleagues[19] conducted a randomized comparison of MECT + risperidone versus risperidone alone in 62 patients with schizophrenia who were ECT responders. MECT was used weekly in the first month, twice in the second month, and monthly thereafter for the remainder of 1 year (16 total treatments). Patients in the MECT group had a significantly lower relapse rate (only 4/27 relapsed) and longer relapse-free survival time (11 months) compared with medication control subjects (14/26 relapsed; seven relapsed in first 6 months and seven in second 6 months).

MANIA

ECT appears in the treatment algorithm for mania within the treatment guidelines of many professional bodies. Mania is recognized by the National Institute for Health and Care Excellence[6] as an indication for ECT, which states that ECT may be used to treat a prolonged or severe manic episode. A recent international survey of professional organizations with published guidelines for the treatment of mania showed that seven of nine organizations listed ECT as an option for the second-line treatment of mania.[20] For those organizations endorsing ECT, it was generally reserved for severe and/or treatment-resistant cases. ECT was not a recommended treatment by any of the international bodies for maintenance therapy for bipolar disorder.

A 2011 review on ECT and bipolar disorder reported on 28 clinical trials (mostly uncontrolled, nonrandomized, and not blinded). The range of clinical response in these trials was broad, from 48.1% to 100%.[21] The variability in response could be explained by nonstandard means of diagnosis, changes over time in the frequency of treatment-resistant mania, lack of blinding, variability in psychometric instruments, and different definitions of response. Given that the cited studies dated back to 1942, there were also important differences in ECT technique. For all these reasons these studies are difficult to interpret. A more recent naturalistic report using prospective systematic measurement in treatment-resistant patients noted 75% response rate for six patients with mania and 72.9% response rate for 55 bipolar patients in mixed state.[22]

We located six RCTs of ECT in mania (**Table 2**).[23–28] These dated from 1987 to 2009 and would meet most definitions of modern ECT and modern clinical trial methodology. None of the studies would meet modern definitions of large RCT, therefore all the results must be interpreted with caution. Inclusion criteria generally required a high severity of illness, and the patients were treated in an inpatient setting, in those instances when setting was specified. The mean number of ECT sessions was in the seven to nine range. Most, but not all studies reported their results categorically as responder versus nonresponder status. Of those studies that reported responder rates, there were 121 patients assigned to various forms of ECT, with an overall 72.7% response rate. Two of the RCTs explicitly required that the patient demonstrate treatment resistance before entering their studies. Notably, response rates were high and comparable with those reports that did not require treatment resistance for inclusion. Response rates were generally calculated at the end of ECT or within a week after the conclusion of the ECT course, so longer-term outcomes were generally not reported from these RCT.

The study by Sikdar and coworkers[26] is the only sham-controlled ECT study in mania, and shows an overwhelming advantage for real ECT + lithium versus sham ECT + lithium. Four of the RCTs performed various comparisons of BF versus BT, versus right unilateral (RUL), versus left unilateral ECT. Although differences in setting invalidate the simple combination of results across the studies, the overall impression is that bilateral forms of ECT are more reliable in their antimanic effect than any form of unilateral ECT. Contrasts of BT versus BF ECT suggest that BF electrode placement works faster and has fewer global cognitive side effects than BT ECT. Finally, the sole RCT contrasting different stimulus doses found no advantage for high-dose versus barely suprathreshold BT ECT. The Schnur and colleagues[30] study also provided data on symptom profiles that predicted ECT response in mania, reporting that signs and symptoms of anger, irritability, and suspiciousness were predictors of nonresponse. However, the authors rightfully note that their small total sample size of 18

Table 2
Randomized, controlled studies of ECT in mania

Study	Randomized Comparison	Sample	Diagnostic Criteria	ECT Technique	Outcome Measures	Main Results
Milstein et al,[23] 1987	BL (n = 11) vs initial RUL a switch to BL (n = 6)	Inpatients with mania or mixed state Score ≥7 on the manic portion of the Severity of Depression and Mania Scale PRN neuroleptic allowed 200–400 PCZ equivalents No requirement for treatment resistance	DSM-III per Research Diagnostic Criteria	Brief pulse 3 times per week No discussion about stimulus dosing	Semiblind ratings of MRS Also, CGI, Global Assessment Scale	Patients who started with BL had numerically superior results at the end of wk 2 for CGI ($P<.05$), Global Assessment Scale ($P<.05$), and MRS Statistical significance not reported for MRS
Small et al,[24] 1988 (This study is derivative of Milstein et al, above)	ECT (n = 17) vs Li$^+$ (n = 17)	Inpatients with mania or mixed state Score ≥7 on the manic portion of the Severity of Depression and Mania Scale PRN neuroleptic allowed 200–400 PCZ equivalents No requirement for treatment resistance	DSM-III per Research Diagnostic Criteria	RUL with possibility switch to BL (average 9 sessions) Brief pulse 3 times per week No discussion about stimulus dosing	Semiblind ratings of MRS Calculated % improvement from baseline	81% improvement in MRS seen in Li$^+$ patients vs 95% improvement in ECT patients, $P<.05$
Mukherjee et al,[25] 1988	BL (n = 4), RUL (n = 8), LUL (n = 5)	MMS ≥30 and met RDC criteria for manic episode All participants had failed ≥3 wk of lithium and/or antipsychotic	DSM-III	Brief pulse at 150% of seizure threshold, 3 d/wk, or 5 d/wk	Blind measurement of MMS; recovery = no longer meets RDC criteria for mania	Rates of response: BL: 4/7 RUL: 5/8 LUL: 2/5 Change in MMS scores: BL: −40.4% RUL: −37.4% LUL: −44.8%

Study	Sample/Design	Diagnosis	Criteria	Intervention	Outcome Measure	Results
Sikdar et al,[26] 1994	ECT + CPZ 600 mg (n = 15) vs sham ECT + CPZ 600 mg (n = 15)	Inpatients with mania, and baseline MRS ≥14	DSM-III-R	Eight sessions of BL sinewave vs anesthesia without ECT	Blind measurement of MRS; recovery = MRS <6	12/15 in ECT group vs 1/15 in sham group recovered P<.001
Hiremani et al,[27] 2008	BF (n = 17) vs BT (n = 19) ECT	Inpatient with mania, including 6 who were treatment resistant Mean haloperidol dose BF group = 43.8 mg, and BT group = 96.4 mg	DSM-IV	Stimulus dose 1.5X seizure threshold, 3 times per week with a brief pulse constant current device (mean of 7.5–7.6 sessions)	Blind ratings of YMRS A 50% reduction from baseline in YMRS = response	BF group improved faster than BT group (P<.03) By end of treatment, response to BF = 87.5% and BT = 72.2%
Barekatain et al,[28] 2008	BF (n = 14) vs BT (n = 14) Participants were allowed lorazepam, 1-mg equivalents per day	Inpatients with DSM-IV mania per Mini International Neuropsychiatric Interview Medication resistance not required for entry	DSM-IV	Stimulus dose 1.5X seizure threshold with a brief pulse device	Blind ratings of YMRS A 50% reduction from baseline in YMRS = response Cognition is measured with MMSE	No difference between groups in YMRS scores (exact rates of response not reported), but MMSE scores were higher at the end of ECT in those assigned to BF
Mohan et al,[29] 2009	Titrated BT ECT, followed by BL ECT at barely suprathreshold (n = 26) and 2.5X threshold (n = 24)	Inpatients older than 18 y with a manic episode, with YMRS ≥26 All patients were treatment resistant, and received risperidone 6–8 mg/d or olanzapine 15–30 mg/d	DSM-IV	BT brief pulse ECT (mean of 7.6 sessions for both groups)	Blind ratings of YMRS and CGI A 50% reduction from baseline in YMRS = response Also measured MMSE, autobiographical memory, and Wechsler Memory Scale	Barely suprathreshold response = 92%, and 2.5X threshold response = 91.7% No difference between groups in any cognitive measure

Abbreviations: BT, Bitemporal; DSM-IV, Diagnostic and Statistical Manual-fourth edition; LUL, left unilateral; MMS, Modified Mania Scale; MMSE, Mini-mental status exam; MRS, Mania Rating Scale; RDC, Research diagnostic criteria; RUL, right unilateral; YMRS, Young Mania Rating Scale.

patients limits the utility of their findings. The impressions from these six RCTs are echoed in other reviews on this topic.[31]

Treatment Considerations

The risk of a switch from depression to mania is always present in the application of ECT in patients with bipolar disorder. The risk is reported at 24%, and although some advocate for continuing ECT and treating through the mania, others have suggested suspending ECT and resuming intensive pharmacotherapy.[32]

There are no logical objections to the use of antipsychotics during a course of ECT for mania, but there are theoretic objections to the use of anticonvulsants and lithium. Remarkably, most patients can experience a successful course of ECT despite ongoing use of an anticonvulsant mood stabilizer.[33] Early reports on the combination of lithium and ECT presented concerns about long ECT seizures and aggravated cognitive problems.[34] However, the rate of lithium-related problems was reported as zero in 90 consecutive patients with mania receiving lithium concurrently with ECT.[35] The modern practice of ECT would expect the administration of at least one antimanic psychotropic in conjunction with a course of ECT for mania.

It is unknown how often treatment resistance develops in an episode of mania. Ciapparelli and colleagues[36] defined treatment-resistant mixed mania as failure to respond to at least 16 weeks of two or more mood stabilizers and antipsychotics. In their recent series of 41 treatment-resistant patients with mixed mania, the authors reported a 56% response rate with a mean of 7.2 sessions of BL pulse ECT.

POST-TRAUMATIC STRESS DISORDER

Many patients with PTSD do not achieve full remission from current pharmacotherapy and psychotherapy and ECT has sometimes been used in these cases.[37] However, there are no RCTs that examine the role of ECT in PTSD and PTSD is still not a recognized indication for ECT in any published treatment guideline.[38] A retrospective chart review by Watts[39] examined the use of ECT for treatment of PTSD in 26 military veterans who had major depression and PTSD. All patients started with RUL ECT (at 2.5 times seizure threshold). Five patients did not respond to RUL ECT and were switched to BT ECT after session 8. Patients had significant reduction in the symptoms of major depression and "some amelioration in PTSD symptoms." There was a mean reduction in PTSD symptoms after treatment ($P<.001$). However, only 35% of patients had greater than or equal to 20% reduction in symptoms. The main limitations of this study were that it was retrospective, a small sample size, and lack of non-ECT control.

In another retrospective study, Ahmadi and colleagues[40] compared patients with comorbid PTSD and major depressive disorder who received BF ECT (n = 92) with matched patients who did not receive ECT (n = 3393). ECT was administered thrice-weekly. Improvement in PTSD and major depressive disorder symptoms was assessed using clinical global impression scale (CGI). There was statistically significant improvement in the ECT (90%) group, compared with the antidepressant medications group (50%; $P = .001$).

The most recent clinical trial is an open-label study by Margoob and coworkers.[41] Twenty civilians were enrolled with severe, chronic, treatment-resistant PTSD (failure to respond to an adequate trial of four antidepressants or more, and 12 sessions of cognitive behavior therapy). Six sessions of bilateral ECT were given to all 20 outpatients twice-weekly. The stimulus intensity was barely suprathreshold. PTSD symptom severity was primarily measured with the Clinician-Administered PTSD Scale (CAPS). Secondary outcome measures were the Montgomery-Asberg Depression Rating

Scale (MADRS) and the clinical global impression-severity scale (CGI-S). Seventeen participants completed the study. Mean CAPS scores for all the sample decreased by 34% (P<.001), and MADRS decreased by 51.1% (P<.001). The authors reported that the correlation between improvement in CAPS and MADRS was low. These data seem encouraging; however, the overall body of evidence is insufficient to support routine use of ECT for PTSD because of limited research, small sample size, and design limitations. These encouraging early studies warrant replication in an RCT, especially for treatment-resistant PTSD.

CATATONIA

Catatonia is a neuropsychiatric condition characterized by wide range of psychomotor abnormalities ranging from stupor to marked agitation that is, referred to as catatonic excitement. Untreated catatonia can lead to poor outcomes because of poor nutritional status of these individuals, increased risk of venous thrombosis, decubitus ulcers, and pneumonia caused by immobility.[42] On the contrary, catatonic excitement and combativeness can pose risk of injury to self and others. Hence, catatonic state frequently represents a psychiatric emergency. Fortunately, benzodiazepines or barbiturates are effective in up to 60% to 80% of cases.[43] Although ECT is an effective treatment of catatonic syndrome there are no RCTs and it is most often considered when there is a poor response to medication or in cases where the condition is at risk of severe physiologic detriment, such as malignant catatonia.[44] McCall[45] demonstrated that only 10 of 20 patients with catatonia demonstrated a significant initial improvement in speech and behavior (score of 4 or 5 on CGI scale; "definite and sustained" or "dramatic") when administered intravenous amobarbital at an average dosage of 4.8 mg/kg. However, 19 of 20 patients ultimately had resolution of catatonic features with continued treatment using a combination of medication and ECT.

Most published studies of ECT for catatonia include patients with demonstrated refractoriness to benzodiazepines. However, in a study with algorithmic approach of treatments offered to patients with catatonic symptoms, ECT emerged as clearly more beneficial than the alternatives. Patients not responding to one treatment were offered the alternatives sequentially with some provision for patient and family preference. The first treatment options were benzodiazepines or ECT, second options were antipsychotic or ECT, third options chlorpromazine or ECT, and the final option was ECT alone. Authors report an overall efficacy rate of 100% for ECT in comparison with chlorpromazine 68%, risperidone 26%, haloperidol 16%, and benzodiazepines 2%.[46] BT ECT was used in this study and the frequency of the treatments was three times weekly with a mean of 8.8 treatments. The low efficacy of benzodiazepines in this study was likely caused by low dosage (eg, 3 mg oral lorazepam) as regulated by the Japan Ministry of Health, Labor and Welfare.

Medda and colleagues[47] treated 26 patients with bipolar disorder with catatonia features with ECT. These patients were resistant to pharmacotherapy including lorazepam at doses of 6 to 24 mg/d. A total of 21 of the 26 patients (80.8%) were classified as responders and required a mean of 10.2 ± 3 treatments. Compared with baseline scores, there was 82% reduction in Bush-Francis Catatonia rating scale scores[48] and 50% reduction in global severity of the illness, general psychopathology, and psychotic symptoms. ECT seemed safe for the patients in this study, with many individuals classified as having high burden of medical comorbidity.

When benzodiazepine treatment does not result in complete remission, they may still be combined with ECT, although concerns have long been raised about their impact on seizure threshold and seizure duration.[49] In a prospectively identified case series of five patients with catatonia, Petrides and colleagues[50] report that loraz-epam became effective at the same or at lower doses after the ECT was initiated because of lack of response with lorazepam treatment. Also, in two cases, addition of lorazepam enhanced the therapeutic response of ECT suggesting a synergistic rela-tionship between lorazepam and ECT when treating catatonic syndrome.

Rasmussen and colleagues[51] noted that benzodiazepine response rate is dimin-ished when catatonia is present with schizophrenia. This may also be true for ECT. In a study of five patients with catatonia secondary to schizophrenia and four patients with catatonia secondary to a mood disorder, patients with mood disorder showed greater clinical improvement and required fewer treatments overall.[52]

Other studies paint a more positive picture of the role of ECT in the care of patients with catatonia associated with schizophrenia. In a 1-year outcome study, Suzuki and colleagues[53] examined 11 consecutive patients with catatonic schizophrenia referred for acute ECT after failing to respond to other treatments, including benzodiazepines in 10 cases. ECT was administered acutely thrice-weekly for a mean of 9.9 ± 1.3 treat-ments. All 11 patients met criteria for a clinical response with a score of less than 25 on BPRS. In a subsequent pharmacotherapy maintenance study, the same ECT re-sponders were assessed weekly using BPRS for 48 weeks or until they met criteria for relapse or recurrence (defined as BPRS score of >37 on 3 consecutive days). Relapse occurred in seven patients (63.6%) and all in the first 6 months.[54] Patients who relapsed in the phase 2 study were retreated with acute ECT treatments and all seven patients responded to the second course of acute ECT (mean of 12.3 ± 3.9 treatments). Finally, the responders were then treated with a fixed regimen of continuation ECT combined with pharmacotherapy. Continuation ECT was admin-istered for 6 months with four ECT sessions at weekly intervals followed by four ECT sessions administered every 2 weeks, and the final three ECT sessions were given every 4 weeks. Four out of these seven patients relapsed in 1-year follow-up including one drop-out.[55]

Catatonia is associated with grave complications and treatment should be prompt. One study provides a glimpse into how this may not be adequately addressed in some settings. In a population of heterogeneous cases, 13 patients with benign catatonia, 11 with malignant catatonia, and 10 patients with neuroleptic malignant syndrome were studied retrospectively.[56] Overall response to treatment was encouraging, because 58% showed complete remission and 18% reached partial remission with benzodiazepines and/or ECT. In medication-resistant patients treated with ECT, 50% of patients recovered completely. Strikingly, the time lag reported in this study between the onset of catatonic symptoms and first-line treatment targeting catatonia was 15 ± 36 days and the time lag between first and the second line of ECT treatment was found to be 27 ± 46 days.

PARKINSON DISEASE

PD is a neurodegenerative movement disorder characterized by resting tremor, rigid-ity, bradykinesia, and postural instability associated with loss of the dopaminergic nigrostriatal neurons and decreased striatal levels of dopamine. Depression is a com-mon nonmotor feature of this illness in up to 40% of patients.[57] Studies of the effect of ECT in animal models[58] and humans[59] consistently suggest enhancement of dopa-mine activity. Benefits of ECT in PD came to light in the 1970s when patients treated with ECT for depression with comorbid PD showed improvement in motor symptoms of PD.[60] Borisovskaya and colleagues[61] recently published a systematic review of 43 published studies and recommended that ECT be included in guidelines for treatment of patients with PD. Their analysis included 116 patients with depression and PD, and found that depression improved in 93.1% and when motor symptom severity was reported, 83% of patients were deemed improved.

In a double-blind controlled study, patients with treatment-resistant PD showing severe "on-off" phenomenon with pronounced "off" periods, patients treated with ECT significantly prolonged the duration of "on" phase compared with the sham ECT. In the open-label part of the study, severity of parkinsonian symptoms as measured on Webster scale and time and number of steps required to walk 10 m improved. However, the benefits of the treatment were short lived between 2 and 3 weeks.[62] The improvement of movement disorders with ECT is sometimes attributed to the improvement in the depression that is frequently comorbid in patients with PD, but in this study the sample consisted of patients with PD without depressive illness.

The durability of antiparkinsonian effects of ECT is variable but time-limited. An open-label study included seven patients ages between 61 and 73 years old with major depression and PD. After two treatments there was significant improvement in motor functions (rigidity, gait, tremor, bradykinesia, and postural instability) in five of the seven patients. Two of the patients developed dyskinetic movements that improved after reduction in doses of dopaminergic drugs. The duration of improvement varied from 1 to 6 months after cessation of ECT.[63] In another open-label study examining 16 patients with advanced PD with comorbid depression, the antiparkinsonian effect lasted a few days to 4 weeks in eight patients, 3 to 5 months in seven patients, and 18 months in one patient.[64]

The existing evidence suggests ECT does have a role in the treatment of PD, not only for the treatment of depression associated with PD, but also for improving the motor symptoms of PD

OVERALL SUMMARY/FUTURE DIRECTIONS

ECT is remarkably effective over a broad spectrum of neuropsychiatric conditions and should not be limited to major depression alone. The ECT research agenda is similarly broad and ultimately will be driven by the developing understanding of its mechanism of action. Where the literature is sparse, and the need is acute, off-label prescribing must proceed with caution, and not overly impeded by regulatory bodies.

REFERENCES

1. McDonald WM, Weiner RD, Fochtmann LJ, et al. The FDA and ECT. J ECT 2016; 32(2):75–7.
2. U.S. Department of Health and Human Services Food and Drug Administration. Electroconvulsive therapy (ECT) devices for class II intended uses. Rockville (MD): 2015. Available at: https://www.gpo.gov/fdsys/pkg/FR-2015-32592.pdf. Accessed May 1, 2018.
3. Radley DC, Finkelstein SN, Stafford RS. Off-label prescribing among office-based physicians. Arch Intern Med 2006;166(9):1021–6.
4. Kreyenbuhl J, Buchanan RW, Dickerson FB, et al. The Schizophrenia Patient Outcomes Research Team (PORT): updated treatment recommendations 2009. Schizophr Bull 2010;36(1):94–103.
5. Hasan A, Falkai P, Wobrock T, et al. World Federation of Societies of Biological Psychiatry (WFSBP) guidelines for biological treatment of schizophrenia, part 1: update 2012 on the acute treatment of schizophrenia and the management of treatment resistance. World J Biol Psychiatry 2012;13(5):318–78.

6. National Institute for Health and Clinical Excellence. NICE technology appraisal guidance No.59: The clinical effectiveness and cost effectiveness of electroconvulsive therapy (ECT) for depressive illness, schizophrenia, catatonia and mania. 2003. Available at: https://www.nice.org.uk/guidance/ta59. Accessed May 1, 2018.

7. Tharyan P, Adams CE. Electroconvulsive therapy for schizophrenia. Cochrane Database Syst Rev 2005;(2):CD000076.

8. Brandon S, Cowley P, McDonald C, et al. Leicester ECT trial: results in schizophrenia. Br J Psychiatry 1985;146:177–83.

9. Sarkar P, Andrade C, Kapur B, et al. An exploratory evaluation of ECT in haloperidol-treated DSM-IIIR schizophreniform disorder. Convuls Ther 1994; 10(4):271–8.

10. Ukpong DI, Makanjuola RO, Morakinyo O. A controlled trial of modified electroconvulsive therapy in schizophrenia in a Nigerian teaching hospital. West Afr J Med 2002;21(3):237–40.

11. Masoudzadeh A, Khalilian AR. Comparative study of clozapine, electroshock and the combination of ECT with clozapine in treatment-resistant schizophrenic patients. Pak J Biol Sci 2007;10(23):4287–90.

12. Abraham KR, Kulhara P. The efficacy of electroconvulsive therapy in the treatment of schizophrenia. A comparative study. Br J Psychiatry 1987;151:152–5.

13. Goswami U, Kumar U, Singh B. Efficacy of electroconvulsive therapy in treatment resistant schizophrenia: a double-blind study. Indian J Psychiatry 2003;45(1): 26–9.

14. Chanpattana W, Chakrabhand ML, Sackeim HA, et al. Continuation ECT in treatment-resistant schizophrenia: a controlled study. J ECT 1999;15(3):178–92.

15. Chanpattana W, Chakrabhand ML. Combined ECT and neuroleptic therapy in treatment-refractory schizophrenia: prediction of outcome. Psychiatry Res 2001;105(1–2):107–15.

16. Petrides G, Malur C, Braga RJ, et al. Electroconvulsive therapy augmentation in clozapine-resistant schizophrenia: a prospective, randomized study. Am J Psychiatry 2015;172(1):52–8.

17. Doongaji DR, Jeste DV, Saoji NJ, et al. Unilateral versus bilateral ECT in schizophrenia. Br J Psychiatry 1973;123(572):73–9.

18. Phutane VH, Thirthalli J, Muralidharan K, et al. Double-blind randomized controlled study showing symptomatic and cognitive superiority of bifrontal over bitemporal electrode placement during electroconvulsive therapy for schizophrenia. Brain Stimul 2013;6(2):210–7.

19. Yang Y, Cheng X, Xu Q, et al. The maintenance of modified electroconvulsive therapy combined with risperidone is better than risperidone alone in preventing relapse of schizophrenia and improving cognitive function. Arq Neuropsiquiatr 2016;74(10):823–8.

20. Parker G, Graham R, Tavella G. Is there consensus across international evidence-based guidelines for the management of bipolar disorder? Acta Psychiatr Scand 2017;135:515–26.

21. Versiani M, Cheniaux E, Landeira-Fernandez J. Efficacy and safety of electroconvulsive therapy in the treatment of bipolar disorder. J ECT 2011;27(2):153–64.

22. Perugi G, Medda P, Toni C, et al. The role of electroconvulsive therapy (ECT) in bipolar disorder: effectiveness in 522 patients with bipolar depression, mixed-state, mania and catatonic features. Curr Neuropharmacol 2017;15:359–71.

23. Milstein V, Small J, Klapper M, et al. Uni- versus bilateral ECT in the treatment of mania. Convulsive Ther 1987;3(1):1–9.

24. Small J, Klapper M, Kellams J, et al. Electroconvulsive treatment compared with lithium in the management of manic states. Arch Gen Psychiatry 1988;45:727–32.
25. Mukherjee S, Sackeim H, Lee C. Unilateral ECT in the treatment of manic episodes. Convulsive Ther 1988;4(1):74–80.
26. Sikdar S, Kulhara P, Avasthi A, et al. Combined chlorpromazine and electroconvulsive therapy in mania. Br J Psychiatry 1994;164:806–10.
27. Hiremani R, Thirthalli J, Tharayil B, et al. Double-blind randomized controlled study comparing short-term efficacy of bifrontal and bitemporal electroconvulsive therapy in acute mania. Bipolar Disord 2008;10:701–7.
28. Barekatain M, Jahangard L, Haghighi M, et al. Bifrontal versus bitemporal electroconvulsive therapy in severe manic patients. J ECT 2008;24(3):199–202.
29. Mohan T, Tharyan P, Alexander J, et al. Effects of stimulus intensity on the efficacy and safety of twice-weekly, unilateral electroconvulsive therapy (ECT) combined with antipsychotics in acute mania: a randomised clinical trial. Bipolar Disord 2009;11:126–34.
30. Schnur D, Mukherjee S, Sackeim H, et al. Symptomatic predictors of ECT response in medication-nonresponsive manic patients. J Clin Psychiatry 1992; 53(2):63–6.
31. Mukherjee S, Sackeim H, Schnur D. Electroconvulsive therapy of acute manic episodes: a review of 50 years' experience. Am J Psychiatry 1994;151(2):169–76.
32. Lee J, Arcand A, Narang P, et al. ECT-induced mania. Innov Clin Neurosci 2014; 11(11–12):27–9.
33. Rubner P, Koppi S, Conca A. Frequency of and rationale for the combined use of electroconvulsive therapy and antiepileptic drugs in Austria and the literature. World J Biol Psychiatry 2009;10:836–45.
34. el-Mallakh R. Complications of concurrent lithium and electroconvulsive therapy: a review of clinical material and theoretical considerations. Biol Psychiatry 1988; 23(6):595–601.
35. Volpe F, Tavares A. Lithium plus ECT in mania in 90 cases: safety issues. J Neuropsychiatry Clin Neurosci 2012;24(2):E33.
36. Ciapparelli A, Dell'Osso L, Tundo A, et al. Electroconvulsive therapy in medication-nonresponsive patients with mixed mania and bipolar depression. J Clin Psychiatry 2001;62:552–5.
37. Berger W, Portella CM, Fontenelle LF, et al. Antipsychotics, anticonvulsants, antiadrenergics and other drugs: what to do when posttraumatic stress disorder does not respond to selective serotonin reuptake inhibitors? Rev Bras Psiquiatr 2007;29(Suppl 2):S61–5 [in Portuguese].
38. Youssef NA, McCall WV, Andrade C. The role of ECT in posttraumatic stress disorder: a systematic review. Ann Clin Psychiatry 2017;29(1):62–70.
39. Watts BV. Electroconvulsive therapy for comorbid major depressive disorder and posttraumatic stress disorder. J ECT 2007;23(2):93–5.
40. Ahmadi N, Moss L, Simon E, et al. Efficacy and long-term clinical outcome of comorbid posttraumatic stress disorder and major depressive disorder after electroconvulsive therapy. Depress Anxiety 2016;33(7):640–7.
41. Marqoob MA, Ali Z, Andrade C. Efficacy of ECT in chronic, severe, antidepressant- and CBT-refractory PTSD: an open, prospective study. Brain Stimul 2010; 3(1):28–35.
42. McCall WV, Mann SC, Shelp FE, et al. Fatal pulmonary embolism in the catatonic syndrome: two case reports and a literature review. J Clin Psychiatry 1995;56(1): 21–5.

43. Wijemanne S, Jankovic J. Movement disorders in catatonia. J Neurol Neurosurg Psychiatry 2015;86(8):825–32.
44. Fink M, Taylor MA. The catatonia syndrome: forgotten but not gone. Arch Gen Psychiatry 2009;66(11):1173–7.
45. McCall WV. The response to an amobarbital interview as a predictor of therapeutic outcome in patients with catatonic mutism. Convuls Ther 1992;8(3): 174–8.
46. Hatta K, Miyakawa K, Ota T, et al. Maximal response to electroconvulsive therapy for the treatment of catatonic symptoms. J ECT 2007;23(4):233–5.
47. Medda P, Toni C, Luchini F, et al. Catatonia in 26 patients with bipolar disorder: clinical features and response to electroconvulsive therapy. Bipolar Disord 2015;17(8):892–901.
48. Bush G, Fink M, Petrides G, et al. Catatonia. I. Rating scale and standardized examination. Acta Psychiatr Scand 1996;93(2):129–36.
49. Boylan LS, Haskett RF, Mulsant BH, et al. Determinants of seizure threshold in ECT: benzodiazepine use, anesthetic dosage, and other factors. J ECT 2000; 16(1):3–18.
50. Petrides G, Divadeenam KM, Bush G, et al. Synergism of lorazepam and electroconvulsive therapy in the treatment of catatonia. Biol Psychiatry 1997;42(5): 375–81.
51. Rasmussen SA, Mazurek MF, Rosebush PI. Catatonia: our current understanding of its diagnosis, treatment and pathophysiology. World J Psychiatry 2016;6(4): 391–8.
52. Escobar R, Rios A, Montoya ID, et al. Clinical and cerebral blood flow changes in catatonic patients treated with ECT. J Psychosom Res 2000;49(6):423–9.
53. Suzuki K, Awata S, Matsuoka H. Short-term effect of ECT in middle-aged and elderly patients with intractable catatonic schizophrenia. J ECT 2003;19(2): 73–80.
54. Suzuki K, Awata S, Matsuoka H. One-year outcome after response to ECT in middle-aged and elderly patients with intractable catatonic schizophrenia. J ECT 2004;20(2):99–106.
55. Suzuki K, Awata S, Takano T, et al. Continuation electroconvulsive therapy for relapse prevention in middle-aged and elderly patients with intractable catatonic schizophrenia. Psychiatry Clin Neurosci 2005;59(4):481–9.
56. Tuerlings JH, van Waarde JA, Verwey B. A retrospective study of 34 catatonic patients: analysis of clinical care and treatment. Gen Hosp Psychiatry 2010;32(6): 631–5.
57. Tandberg E, Larsen JP, Aarsland D, et al. The occurrence of depression in Parkinson's disease. A community-based study. Arch Neurol 1996;53(2):175–9.
58. Landau AM, Chakravarty MM, Clark CM, et al. Electroconvulsive therapy alters dopamine signaling in the striatum of non-human primates. Neuropsychopharmacology 2011;36(2):511–8.
59. Baldinger P, Lotan A, Frey R, et al. Neurotransmitters and electroconvulsive therapy. J ECT 2014;30(2):116–21.
60. Lebensohn ZM, Jenkins RB. Improvement of Parkinsonism in depressed patients treated with ECT. Am J Psychiatry 1975;132(3):283–5.
61. Borisovskaya A, Bryson WC, Buchholz J, et al. Electroconvulsive therapy for depression in Parkinson's disease: systematic review of evidence and recommendations. Neurodegener Dis Manag 2016;6(2):161–76.

62. Andersen K, Balldin J, Gottfries CG, et al. A double-blind evaluation of electro-convulsive therapy in Parkinson's disease with "on-off" phenomena. Acta Neurol Scand 1987;76(3):191–9.
63. Douyon R, Serby M, Klutchko B, et al. ECT and Parkinson's disease revisited: a "naturalistic" study. Am J Psychiatry 1989;146(11):1451–5.
64. Fall PA, Ekman R, Granerus AK, et al. ECT in Parkinson's disease. Changes in motor symptoms, monoamine metabolites and neuropeptides. J Neural Transm Park Dis Dement Sect 1995;10(2–3):129–40.

Deep Brain Stimulation in Psychiatry

Mechanisms, Models, and Next-Generation Therapies

Mustafa Taha Bilge, PhD[a], Aishwarya K. Gosai, BA[a],
Alik S. Widge, MD, PhD[a,b],*

KEYWORDS

- Closed-loop DBS • Network-oriented DBS • DBS in psychiatry
- Mechanisms of DBS • Dimension-oriented psychiatry

KEY POINTS

- The likely mechanism of deep brain stimulation is altered interneuronal communication, which may include alterations in neural firing patterns, oscillatory dynamics, or synaptic plasticity.
- Deep brain stimulation acts at the network level, not on single brain structures.
- Advanced technologies, including closed loop systems, are being deployed in movement disorders. Recent progress in novel applications suggests that they may soon be used in psychiatry.
- The optimal use of deep brain stimulation likely requires a dimensional approach to identify patients with treatment-amenable brain circuit impairment.

Disclosure Statement: A.S. Widge receives consulting income and device donations from Medtronic, which manufactures deep brain stimulation systems. A.S. Widge has also filed multiple patent applications related to closed loop deep brain stimulation, none of which is yet commercially licensed.

Preparation of this work was not sponsored or supported by any commercial entity. A.S. Widge, A.K. Gosai, and M.T. Bilge were supported by grants to A.S. Widge from the Brain & Behavior Research Foundation, National Institutes of Health (MH109722, MH111320, and NS100548), and Defense Advanced Research Projects Agency (Cooperative Agreement W911NF-14-2-0045). The views, opinions, and/or findings expressed are those of the authors and should not be interpreted as representing the official views or policies of any sponsor or funding source.

[a] Department of Psychiatry, Massachusetts General Hospital, Harvard Medical School, 149 13th Street, Charlestown, Boston, MA 02129, USA; [b] Picower Institute for Learning and Memory, Massachusetts Institute of Technology, Cambridge, MA, USA
* Corresponding author. Department of Psychiatry, Massachusetts General Hospital, Harvard Medical School, 149 13th Street, Room 2627, Charlestown, MA 02129.
E-mail address: awidge@partners.org

Psychiatr Clin N Am 41 (2018) 373–383
https://doi.org/10.1016/j.psc.2018.04.003
0193-953X/18/© 2018 Elsevier Inc. All rights reserved.

INTRODUCTION: THE PROMISE AND FRUSTRATIONS OF DEEP BRAIN STIMULATION IN PSYCHIATRY

As discussed in the companion article by Darin D. Dougherty, "Deep Brain Stimulation—Clinical Applications," in this issue, deep brain stimulation (DBS) has promise in intractable obsessive-compulsive disorder (OCD) and major depression (MDD), but has not fared well in traditional randomized trials. This contrasts with the success of DBS in Parkinson disease (PD), where it has become a part of standard care.[1] The difference in outcomes arises because PD and other movement disorders arise from well-explored neural circuitry, with well-understood, reliable measures of symptoms. Psychiatric conditions arise from multiple dysfunctional neural circuits, not all of which are known or well-described.[2,3] Our symptom measures are also less robust, diluting the clinical signal.[4,5] For example, a metaanalysis of depression questionnaires showed that general factors, such as mood, explain more variance than any specific MDD symptom.[6] In the *Diagnostic and Statistical Manual of Mental Disorders, 5th edition*, field trials, comorbidity was more common than "pure" diagnoses, suggesting that diagnostic criteria and rating scales do not measure separable entities.[7]

Studies in both psychiatric and PD patients have yielded proposed mechanisms of DBS, leading to new treatment strategies. Some of these proposals emphasize anatomy; others have both functional and anatomic components. We argue that DBS in psychiatry depends on both function and anatomy, viewed at the circuit/network level. Herein, we review the functional and network-oriented theories of psychiatric DBS. We begin each section with a review of what is known or strongly suspected, then highlight directions the field may soon take.

NEUROPHYSIOLOGIC MECHANISMS OF DEEP BRAIN STIMULATION
Neural Inhibition

DBS often mimics the clinical effect of a brain lesion at the target site. Most of the PD and MDD/OCD targets were chosen because a lesion at that target was known or expected to ameliorate disease.[8,9] Several studies reported decreased neural activity at the DBS site.[10–12] Yet, DBS-like stimulation can also increase neural activity, depending on how the electric field is oriented relative to individual cells.[13,14] DBS also seems to increase brain metabolism at structures connected to the target.[15–17] This finding casts doubt on the inhibition hypothesis.

Informational Lesion

One possible explanation for these contradictions is that DBS may be inhibitory at the level of information flow. The high-frequency pulses (>100 Hz) used in DBS are above the firing frequency of most neurons, meaning that DBS effectively "takes over" the stimulated axons and cell bodies. Normal brain activity is irregular and variable, and that irregularity conveys information. DBS changes this to regularized, less-variant activity,[18] decreasing the amount of information sent between network nodes in a mathematical sense.[19] This decrease might make the overall network function better. For instance, in a hemiparkinsonian rat model of PD, the amount of information (ie, neuronal entropy) in the globus pallidus and substantia nigra increased after the onset of Parkinsonism.[20] DBS of those regions decreased local information but increased the information transmission between these regions.[20] The informational lesion theory has only been evaluated in PD, but with good results. A human study showed that pulse sequences optimized for information blockade are as effective as high-frequency, DBS but require much less energy delivery to the brain.[21]

Disruption of Pathologic Oscillations

Neural network communication requires coordination of activity within and between areas. When networks are functioning efficiently, coordinated oscillations appear in the local field potential (LFP)[22] and scalp electroencephalogram. Neural network dysfunction may be reflected in abnormal oscillatory activity, and rhythmic DBS might restore normal oscillations. For example, beta band (12–30 Hz) power normally decreases during movement.[23] In PD, however, corticobasal circuits remain in synchronized (ie, coherent) beta oscillation, which is believed to produce the core symptoms in PD of bradykinesia and rigidity.[24,25] Patients receiving DBS for the first time showed decreased beta-gamma synchrony (cross-frequency coupling) between the subthalamic nucleus (STN) and motor cortex.[26] Similarly, the extent to which the power of gamma band activity (>40 Hz) was nested within alpha/beta band activity decreased with DBS of ventral striatum/ventral capsule in patients with OCD,[27] although this effect did not replicate in an independent sample.[28] This touches a much broader difficulty with identifying oscillatory biomarkers of psychiatric illness, to which we return elsewhere in this article. The beta findings in PD, replicated by multiple groups, led to an important innovation: DBS systems that can record and store electrophysiologic information from human patients as they undergo treatment.[29] Those systems offer an unparalleled view into brain function.[30]

The effect of DBS on oscillations offers the potential for treatment innovation. Stimulation could be aligned to coincide with the phase of frequency of a band of interest, such as frontal theta in anxiety disorders[31] or beta band in PD.[24,32] This approach was taken in a PD DBS study, where phase dependent DBS (ie, DBS delivered in synchrony with beta band activity) was superior to consistent, high-frequency DBS.[32] In depression, a transcranial magnetic device operating on similar frequency-locked principles has evidence of possible efficacy.[33] The authors have launched a trial specifically designed to modify oscillations in corticostriatal loops of OCD (NCT03184454). As we learn to better identify the oscillatory features of dysfunctional networks, oscillation-based DBS may become useful in psychiatric disorders.

Neuroplasticity

Neuroplasticity underlies the brain's long-term learning and reorganization capabilities.[34] Psychiatric DBS changes symptoms over a slow time course consistent with plasticity effects,[16,25,35] implying that DBS may work through neuroplasticity. This hypothesis is supported by animal studies [36–39] Hamani and colleagues[36] found that a single DBS session increased stressed rats' performance on a working memory task, but only when measured 33 days after the DBS treatment. Chakravarty and colleagues[37] demonstrated that DBS of ventromedial prefrontal cortex, a putative rodent homologue of human subcallosal cingulate, increased synaptic density. Last, Creed and colleagues[39] reversed cocaine-induced plasticity in the nucleus accumbens (NAc) of rodents with DBS. They found that DBS successfully suppressed sensitization responses caused by repeated exposure to cocaine, but only when administered with a D1R antagonist that altered local excitability. These findings demonstrate the potential of DBS to induce neuroplasticity and structural alterations of neural networks. This could be a critical mechanism to exploit, given the role of learning and plasticity impairments in psychiatric conditions.[40,41]

NETWORK MECHANISMS AND TARGETS FOR DEEP BRAIN STIMULATION

Modern neuroscience focuses on networks as units of study.[42] Psychiatric dysfunctions are commonly believed to be dysfunctions of neural networks, and DBS likely acts at the network level. For example, STN and globus pallidus internus are both parts of the cortico–basal ganglia network,[43] and DBS at either site can be effective in PD. DBS of the STN is believed to reduce excitation from STN to globus pallidus, leading to higher firing rates in globus pallidus and a variety of downstream effects.[44] This process ultimately normalizes activity throughout the corticobasal loop, decreasing the motor signs of PD.[45] Similarly, dysfunctions of corticostriatothalamo-cortical[9,46,47] circuits are associated with OCD, and nodes in these loops are targeted for OCD neurosurgery.[46,48,49] With the advent of modern imaging technologies, such as diffusion tensor imaging and functional connectivity MRI, researchers can better study structural and functional networks.[50] This methodology is enabling more rigorous empirical and computational studies of the mechanisms of DBS at a network level.[51]

Network Studies and Functional Mapping

Network effects of DBS are readily observable in regions connected to a DBS target. In their study of the subgenual anterior cingulate (Cg25), Mayberg and colleagues[12] showed reduced cerebral blood flow (CBF) to Cg25 and the neighboring orbitofrontal cortex after DBS. However, long-term responders to DBS also demonstrated CBF changes in other regions involved in depression, such as increases in dorsolateral prefrontal cortex and decreases in hypothalamus.

Similar findings are also seen with acute stimulation. Rauch and colleagues[15] found increased CBF in right medial orbitofrontal cortex and the right dorsolateral putamen from acute high-frequency (clinically effective) DBS. Similarly, Dougherty and colleagues[46] also observed increased regional CBF in patients with OCD in the dorsal anterior cingulate cortex when the stimulation DBS contact was more ventral in ventral capsule/ventral striatum. This effect also significantly correlated with improvements in the depressive symptom severity of patients with OCD. However, with more dorsal stimulation, the network activation changed and regional CBF increases were observed in the thalamus, striatum, and globus pallidus. Taken together, these results suggest that DBS must influence wide networks to be clinically effective. The wide network hypothesis is supported by recent diffusion tensor imaging studies.[50,51] For example, Riva-Posse and colleagues[50] recently identified 4 white matter bundles that were uniquely activated in a cohort of DBS responders. The researchers then used the identified bundles as DBS targets in a new cohort of MDD patients. This advanced targeting yielded response rates of 73% at 6 months and 82% at 1 year in the new prospective (albeit unblinded) cohort,[50] much higher than those in a recent nontargeted DBS trial.[52]

Optogenetics, the use of light in modulating neural activity,[53] is another state-of-the-art technique that informs network-oriented DBS. In animal models, optogenetics allows stimulation of specific connections between brain nuclei, allowing researchers to narrow the mechanisms of DBS to subnetworks. In a recent example, Gradinaru and colleagues[54] tested whether the effect of DBS in PD is due to inhibition of STN, or instead due to disrupted connectivity between STN and the motor cortex. They reported that, in hemiparkinsonian rats, precise inhibition of STN did not lead to improvements in symptoms of PF. The only optogenetic manipulation improving PD symptoms was exciting the afferent motor cortex neurons that projected into STN. Similar studies should be possible in animal models of psychiatric illness; indeed, optogenetic stimulation of specific projections has dramatic effects on a variety of laboratory behaviors that model aspects of mental illness.[55]

Next Steps: From Diagnoses to Dimensions

Changes in brain physiology, including information flow, oscillatory synchrony, and synaptic weighting, may each play a role in the therapeutic effects of DBS. Each of these factors seems to act more at the network level than on any single brain structure. As described elsewhere in this article, specific DBS protocols and/or combinations of DBS with targeted pharmacology can produce equally specific physiologic changes. Novel closed loop and recording systems will soon be able to monitor those changes and adjust stimulation intensity without immediate physician involvement.[30,56,57] This is a powerful toolbox, and its main limitation is that we do not know which physiologic changes may be beneficial for which mental illness. There is an extensive literature on attempts to find physiologic biomarkers, especially in MDD.[58] The results are very mixed, and our group's attempts to independently replicate candidate markers have failed.[59–61] We argue that this problem arises from the heterogeneity of categorical psychiatric diagnoses.[62] MDD, OCD, and other DBS-targetable disorders are too phenotypically diverse to arise from only 1 neurologic impairment. The National Institute of Mental Health's Research Domain Criteria initiative seeks to recast mental illnesses not as diagnoses, but as quantitatively described impairment in specific functional domains.[3,5] This domain- and circuit-oriented approach to illness may be particularly useful for psychiatric DBS. DBS modulates specific circuits, which in turn might lead to focused behavioral changes that cut across traditional diagnoses.[62] Multiple groups are now identifying cross-diagnostic network signatures in psychiatric populations,[63,64] and stimulation based on these signatures may change psychiatrically relevant behaviors.[57]

Next Steps: Closed Loop, Activity-Dependent Stimulation

DBS as practiced to date is "open loop." That is, the physician takes clinical data into account, sets the stimulation parameters, and then a single pattern of stimulation is applied to the patient's brain for the next several weeks to months.[8] This practice is substantially based on trial and error[65] and the decisions are based on physicians' subjective evaluations and indirect behavioral assessment.[3–5] "Closed loop" DBS is an emerging alternative. In this paradigm, a neural biomarker that captures an essential aspect of disease is identified, such as increased beta band activity in the STN in PD.[23,24] The DBS system then directly measures the biomarker and uses this information to adjust stimulation parameters.[30] DBS systems currently in production (eg, Medtronic's PC+S, Medtronic, Minneapolis, MN) can record LFPs from lead contacts at the site of stimulation.[29] Stimulation parameters may be adjusted by predictive algorithms to achieve a desired neurophysiologic signature.[57] Preliminary demonstrations of this approach in PD have equaled and, in some cases, exceeded the performance of traditional DBS.[43,66]

As noted, biomarker development is a major challenge for closed loop DBS algorithm development in psychiatry. We suggest a domain-oriented approach applied in 4 steps (**Fig. 1**). *Diagnostic and Statistical Manual of Mental Disorders, 5th edition,* based diagnoses (eg, general anxiety disorder and major depressive disorder) that may share a common phenotype (eg, cognitive rigidity). These phenotypes may be identified through a combination of self-report questionnaires (eg, for the cognitive rigidity example, the Brief Inventory of Executive Functioning[67]), standardized behavioral assessments (eg, a cognitive interference task[68]), and imaging techniques. Patients who demonstrate the phenotypic impairment of interest could then be studied with high temporal resolution recordings (eg, LFP and electroencephalogram) to identify candidate predictive algorithms.[30,57] The developed algorithms could then aid the DBS physician in adjusting stimulation settings. With full closed loop DBS, the adjustment process could be transferred to an automatic controller in the DBS system itself. It should be noted that closed loop DBS in psychiatry remains more of a vision than a near-term guarantee. There have been successful pilots in Parkinsonism,[43] and reports of early psychiatric closed loop demonstrations in laboratory environments,[57] but the concept remains to be validated in a clinical setting. The essential test for its efficacy is how it performs in comparison with the current open loop approaches.

A recent demonstration by Wu and colleagues[56] exemplifies the approach. The authors selected a phenotypical component of hypersensitivity to reward, then modeled this phenotype by creating a group of mice prone to binge eating. The LFPs from NAc of the mice had higher delta-band (ie, 1–4 Hz) power in NAc when these mice anticipated food. This biomarker was used to trigger a DBS-like neurostimulator in the NAc, disrupting the reward hypersensitivity. This closed loop neurostimulation extinguished animals' tendency to binge on high-fat chow. Additionally, a similar delta band signature of reward anticipation was identified in NAc LFPs of a pilot human subject, demonstrating this biomarker's potential translational relevance. Based on this result, the authors hope to implement delta-locked closed loop DBS in disorders of human reward hypersensitivity, including binge eating and drug addiction.

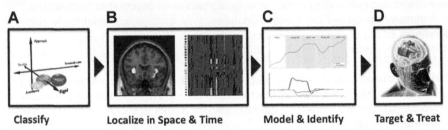

A	**B**	**C**	**D**
Classify	Localize in Space & Time	Model & Identify	Target & Treat

Fig. 1. A closed loop deep brain stimulation pipeline example. (*A*) The patients' dysfunction is individually assessed. The emphasis is in measuring patients' (dys)function in multiple cross-diagnostic domains. (*B*) Activity correlated with domain/function impairment is localized to brain structures that are amenable to neurostimulation. (*C*) Computational modeling quantifies the relationship of behavior to brain activity and formulates a control relationship between brain and behavior. (*D*) Based on this quantification, closed loop treatment specific to individual patients is administered. GAD, generalized anxiety disorder; MDD, major depressive disorder; TBI, traumatic brain injury. (*From* Widge AS, Ellard KK, Paulk AC, et al. Treating refractory mental illness with closed loop brain stimulation: progress towards a patient-specific transdiagnostic approach. Exp Neurol 2017;287(Part 4):470; with permission.)

Next Steps: Ethical Foundations for Deep Brain Stimulation in Psychiatry

DBS aims to improve psychiatric outcomes by altering emotion-related brain function. This DBS effect raises concerns around patient autonomy,[69] decisional capacity,[70] subject selection,[71] control over the device's function, and informed consent.[72] DBS may alter a patient's sense of authenticity, create a sense of alienation from that "authentic self," or change interpersonal dynamics.[73] For instance, Klein and colleagues[74] conducted a study of MDD and patients with OCD who had undergone DBS surgery. Although many patients found it a challenge to decipher how much of their emotional state was the direct result of DBS, a few stated that DBS had, indeed, helped them return to their "true self."[75] In line with those results, de Haan and colleagues[76] found that the clinical experience of DBS is not limited to psychopathologic symptoms. It instead pervades the participants' sense of self-reliance and basic trust. The authors suggested offering participants options to contact other DBS participants, because the unusual nature of the intervention may lead them to experience isolation. Another potential issue with DBS consent is subjects' impaired ability to make informed decisions. For instance, Fisher and colleagues[77] found that, despite an intact decisional capacity in patients with Treatment resistant-depression (TRD), 64% displayed therapeutic misconception, an inability to differentiate between treatment and clinical research. Remedying this issue requires educating participants, preferably, by individuals who are not directly involved in the study.[77] These considerations will become more important as advanced technologies, including those with some capacity for self-adjustment, become available. The next generation of DBS studies will likely incorporate ethical review and/or research ethicists directly into their design.

SUMMARY

Based on the experimental evidence reviewed herein,[12,15,54,65] DBS likely exerts its effect at the network level. Probable mechanisms include affecting information transmission between brain structures,[20] disrupting pathologic oscillations,[26] and inducing long-term plasticity.[36,37,39] These mechanisms are all aspects of the phenomenon of interneuronal communication. Accordingly, conceiving of DBS as a network therapy may help understand its effects and uses.[57]

Manual programming of DBS parameters by clinicians may not be an effective way to modulate networks. Closed loop DBS technology, which uses neural signal-based algorithms to adjust treatment parameters dynamically,[29,30] has demonstrated early efficacy in movement disorders.[43] Pilot closed loop investigations are also underway in psychiatric disorders.[57] A more dimensional approach to psychiatry should help to identify the circuit bases of mental illness, in turn indicating which patients may benefit most from DBS at a given target site. Understanding these mechanisms and the basis for patient-specific DBS is critical to achieve the clinical promise of this innovative, but still nascent therapy.

REFERENCES

1. Krack P, Martinez-Fernandez R, del Alamo M, et al. Current applications and limitations of surgical treatments for movement disorders: surgical treatments for movement disorders. Mov Disord 2017;32(1):36–52.
2. Lichtman JW, Denk W. The big and the small: challenges of imaging the brain's circuits. Science 2011;334(6056):618–23.
3. Cuthbert BN, Insel TR. Toward the future of psychiatric diagnosis: the seven pillars of RDoC. BMC Med 2013;11(1):126.

4. Kramer M. Cross-national study of diagnosis of the mental disorders: origin of the problem. Am J Psychiatry 1969;125(10S):1–11.
5. Cuthbert B, Insel T. The data of diagnosis: new approaches to psychiatric classification. Psychiatry 2010;73(4):311–4.
6. Shafer AB. Meta-analysis of the factor structures of four depression questionnaires: Beck, CES-D, Hamilton, and Zung. J Clin Psychol 2006;62(1):123–46.
7. Regier DA, Narrow WE, Clarke DE, et al. DSM-5 field trials in the United States and Canada, Part II: test-retest reliability of selected categorical diagnoses. Am J Psychiatry 2013;170(1):59–70.
8. Dougherty DD, Widge AS. Neurotherapeutic interventions for psychiatric illness. Harv Rev Psychiatry 2017;25(6):253–5.
9. Widge AS, Dougherty DD. Deep brain stimulation for treatment-refractory mood and obsessive-compulsive disorders. Curr Behav Neurosci Rep 2015;2(4): 187–97.
10. Vitek JL. Mechanisms of deep brain stimulation: excitation or inhibition. Mov Disord 2002;17(S3):S69–72.
11. Welter ML, Houeto JL, Bonnet AM, et al. Effects of high-frequency stimulation on subthalamic neuronal activity in parkinsonian patients. Arch Neurol 2004;61(1): 89–96.
12. Mayberg HS, Lozano AM, Voon V, et al. Deep brain stimulation for treatment-resistant depression. Neuron 2005;45(5):651–60.
13. McIntyre CC, Grill WM, Sherman DL, et al. Cellular effects of deep brain stimulation: model-based analysis of activation and inhibition. J Neurophysiol 2004; 91(4):1457–69.
14. Florence G, Sameshima K, Fonoff ET, et al. Deep brain stimulation: more complex than the inhibition of cells and excitation of fibers. Neuroscientist 2016;22(4): 332–45.
15. Rauch SL, Dougherty DD, Malone D, et al. A functional neuroimaging investigation of deep brain stimulation in patients with obsessive–compulsive disorder. J Neurosurg 2006;104(4):558–65.
16. Dougherty DD, Rezai AR, Carpenter LL, et al. A randomized sham-controlled trial of deep brain stimulation of the ventral capsule/ventral striatum for chronic treatment-resistant depression. Biol Psychiatry 2015;78(4):240–8.
17. Mayberg HS. Targeted electrode-based modulation of neural circuits for depression. J Clin Invest 2009;119(4):717–25.
18. Grill WM, Snyder AN, Miocinovic S. Deep brain stimulation creates an informational lesion of the stimulated nucleus. Neuroreport 2004;15(7):1137–40.
19. Dorval AD, Russo GS, Hashimoto T, et al. Deep brain stimulation reduces neuronal entropy in the MPTP-primate model of Parkinson's disease. J Neurophysiol 2008;100(5):2807–18.
20. Dorval AD, Grill WM. Deep brain stimulation of the subthalamic nucleus reestablishes neuronal information transmission in the 6-OHDA rat model of parkinsonism. J Neurophysiol 2014;111(10):1949–59.
21. Brocker DT, Swan BD, So RQ, et al. Optimized temporal pattern of brain stimulation designed by computational evolution. Sci Transl Med 2017;9(371):eaah3532.
22. Buzsáki G, Draguhn A. Neuronal oscillations in cortical networks. Science 2004; 304(5679):1926–9.
23. Cassidy M, Mazzone P, Oliviero A, et al. Movement-related changes in synchronization in the human basal ganglia. Brain 2002;125:1235–46.
24. Little S, Pogosyan A, Kuhn AA, et al. Beta band stability over time correlates with Parkinsonian rigidity and bradykinesia. Exp Neurol 2012;236(2):383–8.

25. Herrington TM, Cheng JJ, Eskandar EN. Mechanisms of deep brain stimulation. J Neurophysiol 2016;115(1):19–38.
26. de Hemptinne C, Swann NC, Ostrem JL, et al. Therapeutic deep brain stimulation reduces cortical phase-amplitude coupling in Parkinson's disease. Nat Neurosci 2015;18(5):779–86.
27. Bahramisharif A, Mazaheri A, Levar N, et al. Deep brain stimulation diminishes cross-frequency coupling in obsessive-compulsive disorder. Biol Psychiatry 2016;80(7):e57–8.
28. Widge AS, Zorowitz S, Link K, et al. Ventral capsule/Ventral striatum deep brain stimulation does not consistently diminish occipital cross-frequency coupling. Biol Psychiatry 2016;80(7):e59–60.
29. Stanslaski S, Afshar P, Cong P, et al. Design and validation of a fully implantable, chronic, closed-loop neuromodulation device with concurrent sensing and stimulation. IEEE Trans Neural Syst Rehabil Eng 2012;20(4):410–21.
30. Lo M-C, Widge AS. Closed-loop neuromodulation systems: next-generation treatments for psychiatric illness. Int Rev Psychiatry 2017;29(2):191–204.
31. Cavanagh JF, Shackman AJ. Frontal midline theta reflects anxiety and cognitive control: meta-analytic evidence. J Physiol Paris 2015;109(1–3):3–15.
32. Cagnan H, Pedrosa D, Little S, et al. Stimulating at the right time: phase-specific deep brain stimulation. Brain 2017;140(1):132–45.
33. Jin Y, Phillips B. A pilot study of the use of EEG-based synchronized Transcranial Magnetic Stimulation (sTMS) for treatment of major depression. BMC Psychiatry 2014;14(1):13–9.
34. Bennett EL, Diamond MC, Krech D, et al. Chemical and anatomical plasticity of brain. Science 1964;146(3644):610–9.
35. Greenberg BD, Gabriels LA, Malone DA Jr, et al. Deep brain stimulation of the ventral internal capsule/ventral striatum for obsessive-compulsive disorder: worldwide experience. Mol Psychiatry 2010;15(1):64–79.
36. Hamani C, Stone SS, Garten A, et al. Memory rescue and enhanced neurogenesis following electrical stimulation of the anterior thalamus in rats treated with corticosterone. Exp Neurol 2011;232(1):100–4.
37. Chakravarty MM, Hamani C, Martinez-Canabal A, et al. Deep brain stimulation of the ventromedial prefrontal cortex causes reorganization of neuronal processes and vasculature. Neuroimage 2016;125:422–7.
38. Do-Monte FH, Rodriguez-Romaguera J, Rosas-Vidal LE, et al. Deep brain stimulation of the ventral striatum increases BDNF in the fear extinction circuit. Front Behav Neurosci 2013;7:1–9.
39. Creed M, Pascoli VJ, Lüscher C. Refining deep brain stimulation to emulate optogenetic treatment of synaptic pathology. Science 2015;347(6222):659–64.
40. Vinogradov S, Fisher M, de Villers-Sidani E. Cognitive training for impaired neural systems in neuropsychiatric illness. Neuropsychopharmacology 2012;37(1):43–76.
41. Subramaniam K, Luks TL, Garrett C, et al. Intensive cognitive training in schizophrenia enhances working memory and associated prefrontal cortical efficiency in a manner that drives long-term functional gains. Neuroimage 2014;99:281–92.
42. McClelland JL, Rumelhart DE. Distributed memory and the representation of general and specific information. J Exp Psychol Gen 1985;114(2):159.
43. Rosin B, Slovik M, Mitelman H, et al. Closed-loop deep brain stimulation is superior in ameliorating parkinsonism. Neuron 2011;72(2):370–84.
44. Hashimoto T, Elder CM, Okun MS, et al. Stimulation of the subthalamic nucleus changes the firing pattern of pallidal neurons. J Neurosci 2003;23(5):1916–23.

45. Davis KD, Taub E, Houle S, et al. Globus pallidus stimulation activates the cortical motor system during alleviation of parkinsonian symptoms. Nat Med 1997;3(6): 671–4.
46. Dougherty DD, Chou T, Corse AK, et al. Acute deep brain stimulation changes in regional cerebral blood flow in obsessive-compulsive disorder. J Neurosurg 2016;125(5):1087–93.
47. Milad MR, Rauch SL. Obsessive-compulsive disorder: beyond segregated cortico-striatal pathways. Trends Cogn Sci 2012;16(1):43–51.
48. Kohl S, Schönherr DM, Luigjes J, et al. Deep brain stimulation for treatment-refractory obsessive compulsive disorder. BMC Psychiatry 2014;14(214):1–10.
49. Malone DA, Dougherty DD, Rezai AR, et al. Deep brain stimulation of the ventral capsule/ventral striatum for treatment-resistant depression. Biol Psychiatry 2009; 65(4):267–75.
50. Riva-Posse P, Choi KS, Holtzheimer PE, et al. A connectomic approach for sub-callosal cingulate deep brain stimulation surgery: prospective targeting in treatment-resistant depression. Mol Psychiatry 2018;23(4):843–9.
51. McIntyre CC, Hahn PJ. Network perspectives on the mechanisms of deep brain stimulation. Neurobiol Dis 2018;23(4):843–9.
52. Holtzheimer PE, Husain MM, Lisanby SH, et al. Subcallosal cingulate deep brain stimulation for treatment-resistant depression: a multisite, randomised, sham-controlled trial. Lancet Psychiatry 2017;4:839–49.
53. Deisseroth K, Feng G, Majewska AK, et al. Next-generation optical technologies for illuminating genetically targeted brain circuits. J Neurosci 2006;26(41): 10380–6.
54. Gradinaru V, Mogri M, Thompson KR, et al. Optical deconstruction of parkinsonian neural circuitry. Science 2009;324(5925):354–9.
55. Steinberg EE, Christoffel DJ, Deisseroth K, et al. Illuminating circuitry relevant to psychiatric disorders with optogenetics. Curr Opin Neurobiol 2015;30:9–16.
56. Wu H, Miller KJ, Blumenfeld Z, et al. Closing the loop on impulsivity via nucleus accumbens delta-band activity in mice and man. Proc Natl Acad Sci U S A 2018; 115(1):192–7.
57. Widge AS, Ellard KK, Paulk AC, et al. Treating refractory mental illness with closed-loop brain stimulation: progress towards a patient-specific transdiagnostic approach. Exp Neurol 2017;287:461–72.
58. Wade EC, Iosifescu DV. Using electroencephalography for treatment guidance in major depressive disorder. Biol Psychiatry Cogn Neurosci Neuroimaging 2016; 1(5):411–22.
59. Widge AS, Avery DH, Zarkowski P. Baseline and treatment-emergent EEG biomarkers of antidepressant medication response do not predict response to repetitive transcranial magnetic stimulation. Brain Stimul 2013;6(6):929–31.
60. Widge AS, Bilge MT, Montana R, et al. Electroencephalographic biomarkers for treatment response prediction in major depressive illness: a meta-analysis.
61. McLoughlin G, Makeig S, Tsuang MT. In search of biomarkers in psychiatry: EEG-based measures of brain function. Am J Med Genet B Neuropsychiatr Genet 2014;165(2):111–21.
62. Widge AS, Deckersbach T, Eskandar EN, et al. Deep brain stimulation for treatment-resistant psychiatric illnesses: what has gone wrong and what should we do next? Biol Psychiatry 2016;79(4):e9–10.
63. Drysdale AT, Grosenick L, Downar J, et al. Resting-state connectivity biomarkers define neurophysiological subtypes of depression. Nat Med 2016;23(1):28–38.

64. Grisanzio KA, Goldstein-Piekarski AN, Wang MY, et al. Transdiagnostic symptom clusters and associations with brain, behavior, and daily function in mood, anxiety, and trauma disorders. JAMA Psychiatry 2017. https://doi.org/10.1001/jamapsychiatry.2017.3951.

65. Choi KS, Riva-Posse P, Gross RE, et al. Mapping the "depression switch" during intraoperative testing of subcallosal cingulate deep brain stimulation. JAMA Neurol 2015;72(11):E1–9.

66. Herron JA, Thompson MC, Brown T, et al. Cortical brain–computer interface for closed-loop deep brain stimulation. IEEE Trans Neural Syst Rehabil Eng 2017; 25(11):2180–7.

67. Gioia GA, Isquith PK, Guy SC, et al. Test review behavior rating inventory of executive function. Child Neuropsychol 2000;6(3):235–8.

68. Bush G, Shin LM, Holmes J, et al. The multi-source interference task: validation study with fMRI in individual subjects. Mol Psychiatry 2003;8(1):60–70.

69. Johansson V, Garwicz M, Kanje M, et al. Authenticity, depression, and deep brain stimulation. Front Integr Neurosci 2011;5:1–3.

70. Rabins P, Appleby BS, Brandt J, et al. Scientific and ethical issues related to deep brain stimulation for disorders of mood, behavior, and thought. Arch Gen Psychiatry 2009;66(9):931–7.

71. Lipsman N, Bernstein M, Lozano AM. Criteria for the ethical conduct of psychiatric neurosurgery clinical trials. Neurosurg Focus 2010;29(2):E9.

72. Schermer M. Ethical issues in deep brain stimulation. Front Integr Neurosci 2011; 5:1–5.

73. Kraemer F. Me, myself and my brain implant: deep brain stimulation raises questions of personal authenticity and alienation. Neuroethics 2013;6(3):483–97.

74. Klein E, Goering S, Gagne J, et al. Brain-computer interface-based control of closed-loop brain stimulation: attitudes and ethical considerations. Brain Computer Interfaces 2016;3(3):140–8.

75. Nyholm S, O'Neill E. Deep brain stimulation, continuity over time, and the true self. Camb Q Healthc Ethics 2016;25(4):647–58.

76. de Haan S, Rietveld E, Stokhof M, et al. Effects of deep brain stimulation on the lived experience of obsessive-compulsive disorder patients: in-depth interviews with 18 patients. PLoS One 2015;10(8):e0135524.

77. Fisher CE, Dunn LB, Christopher PP, et al. The ethics of research on deep brain stimulation for depression: decisional capacity and therapeutic misconception. Ann N Y Acad Sci 2012;1265(1):69–79.

Deep Brain Stimulation
Clinical Applications

Darin D. Dougherty, MD, MMSc

KEYWORDS

- Deep brain stimulation • DBS in Psychiatry • Mechanisms of DBS
- Treatment resistant depression • Treatment-refractory OCD

KEY POINTS

- Deep brain stimulation has a longer history of use in neurology for movement disorders, but work has been performed for psychiatric indications.
- Deep brain stimulation of the ventral/capsule/ventral striatum is approved by the US Food and Drug Administration for the treatment of treatment-refractory obsessive-compulsive disorder.
- Although open-label trials of deep brain stimulation for treatment-resistant depression at multiple targets have been encouraging, controlled trials for approval from the US Food and Drug Administration have been negative.
- Future approaches may include refined targeting using tractography, alternate clinical trial designs, or closed loop approaches.

INTRODUCTION

Deep brain stimulation (DBS) has been used since the 1980s for the treatment of movement disorders. First used for Parkinson's disease, DBS is now approved by the US Food and Drug Administration (FDA) the for treatment of Parkinson's disease, essential tremor, and dystonia, and it is estimated that approximately 150,000 patients with movement disorders have been implanted with DBS devices in the United States

Disclosure Statement: The author has received honoraria, research support and device donation from Medtronic, which manufactures deep brain stimulation systems. D.D. Dougherty has also filed multiple patents related to closed-loop deep brain stimulation, none of which is yet commercially licensed. Preparation of this work was not sponsored or supported by any commercial entity. D.D. Dougherty was supported by grants to D.D. Dougherty from the National Institutes of Health (MH109722, MH111320, and NS100548), and Defense Advanced Research Projects Agency (Cooperative Agreement W911NF-14-2-0045). The views, opinions, and/or findings expressed are those of the authors and should not be interpreted as representing the official views or policies of any sponsor or funding source.
Division of Neurotherapeutics, Department of Psychiatry, Massachusetts General Hospital, Harvard Medical School, CNY2612, 149 13th Street, Boston, MA 02129, USA
E-mail address: ddougherty@partners.org

Psychiatr Clin N Am 41 (2018) 385–394
https://doi.org/10.1016/j.psc.2018.04.004

Abbreviations	
DBS	Deep brain stimulation
FDA	US Food and Drug Administration
HDE	Humanitarian device exemption
HDRS-17	Hamilton Depression Rating Scale
MADRS	Montgomery-Åsberg Rating Scale
OCD	Obsessive-compulsive disorder
sgACC	Subgenual anterior cingulate cortex
slMFB	Superolateral branch of the medial forebrain bundle
STN	Subthalamic nucleus
TRD	Treatment-resistant depression
VC/VS	Ventral capsule/ventral striatum
YBOCS	Yale-Brown Obsessive Compulsive Scale.

alone.[1] DBS works, as the name suggests, via electrodes stereotactically implanted in specific targets within the brain. A subcutaneous wire travels from the electrode to a pacemaker-like device, called an implantable pulse generator that is implanted subcutaneously on the chest wall (usually subclavicular). After DBS implantation, clinicians use a computer that communicates with the implantable pulse generator transcutaneously to set the stimulation parameters. Stimulation parameters include which contacts on the electrode (there are usually 4) deliver stimulation (thus, precisely where in the brain stimulation is delivered), amplitude, frequency, and pulse width. Targets most commonly used for DBS for movement disorders are the subthalamic nucleus (STN) and globus pallidus interna.

The first use of DBS for a psychiatric indication was published by Nuttin and colleagues[2] in 1999. Based on an extant literature suggesting that ablation of the anterior limb of the internal capsule (called an anterior capsulotomy) is an effective treatment for treatment-refractory obsessive-compulsive disorder (OCD), the investigators implanted bilateral DBS electrodes in the anterior limb of the internal capsule in 4 patients with treatment-refractory OCD and reported that 3 of the 4 patients received clinical benefit. Since then, many studies of DBS for treatment-refractory psychiatric illness have been performed. It is essential to note that DBS is only indicated for severe, chronic, treatment-refractory psychiatric illness and that DBS for treatment-refractory psychiatric illness should be overseen by an experienced multidisciplinary team of clinicians. The object of this review is to review the experience of DBS for treatment-refractory psychiatric illness up until now and then to discuss future directions for the field (**Fig. 1**).

OBSESSIVE-COMPULSIVE DISORDER
Ventral Capsule/Ventral Striatum

After the positive results reported by Nuttin and colleagues, multiple groups of investigators began to explore the use of DBS for treatment-refractory OCD. The worldwide experience of DBS for treatment-refractory OCD was described in a landmark paper by Greenberg and colleagues[3] in 2010. Their article describes the results of the use of DBS at the ventral capsule/ventral striatum (VC/VS) target for treatment-refractory OCD from teams in the United States and Europe. In a total of 26 patients with treatment-refractory OCD, the mean baseline Yale-Brown Obsessive Compulsive Scale (YBOCS) score of 34.0 decreased to a mean of 21.0 after 3 months of active DBS treatment.[4] As a categorical measure, a total of 73% of the patients with treatment-refractory OCD experienced at least a 25% improvement on the YBOCS at last follow-up, and 61.5% experienced at least a 35% improvement on the YBOCS

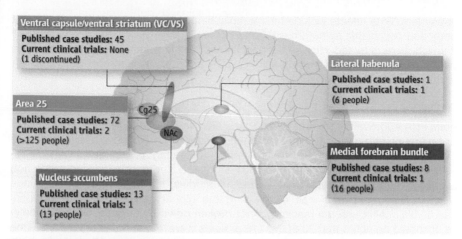

Fig. 1. Deep brain stimulation targets for psychiatric illness. (*From* Underwood E. Short-circuiting depression. Science 2013;342(6158):548–51; with permission.)

at last follow-up. Additionally, after 36 months of DBS treatment, the mean Hamilton Depression Rating Scale (HDRS-17) score decreased by 43.2% and 14 of the 26 patients experienced remission of their depressive symptoms (defined as a HAM-D score of <7).[5] Note that, over time, the anterior limb of the internal capsule target migrated slowly posteriorly to the current target, the VC/VS. As the target migrated posteriorly, the response rate increased and less energy was required to achieve therapeutic benefit, suggesting that the more posterior target is closer to the key circuitry implicated in therapeutic benefit. Last, adverse events were noted. Surgical severe adverse events included implantation-related hemorrhage, a single seizure, and an infected surgical incision. Acute stimulation effects included increased anxiety and/or depression, mood elevation (including hypomania), impaired cognition, and sensorimotor (usually orofacial) effects. All of these side effects were reversed via changes in stimulation parameters. In 2009, the FDA approved VC/VS DBS for treatment-refractory OCD under a humanitarian device exemption (HDE), a mechanism that functions much like orphan drug approval, but for medical devices. Importantly, the HDE approval mechanism was based on open-label data (controlled data were not required).

Subthalamic Nucleus

Mallet and colleagues[6] published the results of the first 2 case reports of DBS in the STN for treatment-refractory OCD in 2002, reporting that both patients were responders. Since then, the STN has emerged as another promising target for DBS for treatment-refractory OCD. In 2008, Mallet and colleagues[7] published the results of a 10-month, crossover, double-blind multicenter study of STN DBS for 16 patients with treatment-refractory OCD. Eight of the patients received active stimulation for 6 months followed by sham stimulation for 6 months and 8 patients received sham stimulation for 6 months followed by active stimulation for 6 months. The mean baseline YBOCS score for the cohorts ranged from 28 to 31, depending on which trial block they were beginning. Overall, the mean YBOCS score after active stimulation was 19, whereas the mean YBOCS score After sham stimulation was 28 (*P* = .01). Additionally, 6 of 8 patients who first received active stimulation were defined as responders, whereas only 3 of 8 patients who first received sham stimulation were defined as responders. Side effects included intracranial hemorrhage in 1 patient and transient motor and psychiatric symptoms in 7 patients, including hypomania in 3 patients, all of which were reversed after adjustment of stimulation parameters. Although these results are encouraging, there is still not FDA approval in place for STN DBS for treatment-refractory OCD.

Summary

Since FDA approval for treatment-refractory OCD in 2009, additional studies of DBS for treatment-refractory OCD (at the targets described herein) have been conducted and some have been controlled trials. A recent metaanalysis provides a valuable review of these studies but, in short, in 31 studies (some controlled and some not) involving 116 patients found that, across all studies, the mean global percentage of YBOCS improvement was 45.1% and the global percentage of responders was 60.0%.[8] Although the results are not broken down by target in the metaanalysis, it should be noted that 83 of the 116 patients were implanted in the anterior limb of the internal capsule, VC/VS, or nucleus accumbens, and 27 patients were implanted in the STN. The remaining 6 patients were implanted in the inferior thalamic peduncle, a target without enough data to adequately assess efficacy at this time.

TREATMENT-RESISTANT DEPRESSION
Subgenual Anterior Cingulate Cortex

The first reported use of DBS for treatment-resistant depression (TRD) was reported by Mayberg and colleagues[9] in 2005. Based on neuroimaging studies that this group and others performed, Mayberg and colleagues chose the subgenual anterior cingulate cortex (sgACC) white matter located adjacent to Brodmann's area 25. Neuroimaging studies demonstrated that the sgACC is activated during sadness induction in healthy volunteers, the sgACC is hyperactive in patients with depression when compared with healthy volunteers, and successful treatment of depression is associated with normalization of sgACC function.[10–16] After 6 months of sgACC DBS, 4 of the 6 patients with TRD were classified as responders (defined as a ≥50% decrease in their HDRS-17 score compared with baseline). Although 3 of the patients in this study experienced infections (which were rectified by surgical and/or antibiotic interventions), the authors reported no motor of psychiatric side effects associated with stimulation.

After these initially promising results, multiple larger open-label trials of sgACC DBS for TRD were conducted with reported response rates ranging from 55% to 92%.[17–20] Side effects included infection, seizure, worsening mood/irritability, worsening depression, suicidal ideation, and suicide. Based on these encouraging data, a large, multicenter, controlled trial of sgACC DBS for TRD was conducted with aim of demonstrating efficacy for potential FDA approval for TRD.[21] Ninety patients with TRD were randomly assigned to active (n = 60) or sham (n = 30) stimulation with the primary outcome measure being frequency of response (defined in this trial as a ≥40% decrease in severity of depressive symptoms instead of the usually required ≥50% reduction in symptom severity). The results of the trial were negative (ie, no statistically significant advantages observed between groups), with 20% of the patients receiving active stimulation being defined as responders at 6 months and 17% of the patients receiving sham stimulation being defined as responders at 6 months. Additionally, 5% of the patients receiving active stimulation were defined as remitters at 6 months and 7% of the patients receiving sham stimulation were defined as remitters at

6 months. Side effects included infection, skin erosion at the surgical site, seizure, worsening depression, and 2 competed suicides.

Ventral Capsule/Ventral Striatum

Based on the marked improvement of depressive symptoms in the open-label trials of VC/VS DBS for treatment-refractory OCD, investigators conducted an open-label trial of VC/VS DBS for TRD.[22] Fifteen patients with TRD were enrolled and received open-label VC/VS for a minimum of 6 months (and as long as 4 years). For the cohort, the mean HAM-D score decreased from 33.1 at baseline to 17.5 at 6 months and 14.3 at last follow-up (mean of 23.5 months). The mean Montgomery-Åsberg Rating Scale (MADRS) score decreased from 34.8 at baseline to 17.9 at 6 months and 15.7 at last follow-up.[23] Responder rates for the HDRS were 40% at 6 months and 53.3% at last follow-up, whereas for the MADRS the response rates were 46.7% at 6 months and 53.3% at last follow-up. Last, remission rates for the HDRS were 20% at 6 months and 40% at last follow-up, whereas for the MADRS the remission rates were 26.6% at 6 months and 33.3% at last follow-up. Side effects included worsening depression, suicidal ideation, insomnia, and hypomania. Both instances of hypomania (which occurred in a single patient) resolved with adjustment of the stimulation parameters.

These initially encouraging findings led to a multicenter controlled trial of VC/VS for TRD to demonstrate efficacy and to potentially obtain FDA approval for TRD.[24] This trial included 30 patients with TRD who were randomly assigned to blinded active versus sham stimulation for 16 weeks followed by an open-label continuation phase with the primary outcome measure being response as defined by a 50% or greater decrease on the MADRS score from baseline at 16 weeks. The results of the trial were negative; at 16 weeks, the response rate for those patients receiving active stimulation was 20%, whereas the response rate for those patients receiving sham stimulation was 14.3%. Additionally, the response rates during the open-label continuation phase were lower than the previous study with the response rates at 12, 18, and 24 months of 20%, 26.7%, and 23.3% respectively. Side effects included worsening depression, suicidal ideation, suicide attempts, insomnia, hypomania, irritability, mania, and 1 completed suicide.

Although the United States controlled trial of VC/VS DBS for TRD was negative, a controlled trial of DBS in the ventral anterior limb of the internal capsule, a target nearly identical to the VC/VS target, was conducted using an alternative clinical trial design and is the only positive controlled trial of DBS for TRD to date.[25] Twenty-five patients with TRD underwent open-label ventral anterior limb of the internal capsule DBS for 52 weeks. After the 52-week open-label treatment, patients were randomized in a double-blind fashion to a 12-week phase where patients were assigned to active and sham stimulation in a crossover fashion with the primary outcome being the difference in HAM-D-17 scores between the active and sham DBS. During the initial open-label phase, the mean HAM-D-17 score decreased from 22.2 to 15.9 with 40% classified as responders. Sixteen patients participated in the randomized crossover phase (9 responders and 7 nonresponders). During the crossover phase, active DBS was associated with a lower mean HAM-D-17 score (13.6) than sham DBS (23.1). The authors reported 5 suicide attempts in 4 patients, 2 completed suicides, transient mania in 2 patients, and transient hypomania in 1 patient.

Nucleus Accumbens

Although the nucleus accumbens is the location where the tip of the electrode is located after VC/VS procedures (the VS, or ventral striatum, component), investigators in Europe have explored this target under the rubric of nucleus accumbens as a target.

An initial open-label study of nucleus accumbens DBS for TRD involving 10 patients found a response rate (defined as a $\geq$50% reduction of the HAM-D) of 50% at 6 months.[26] Side effects included transient increase in anxiety, 1 attempted suicide, and 1 completed suicide. Although not clear whether the results are a separate cohort or continued follow-up of the 10 patients with TRD in the previous study, a long-term follow-up of 11 patients with TRD receiving nucleus accumbens DBS found that 5 (45.5%) were responders at 12 months and remained responders at 24 months, and at last the follow-up at a maximum of 4 years.[27] Side effects were identical to the previously described study, suggesting that this study does represent a continued follow-up of the cohort in the previous study. Although these open-label results are comparable with those seen in many of the sgACC and VC/VS open-label studies for TRD, it is important to note that no controlled trials of the nucleus accumbens target for TRD have been reported to date.

Medial Forebrain Bundle

The medial forebrain bundle has long been known to be an important node in the brain's reward circuitry and animal studies have demonstrated hedonic responses to medial forebrain stimulation. Given that anhedonia is a core feature of major depression, the same German group of researchers who conducted the nucleus accumbens DBS studies described elsewhere in this article have more recently conducted studies of the medial forebrain bundle, specifically the superolateral branch of the medial forebrain bundle (slMFB), DBS for TRD. In an initial open-label pilot study, 7 patients with TRD received slMFB DBS and 6 of the patients with TRD were responders (as defined by a $\geq$50% decrease of the MADRS score from baseline) after 7 days of stimulation.[28] Longer term follow-up of this cohort (and the addition of 1 more patient) revealed sustained results with 6 of the 8 patients (75%) classified as responders and 4 of the 8 (50%) classified as remitters at 12 months.[29] Side effects from this cohort included oculomotor effects (blurred vision, double vision) due to the proximity of the target to the optic nerve and intracranial hemorrhage. Although there no data from controlled trials of slMFB DBS for TRD, the rapidity of response (within 7 days) seems to differentiate slMFB DBS from other targets (which may require months for benefits to accrue).

Other Targets

Based on the hypothesis that overactivation of the lateral habenula may suppress monoaminergic function and stimulate hypothalamic–pituitary–adrenal axis function the lateral habenula has been proposed as a potential DBS target for TRD.[30] A case report of 1 patient with TRD who achieved remission after lateral habenula has been published but no other clinical data regarding lateral habenula DBS are currently available.[31] Lastly, 1 patient with TRD was treated with DBS in the inferior thalamic peduncle with a resultant decrease of their HDRS score from 42 to 6 without relapse for 9 years.[32]

Other Indications

Although studies of DBS for OCD and TRD are reviewed herein, other psychiatric indications are being explored as well, although there are few data available. Although a full review of each indication being studied in early stages is beyond the scope of this review, DBS for other psychiatric indications includes Tourette's syndrome, addiction, anorexia nervosa, autism, schizophrenia, and anxiety disorders. See Graat and colleagues[33] for a recent extensive review.

FUTURE DIRECTIONS

Before a discussion of future directions for the use of DBS for psychiatric illness, the current state of the field should be briefly reviewed. First, DBS has been widely successful for multiple movement disorders, has been an available treatment for decades, and has been used in as many as 150,000 Americans with movement disorders. Second, DBS does have FDA approval for the treatment of 1 psychiatric disorder, namely, treatment-refractory OCD. It should be noted, however, that FDA approval was granted under the HDE mechanism, which does not necessarily require data from controlled trials for approval. Third, because of the higher prevalence of TRD, the HDE mechanism for FDA approval has not been an option for DBS for TRD so controlled data are required. Unfortunately, both US-based controlled trials of DBS, at separate targets, were negative.

New Approaches

Current approaches for DBS surgical implantation typically involve targets defined as x, y, and z coordinates in standardized stereotactic space. This approach does not take individual anatomic variability into account but, rather, takes a one-spot-fits-all approach. However, it is clear that there is marked interindividual variability in where fibers of passage lie in relation to a standard DBS target. As just 1 example, a study by our group showed that the desired fibers of passage that one would want to stimulate for therapeutic benefit (namely, orbitofrontothalamic fibers) may sometimes lie as far as 8 mm in any either direction from the standard VC/VS DBS target.[34] Therefore, using preoperative tractography data to individualize targeting could have a substantial impact on clinical outcome. Riva-Posse and colleagues[35] examined tractography data retrospectively from sixteen patients with TRD who received sgACC DBS and found that all responders shared fiber pathways being affected by the implanted sgACC electrode, although this finding was not consistent in nonresponders. The investigators then took the logical next step, which was to use tractography prospectively for sgACC DBS targeting. The small study using 11 patients yielded response rates of 72.7% and 81.8% at 6 months and 1 year, respectively. Five of the patients with TRD were in remission at 6 months and 6 of the patients with TRD were in remission at 1 year.[36] Although it is difficult to compare clinical outcomes from previous studies using standard anatomic space for DBS targeting to the use of preoperative tractography for prospective targeting without head-to-head studies, this initial small open-label study demonstrates the promise of this approach.

Another important consideration is clinical trial design. Of the 3 published controlled trials of DBS for TRD, both trials that compared active versus sham stimulation soon after DBS electrode implantation were negative; the sole trial that compared active versus sham during a blinded withdrawal phase after a long ($\leq$52 weeks) period of open-label treatment was positive.[21,24,25] Given the variability of time to response (as demonstrated by changes in response rates with time in the studies described above), trying to capture an efficacious clinical signal at the "front end" of a clinical trial, shortly after DBS electrode implantation, during a 4- to 6-month window may be more difficult than allowing for optimization of DBS for maximal clinical benefit for up to 1 year followed by a randomized blinded withdrawal.

It may be that no one DBS target addresses all of the phenotypes associated with the broad categorical diagnosis being studied. For example, for TRD studies the sgACC target was chosen based on its role in negative mood, the VC/VS target was first studied for OCD suggesting an effect on perseverative thinking, and the slMFB target was proposed for anhedonia. Given the phenotypic variability within a categorical diagnosis like depression, perhaps we should not be surprised that any single DBS target is not effective for all patients. An alternative approach may be to target measurable transdiagnostic behaviors embedded within a categorical diagnosis. Using performance on behavioral assays (tasks) as a primary outcome measure, while still embedded within a categorical diagnosis, also makes sense, because we have a better understanding of the circuitry underlying these behavioral domain (eg, fear, reward) than we do for any categorical diagnosis. Study entry based on these criteria may allow for a more precision medicine approach with better outcomes than the current all comers approach.[37]

Last, closed-loop DBS approaches (see M. Taha Bilge and colleagues' article, "Deep Brain Stimulation in Psychiatry: Mechanisms, Models, and Next-Generation Therapies," in this issue) may ultimately be necessary to treat psychiatric disorders with more complex underlying circuitry.[38–41]

REFERENCES

1. Benabid A, Pollak P, Louveau A, et al. Combined (thalamotomy and stimulation) stereotactic surgery of the VIM thalamic nucleus for bilateral Parkinson disease. Stereotact Funct Neurosurg 1987;50(1–6):344–6.

2. Nuttin B, Cosyns P, Demeulemeester H, et al. Electrical stimulation in anterior limbs of internal capsules in patients with obsessive-compulsive disorder. Lancet 1999;354(9189):1526.

3. Greenberg B, Gabriels L, Malone D, et al. Deep brain stimulation of the ventral internal capsule/ventral striatum for obsessive-compulsive disorder: worldwide experience. Mol Psychiatry 2008;15(1):64–79.

4. Goodman WK, Price LH, Rasmussen SA, et al. The Yale-Brown Obsessive Compulsive Scale. I. Development, use, and reliability. Arch Gen Psychiatry 1989;46(11):1006–11.

5. Hamilton M. A rating scale for depression. J Neurol Neurosurg Psychiatry 1960; 23(1):56–62.

6. Mallet L, Mesnage V, Houeto JL, et al. Compulsions, Parkinson's disease, and stimulation. Lancet 2002;360(9342):1302–4.

7. Mallet L, Polosan M, Jaafari N, et al. Subthalamic nucleus stimulation in severe obsessive–compulsive disorder. N Engl J Med 2009;360(9):931–2.

8. Alonso P, Cuadras D, Gabriëls L, et al. Deep brain stimulation for obsessive-compulsive disorder: a meta-analysis of treatment outcome and predictors of response. PLoS One 2015;10(7):e0133591.

9. Mayberg HS, Lozano AM, Voon V, et al. Deep brain stimulation for treatment-resistant depression. Neuron 2005;45(5):651–60.

10. Mayberg HS, Liotti M, Brannan SK, et al. Reciprocal limbic-cortical function and negative mood: converging PET findings in depression and normal sadness. Am J Psychiatry 1999;156(5):675–82.

11. Seminowicz D, Mayberg H, McIntosh A, et al. Limbic–frontal circuitry in major depression: a path modeling metanalysis. Neuroimage 2004;22(1):409–18.

12. Dougherty D, Weiss A, Cosgrove G, et al. Cerebral metabolic correlates as potential predictors of response to anterior cingulotomy for treatment of major depression. J Neurosurg 2003;99(6):1010–7.

13. Goldapple K, Segal Z, Garson C, et al. Modulation of cortical-limbic pathways in major depression: treatment-specific effects of cognitive behavior therapy. Arch Gen Psychiatry 2004;61(1):34–41.

14. Mayberg H, Brannan S, Tekell J, et al. Regional metabolic effects of fluoxetine in major depression: serial changes and relationship to clinical response. Biol Psychiatry 2000;48(8):830–43.
15. Nobler M, Oquendo M, Kegeles L, et al. Decreased regional brain metabolism after ECT. Am J Psychiatry 2001;158(2):305–8.
16. Mottaghy F, Keller C, Gangitano M, et al. Correlation of cerebral blood flow and treatment effects of repetitive transcranial magnetic stimulation in depressed patients. Psychiatry Res 2002;115(1–2):1–14.
17. Lozano A, Mayberg H, Giacobbe P, et al. Subcallosal cingulate gyrus deep brain stimulation for treatment-resistant depression. Biol Psychiatry 2008;64(6):461–7.
18. Kennedy S, Giacobbe P, Rizvi S, et al. Deep brain stimulation for treatment-resistant depression: follow-up after 3 to 6 years. Am J Psychiatry 2011;168(5):502–10.
19. Lozano A, Giacobbe P, Hamani C, et al. A multicenter pilot study of subcallosal cingulate area deep brain stimulation for treatment-resistant depression. J Neurosurg 2012;116(2):315–22.
20. Holtzheimer P. Subcallosal cingulate deep brain stimulation for treatment-resistant unipolar and bipolar depression. Arch Gen Psychiatry 2012;69(2):150–8.
21. Holtzheimer P, Husain M, Lisanby S, et al. Subcallosal cingulate deep brain stimulation for treatment-resistant depression: a multisite, randomised, sham-controlled trial. Lancet Psychiatry 2017;4(11):839–49.
22. Malone D, Dougherty D, Rezai A, et al. Deep brain stimulation of the ventral capsule/ventral striatum for treatment-resistant depression. Biol Psychiatry 2009;65(4):267–75.
23. Montgomery SA, Asberg M. A new depression scale designed to be sensitive to change. Br J Psychiatry 1979;134(4):382–9.
24. Dougherty D, Rezai A, Carpenter L, et al. A randomized sham-controlled trial of deep brain stimulation of the ventral capsule/ventral striatum for chronic treatment-resistant depression. Biol Psychiatry 2015;78(4):240–8.
25. Bergfeld I, Mantione M, Hoogendoorn M, et al. Deep brain stimulation of the ventral anterior limb of the internal capsule for treatment-resistant depression: a randomized clinical trial. JAMA Psychiatry 2016;73(5):456.
26. Bewrnick B, Hurlemann R, Matusch A, et al. Nucleus accumbens deep brain stimulation decreases ratings of depression and anxiety in treatment-resistant depression. Biol Psychiatry 2010;67(2):110–6.
27. Bewernick B, Kayser S, Sturm V, et al. Long-term effects of nucleus accumbens deep brain stimulation in treatment-resistant depression: evidence for sustained efficacy. Neuropsychopharmacology 2012;37(9):1975–85.
28. Schlaepfer T, Bewernick B, Kayser S, et al. Rapid effects of doop brain stimulation for treatment-resistant major depression. Biol Psychiatry 2013;73(12):1204–12.
29. Bewernick B, Kayser S, Gippert S, et al. Deep brain stimulation to the medial forebrain bundle for depression- long-term outcomes and a novel data analysis strategy. Brain Stimul 2017;10(3):664–71.
30. Sartorius A, Henn F. Deep brain stimulation of the lateral habenula in treatment resistant major depression. Mod Hypotheses 2007;69(6):1305–8.
31. Sartorius A, Kiening K, Kirsch P, et al. Remission of major depression under deep brain stimulation of the lateral habenula in a therapy-refractory patient. Biol Psychiatry 2010;67(2):e9–11.

32. Jiménez F, Nicolini H, Lozano A, et al. Electrical stimulation of the inferior thalamic peduncle in the treatment of major depression and obsessive compulsive disorders. World Neurosurg 2013;80(3–4):S30.e17-25.
33. Graat I, Figee M, Denys D. The application of deep brain stimulation in the treatment of psychiatric disorders. Int Rev Psychiatry 2017;29(2):178–90.
34. Makris N, Rathi Y, Mouradian P, et al. Variability and anatomical specificity of the orbitofrontothalamic fibers of passage in the ventral capsule/ventral striatum (VC/VS): precision care for patient-specific tractography-guided targeting of deep brain stimulation (DBS) in obsessive compulsive disorder (OCD). Brain Imaging Behav 2016;10(4):1054–67.
35. Riva-Posse P, Choi K, Holtzheimer P, et al. Defining critical white matter pathways mediating successful subcallosal cingulate deep brain stimulation for treatment-resistant depression. Biol Psychiatry 2014;76(12):963–9.
36. Riva-Posse P, Choi K, Holtzheimer P, et al. A connectomic approach for subcallosal cingulate deep brain stimulation surgery: prospective targeting in treatment-resistant depression. Mol Psychiatry 2017;23(4):843–9.
37. Widge A, Deckersbach T, Eskandar E, et al. Deep brain stimulation for treatment-resistant psychiatric illnesses: what has gone wrong and what should we do next? Biol Psychiatry 2016;79(4):e9–10.
38. Widge A, Ellard K, Paulk A, et al. Treating refractory mental illness with closed-loop brain stimulation: progress towards a patient-specific transdiagnostic approach. Exp Neurol 2017;287:461–72.
39. Meidahl A, Tinkhauser G, Herz D, et al. Adaptive deep brain stimulation for movement disorders: the long road to clinical therapy. Mov Disord 2017;32(6):810–9.
40. Marceglia S, Rosa M, Servello D, et al. Adaptive Deep Brain Stimulation (ADBS) for Tourette syndrome. Brain Sci 2017;8(1):4.
41. Underwood E. Short-circuiting depression. Science 2013;342(6158):548–51.

The Mechanism of Action of Vagus Nerve Stimulation in Treatment-Resistant Depression

Current Conceptualizations

Charles R. Conway, MD*, Willa Xiong, MD

KEYWORDS

- Major depression • Treatment-resistant major depression • Vagus nerve stimulation
- Neurostimulation

KEY POINTS

- Vague nerve stimulation (VNS) is a neuromodulatory treatment of depression with various proposed mechanisms of action underlying its efficacy, although further studies are still needed.
- Complex afferent vagal pathways target regions known to affect depression, including the monoamine brainstem nuclei, insular cortex, thalamus, and prefrontal cortex.
- Neuroimaging data have demonstrated VNS's potential acute, subacute, and chronic effects on cortical and subcortical brain regions involved in affective regulation.
- VNS also may have effects on monoamine release, with neuroplasticity serving as the link between increased neurotransmitter levels and actual antidepressant effects.

ANATOMY OF THE VAGUS NERVE

The vagus nerve (cranial nerve X) is the longest of the cranial nerves. True to its name, the vagus, derived from the Latin term for "wandering," has an extensive web of innervation spreading throughout the thoracic, abdominal, and pelvic cavities. The nerve subserves numerous critical bodily functions and is composed of various nerve fibers, including afferent (ie, to the brain) somatic sensory, special sensory (taste), visceral sensory, and efferent (ie, away from the brain) visceral motor and somatic motor fibers.[1]

Disclosure Statement: Dr C.R. Conway is a research design consultant to LivaNova, the makers of the vagus nerve stimulation device.
Department of Psychiatry, Washington University School of Medicine, 660 South Euclid Avenue, Campus Box 8134, St Louis, MO 63110, USA
* Corresponding author.
E-mail address: conwaycr@wustl.edu

Psychiatr Clin N Am 41 (2018) 395–407
https://doi.org/10.1016/j.psc.2018.04.005
0193-953X/18/Published by Elsevier Inc.

The efferent fibers originate from 2 brainstem nuclei: the dorsal motor nucleus and nucleus ambiguous. In contrast, the afferent fibers targeted during vagal nerve stimulation (VNS) originate from the nodose and jugular ganglia localized just below the foramen magnum, or the opening in the skull between brainstem and spinal cord.[1,2] Afferent fibers carry visceral, somatic (tragus of the earlobe), and special sensory (taste) to the brainstem.[3]

During vagal nerve stimulation, the electrical leads are attached to the left vagus in the midinferior cervical region. In the cervical region, the vagus is positioned between and slightly posterior to the carotid artery and jugular vein, all of which are enmeshed in deep cervical fascia known as the carotid sheath. The majority (approximately 85%) of the cervical vagus nerve is composed of afferent unmyelinated C fibers.[4] These fibers have lower stimulation thresholds, which allow VNS's low-current stimulation to be transmitted primarily afferent, or upstream, to the brain and not downstream to thoracic/abdominal organs, thereby minimizing effects on the heart, lungs, or gastrointestinal tract.[4] With higher currents, myelinated efferent fibers can be activated; this is manifested by activation of the laryngeal and pharyngeal muscles as well as associated hoarseness and stridor—symptoms observed in approximately two-thirds of patients during active VNS stimulation. For this reason, patients receiving VNS therapy may elect to temporarily shut the device off by placing a magnet on the skin over the VNS generator when they are engaging in activities requiring speaking or respiratory exertion.

In humans, the left and right vagal nerves supply parasympathetic visceral motor activity to the sinoatrial and atrioventricular nodes, respectively. Hence, to prevent intracardiac conduction abnormalities, VNS is typically implanted on the left vagus nerve.[5] Studies to date have demonstrated that use of the VNS device in the therapeutic range has limited effects on downstream thoracic and abdominal target tissues (eg, pulmonary, cardiac, and gastrointestinal systems). Given that most therapeutic studies of VNS have not enrolled patients with significant cardiopulmonary disease, however, caution is advised in consideration of such patients, especially those with obstructive sleep apnea.[6,7]

AFFERENT BRAIN AND BRAINSTEM VAGAL PATHWAYS

Although well studied in lower mammals, the afferent vagal brainstem and brain pathways are complex and not completely understood. A summary of these pathways is provided later, and a more complete description can be found in Henry.[8]

As discussed previously, the afferent pathways, which are accessed by VNS, carry somatic sensory information from the skin, special gustatory sensation, and sensation from the larynyx, pharynx, and thoracoabdominal organs. These afferent fibers enter the brainstem at the medullary level, decussate, and then synapse at several nuclei (**Fig. 1**). The most critical pathway for VNS treatment is the tractus solitarius, which terminates in the nucleus tractus solitarius (NTS).[9–11] Fibers from the NTS primarily project upstream to the pontine parabrachial nucleus (PBN) but also project to various other medullary and pontine nuclei, the cerebellar nuclei, and the periaqueductal gray. The periaqueductal gray region is critical for central pain modulation, and limited studies of VNS's analgesic effects may be taking advantage of this regional innervation[12] (see **Fig. 1**).

The NTS projects to both the medullary and pontine raphe nuclei (RN) (ie, the primary brainstem sites for serotonergic nuclei)[13] as well as the pontine locus ceruleus (LC) (ie, the primary brainstem site for noradrenergic nuclei)[13] (**Fig. 2**). These upstream monoamine projections are likely critical in the mood regulation aspects of VNS. In

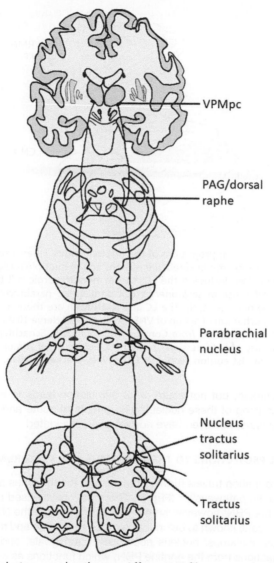

VPMpc

PAG/dorsal
raphe

Parabrachial
nucleus

Nucleus
tractus
solitarius

Tractus
solitarius

Fig. 1. Afferent brainstem vagal pathways. Afferent VN fibers enter the CNS at the level of the medulla and travel in the tractus solitarius, largely terminating in the NTS.[8,10,11,16] On entering the brainstem, some vagal fibers decussate immediately; hence, afferent vagal information travels bilaterally in the CNS. Ascending fibers of the NTS terminate primarily in the PSN; however, some NTS bypass the PBN (not depicted in figure) and ascend uninterrupted to the periaqueductal gray (PAG) as well as the parvocellular ventroposteromedial thalamic nucleus (VPMpc),[16] a site responsible for taste/visceral sensory information. The VPMpc also receives vagal afferent information directly from the PBN. (*Adapted from* Conway CR, Colijn MA, Schachter SC. Vagus nerve stimulation for epilepsy and depression. In: Reti IM, editor. Brain stimulation: methodologies and interventions. 1st edition. Hoboken (NJ): Wiley-Blackwell; 2015. p. 310)

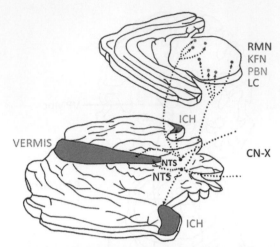

Fig. 2. Pontine and cerebellar projections of the afferent vagus. Fibers from the NTS project to the medial (vermis) and inferior cerebellar regions and to multiple nuclei upstream in the pons and mesencephalon, including the LC; site of noradrenergic cell bodies, the raphe magnus nucleus (RMN); site of serotonergic cell bodies, the parabrachial nucleus (PBN), and the Kölliker-Fuse nucleus (KFN). The LC and RMN both are thought to be relevant to the antidepressant mechanism of action of VNS. CN-X, Cranial Nerve 10 (Vagus); ICH, inferior cerebellar hemisphere. (*Adapted from* Conway CR, Colijn MA, Schachter SC. Vagus nerve stimulation for epilepsy and depression. In: Reti IM, editor. Brain stimulation: methodologies and interventions. 1st edition. Hoboken (NJ): Wiley-Blackwell; 2015. p.311)

animal studies, chronic, but not acute, VNS stimulation leads to increased resting state autonomous firing of these nuclei.[14] The effects of acute and chronic VNS on these nuclei in humans, however, have not yet been elucidated.

AFFERENT VAGAL PROJECTIONS TO THE THALAMUS AND CEREBRUM

Afferent vagal information travels further upstream to the thalamus and cerebrum via several multisynaptic pathways[8,15] (**Fig. 3**). The most heavily used pathways extend from the NTS to the PBN; however, some NTS fibers bypass the NTS[2,8,16] and proceed directly to regions known to be critical in mood regulation and major depression: the hypothalamus, thalamus, nucleus accumbens, amygdala, and stria terminalis. Additionally, projections from the pontine PBN, which functions as a brainstem "relay center" for autonomic and taste information, proceed to upstream regions known to be influential in mood disorders, including the amygdala (central and basolateral nuclei), hypothalamus, and cortical regions, including the anterior insula, lateral prefrontal cortex, infralimbic cortex and other cortical regions.[8,17–21] The insular cortex provides communication with more anterior cortical regions, such as the ventrolateral and orbital prefrontal cortex, and indirectly communicates with the medial prefrontal cortex.[21,22] As discussed later, these regions seem to undergo considerable acute and chronic changes with VNS and may also be critical in determining which depressed patients may respond to VNS treatment.

Additionally, several clinicians and researchers have observed that VNS is associated with increased alertness. This may be due to the PBN projections to the medial reticular formation, a brainstem region associated with alertness and generation of sleep waves.[23,24] Researchers have shown that epilepsy patients receiving VNS

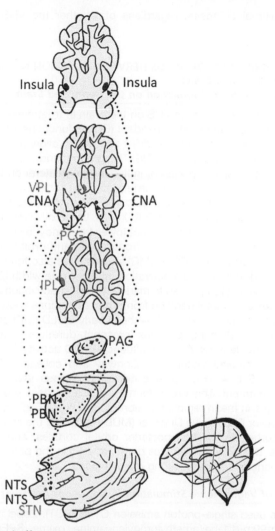

Fig. 3. Brainstem and afferent projections to the cerebrum and limbic system. Afferent vagal projections, originating in the NTS, ascend bilaterally primarily synapsing at the PBN. Some NTS fibers bypass the PBN and proceed upstream directly to more superior brain structures including the ventroposteromedial thalamic nucleus (VPMpc),[16] which also receives afferent vagal information from the PBN. The PBN sends afferent vagal information to multiple locations, including the central nucleus of the amygdala (CNA), the insular cortex, the periaqueductal gray (PAG), all depicted in the figure. The PBN also sends afferent vagal information to the VPMpc and intralaminar thalamic nuclei, the bed nucleus of the stria terminalis, and the hypothalamus (not depicted in figure).[8,18,20] Left vagal projections carrying information regarding conscious sensation of deep pharyngeal tissues, project to the left spinal trigeminal nucleus (STN) and further ascend to the ventral posterior lateral thalamic nuclei (VPL). Hence, with increasing electrical current of VNS, this vago-trigemino-thalamo pathway signals laryngeal pain, which is typically resolved by lowering the current or frequency of the stimulation. IPL, inferior parietal lobule; PCG, postcentral gyrus. (*Adapted from* Conway CR, Colijn MA, Schachter SC. Vagus nerve stimulation for epilepsy and depression. In: Reti IM, editor. Brain stimulation: methodologies and interventions. 1st edition. Hoboken (NJ): Wiley-Blackwell; 2015. p. 312)

have improved diurnal alertness, regardless of whether the VNS lowers seizure frequency.[25]

BRAIN IMAGING CORRELATES OF VAGUS NERVE STIMULATION NEUROANATOMY IN TREATMENT-RESISTANT DEPRESSION

Acute Effects of Vagus Nerve Stimulation on the Depressed Brain

The earliest studies of the effects of VNS on the brain in treatment-resistant depression (TRD) were blood oxygen level–dependent (BOLD) functional MRI (fMRI) studies. Bohning and colleagues[26] fashioned an fMRI scanner to allow real-time, in-scanner images of TRD patients receiving acute VNS. This group found multiple regions known to be associated with major depression, including the bilateral orbitofrontal cortex, parieto-occipital cortex, hypothalamus, the left temporal cortex, and amygdala. Other studies have looked at the effects of varying VNS electrical parameters on regional brain activation and deactivation. Using BOLD fMRI, Lomarev and colleagues[27] determined that higher frequency (20 Hz), but not lower frequency (5 Hz), acute VNS produced regional activation (hypothalamus, frontal pole, and orbitofrontal cortex, and left globus pallidus). Subsequent BOLD fMRI studies have also found that alterations in pulse width altered regional brain activation; higher pulse width (250 and 500 μs), but not lower pulse width (130 μs), led to markedly greater activation of the ventromedial prefrontal cortex and dorsolateral prefrontal cortex, regions known to be critical in the antidepressant effects of VNS.[28,29] All these early BOLD fMRI studies were performed in subjects with differing, previous (prescan), durations of exposure to VNS therapy, subsequently determined to be influence BOLD activity.[30]

Using oxygen 15–labeled water PET, Conway and colleagues[31] assessed the acute effects of VNS in 4 TRD patients naïve to previous VNS therapy via real-time, in-scanner treatment. This group found significant (t test scores ranging from 5.7 to 8.12) changes in mean regional cerebral blood flow (rCBF) in multiple regions associated with Major Depressive Disorder (MDD), including the inferior frontal gyrus, anterior insular cortex, frontal and posterior orbital cortices, and bilateral anterior cingulate cortices. Decreased rCBF was demonstrated in the precuneus, and superior and inferior parietal cortices, among other regions.

Subacute Effects of Vagus Nerve Stimulation in Treatment-Resistant Depression

Two early studies used single-photon emission CT (SPECT). Zobel and colleagues[32] used technetium-99m-d,1-hexamethylpropyleneamine oxime SPECT to measure changes in rCBF after 4 weeks in 12 TRD subjects. This group found decreased rCBF in the cortical regions (eg, medial frontal, precentral, parahippocampal gyri, posterior cingulate, and middle temporal gyrus) as well as subcortical regions (eg, caudate and amygdala). Only 3 of the 12 TRD subjects subsequently responded to VNS. In contrast, Kosel and colleagues[33] also used technetium Tc 99m hexamethylpropyleneamine oxime SPECT in 15 TRD patients after 10 weeks of VNS. This group found largely decreased rCBF localized to the right precuneus, cuneus, lingual gyrus, and left anterior insular cortex as well as increased rCBF in the left inferior frontal gyrus.

Nahas and colleagues[30] bridged both acute and subacute brain imaging studies using BOLD fMRI to study the effects of sustained VNS (0–100 weeks) on TRD patients using real-time, in-scanner techniques. Initially, acute VNS led to activation in the right medial prefrontal gyrus; however, with additional stimulation, the same acute stimulation predominantly led to deactivation. The switch from activation to deactivation occurred after 30 weeks of VNS, which coincided with the patients experiencing an improvement in depressive symptoms. A similar activation greater than deactivation pattern was observed in the right anterior insular cortex. Using linear regression, this group demonstrated a powerful correlation between reduction in depression score and activation of the right anterior insular cortex (r^2 = 0.76, P = .0001). Furthermore, there was a significant correlation between the early right anterior insular activation and severity of depression, as measured by a standard depression scale.

Chronic Effects of Vagus Nerve Stimulation in Treatment-Resistant Depression

Pardo and colleagues[34] used fluorodeoxyglucose F 18 (FDG) PET to assess regional metabolic changes after 6 months and 12 months of VNS in TRD. This group found a trend of decreased mean cerebral metabolic glucose (CMRGlu) in the ventromedial cerebral cortex. Conway and colleagues[29] also used resting state FDG PET to perform serial imaging of TRD patients receiving VNS at 0 months, 3 months, and 12 months of stimulation; 9 of 13 patients in this trial responded to treatment, and 5 of 13 patients fully remitted. A statistically significant decrease in mean CMRGlu was observed in the right dorsolateral prefrontal cortex (Brodmann area 46) after 3 months of stimulation in the patients who eventually responded to treatment at 12 months. This prefrontal decrease in CMRGlu was not observed at 12 months, suggesting that during the course of treatment of TRD with VNS, the brain undergoes a transitional state in the subacute period.

Conway and colleagues[29] findings are consistent with Nahas and colleagues'[30] findings of differing brain responses to VNS at 30 weeks of stimulation, coinciding with the emergence of an antidepressant response. Although Conway and colleagues could no longer observe dorsolateral prefrontal cortex changes at 12 months of stimulation, this group did find increased CMRGlu in the left substantia nigra/ventral tegmental area (VTA) brainstem region at 12 months in VNS antidepressant responders, whereas the opposite pattern (ie, decreased regional CMRGlu in the VTA) was noted in nonresponders. This response-specific increase in VTA activity supports the premise that the antidepressant effects of VNS are dopaminergically mediated, because the VTA is the primary brainstem site of dopamine. This is consistent with the finding that VNS stimulation in TRD increases cerebrospinal fluid concentrations of homovanillic acid, the primary metabolite of dopamine.[35] Dopamine may well play a critical role in many treatments of TRD, including deep brain stimulation,[36] electroconvulsive therapy,[37,38] and repetitive transcranial magnetic stimulation.[39,40]

Are There Biological Markers Predicting Response to Vagus Nerve Stimulation in Treatment-Resistant Depression?

Given the permanent nature of VNS implantation as well as the considerable personal and financial costs of treatment, the ability to be able to predict the likelihood of response to VNS would prove invaluable. In an effort to determine if specific subtypes of TRD may respond to VNS, Conway and colleagues[41] performed baseline resting state FDG PET scans poststimulator implantation and prestimulation and demonstrated that the combination of lower anterior insular cortex CMRGlu (P = .004) and higher orbitofrontal cortex CMRGlu (P = .047) predicted depression rating scale improvements ($R2$ = 0.58, P = .005). In a whole-brain, voxel-wise analysis, baseline CMRGlu in the right anterior insular cortex was strongly correlated with the likelihood of depressive symptom change (r = 0.78, P = .001). These findings suggest that baseline anterior insular and orbitofrontal cortex metabolic activity may influence antidepressant outcomes at 12 months. Recent studies point toward the insular cortex as being a critical region in mood regulation.[42]

OTHER FACTORS CONTRIBUTING TO THE ANTIDEPRESSANT EFFECTS OF VAGUS NERVE STIMULATION

Vagus Nerve Stimulation Effects on Noradrenergic and Serotonergic Neurons

As discussed previously, the afferent vagus has neuroanatomic connections with the brainstem regions, which serve as the primary brain centers for norepinephrine and serotonin—the LC and RN, respectively. Animal studies have demonstrated that VNS enhances noradrenergic and serotonergic neurotransmission in brain areas crucial for mood regulation (eg, prefrontal cortex, amygdala, and hippocampus). Several studies have shown increases in noradrenaline concentrations in the cortex, hippocampus, and medial prefrontal cortex with VNS treatment.[43–46] Not only does sustained VNS seem to increase the firing rate of noradrenergic neurons in the LC but also it suppresses inhibition from GABAergic interneurons,[47–49] leading to further increased noradrenaline release. Sustained VNS has also been found to enhance serotonergic firing in the RN but only after 14 days of treatment.[14,47] Manta and colleagues[47] discovered that serotonergic firing enhancement by VNS was prevented by lesioning noradrenergic neurons, suggesting that the treatment's effects on serotonergic neurons is indirectly mediated via noradrenergic pathways.

Considering that VNS has proved beneficial even in patients with medication-resistant depression, its antidepressant effects have been theorized to be distinct from that of traditional medication treatment.[14] Although antidepressants restore neuronal firing by increasing neurotransmitter release and altering the sensitivity of inhibitory autoreceptors,[50] the aforementioned animal studies propose that VNS increases the baseline firing rate of the LC and RN neurons themselves. Dorr and Debonnel[14] also found that serotonergic and noradrenergic autoreceptors are not desensitized with long-term VNS treatment, as they are with antidepressants, further supporting the theory that VNS has a distinct mechanism of action.

Vagus Nerve Stimulation Effects on Neural Plasticity

VNS has also been implicated in neuroplasticity, or the heterogeneous mechanisms of neuronal birth, survival, migration, and synaptogenesis. A growing body of evidence posits that VNS's neuroplasticity effects may explain the therapeutic lag between acute increases in monoamines and the treatment's antidepressant effects weeks to months later in patients.[51] Neurogenesis, or the generation of fully functional neurons from progenitor cells, takes place in the dentate gyrus of the hippocampus.[52] Biggio and colleagues[53] showed that both short-term and long-term VNS increased dendritic length and complexity of hippocampal neurons. Other animal studies have demonstrated increases in neural progenitor cell proliferation with VNS.[53–55] Moreover, VNS may affect cellular survival and differentiation through expression of brain-derived neurotrophic factor (BDNF) and basic fibroblast growth factor (FGF)[45,53]—factors known to be decreased in mood disorders[56,57] and up-regulated by antidepressant medications.[58–60]

The correlation between VNS-induced neuroplasticity and antidepressant-like effects in behavioral testing is still nebulous. The hippocampal neuronal changes found by Biggio and colleagues[53] did not correlate with any antidepressant actions in animals undergoing the forced swim test. Conversely, Gebhardt and colleagues[55] found associated restorative cognitive effects with VNS-induced progenitor cell proliferation. It is thus unclear at this point whether neuroplasticity changes contribute to VNS's clinical effects on depression or whether they are simply a byproduct of other mechanisms of action resulting in sustained antidepressant action. Regardless, neuroplasticity mechanisms present a plausible hypothesis for VNS's gradual effects, because it takes weeks to months for newborn cells to become fully functional, mature cells capable of restoring the disturbed corticolimbic networks in depressed patients.[61,62]

Neuroplasticity and Monoamine Link

The monoamine and neuroplasticity hypotheses may be interlinked in the mechanism behind VNS' efficacy. The hippocampus is rich in noradrenergic and serotonergic innervation so changes in neurotransmitter concentrations may affect regional plasticity, as demonstrated with antidepressant treatment in rodents.[63,64] Noradrenergic and serotonergic neurons have also been shown to contain FGF-2 known to enhance hippocampal neurogenesis,[65,66] although FGF-2 levels correlated with VNS treatment has yet to be studied. Overall, all evidence for mediation of plasticity via changes in neurotransmitter activity has been indirect in nature, and clinical studies are clearly needed to elucidate this link.

Vagus Nerve Stimulation Effects on Dopamine

Recent studies involving other neurostimulation techniques, specifically repetitive transcranial magnetic stimulation and deep brain stimulation, point to the dopaminergic system as playing a potentially significant role in these treatments' antidepressant effects.[67,68] Several emerging lines of evidence support that VNS's effects may have substantial dopaminergic effects as well. Conway and colleagues found increased regional glucose uptake in the brainstem VTA in TRD patients who responded to 12 months of active VNS, whereas nonresponders did not demonstrate this. In addition, Carpenter and colleagues[35] found increased homovanillic acid, a metabolite of dopamine, in the cerebrospinal fluid of TRD patients. These results linking the dopaminergic system to VNS require further exploration and replication.

SUMMARY

Over the course of the past 2 decades, VNS has been increasingly studied in patients with depression, in particular TRD. Various functional brain imaging techniques, such as fMRI, PET, and SPECT, have identified both acute and chronic (over many months) localized regional brain changes associated with VNS in TRD. Some of the regions implicated include the ventromedial and dorsolateral prefrontal cortices, inferior frontal gyrus, anterior insular cortex, frontal and posterior orbital cortices, anterior cingulate, and brainstem VTA. Additional studies have suggested that baseline anterior insular and orbitofrontal cortex metabolic activity may predict response to VNS. Animal studies have further demonstrated that VNS enhances noradrenergic and serotonergic neurotransmission in brain areas crucial for mood regulation (eg, prefrontal cortex, amygdala, and hippocampus) and may enhance neuroplasticity as well. Similarly, human studies (neuroimaging and cerebral spinal fluid) have demonstrated evidence of dopaminergic changes occurring with VNS in TRD. Much of the mechanism behind VNS's unique effects in TRD continues to remain unknown and further studies in clinical populations are warranted.

REFERENCES

1. Nieuwenhuys R, Voogd J, van Huijzen C. The human central nervous system: a synopsis and atlas. 3rd edition. Berlin: Springer-Verlag; 1988.
2. Parent A, Carpenter's human neuroanatomy. 9th edition. Baltimore (MD): Williams & Wilkins; 1996.
3. Peuker ET, Filler TJ. The nerve supply of the human auricle. Clin Anat 2002;15(1): 35–7.

4. Foley JO, DuBois FS. Quantitative studies of the vagus nerve in the cat. I. The ratio of sensory to motor fibers. J Comp Neurol 1937;67(1):49–67.
5. San Mauro MP, Patronelli F, Spinelli E, et al. Nerves of the heart: a comprehensive review with a clinical point of view. Neuroanatomy 2009;8:26–31.
6. Binks AP, Paydarfar D, Schachter SC, et al. High strength stimulation of the vagus nerve in awake humans: a lack of cardiorespiratory effects. Respir Physiol 2001; 127(2–3):125–33.
7. Banzett RB, Guz A, Paydarfar D, et al. Cardiorespiratory variables and sensation during stimulation of the left vagus in patients with epilepsy. Epilepsy Res 1999; 35(1):1–11.
8. Henry TR. Therapeutic mechanisms of vagus nerve stimulation. Neurology 2002; 59(6 Suppl 4):S3–14.
9. Beckstead RM. An autoradiographic examination of corticocortical and subcortical projections of the mediodorsal-projection (prefrontal) cortex in the rat. J Comp Neurol 1979;184(1):43–62.
10. Kalia M, Sullivan JM. Brainstem projections of sensory and motor components of the vagus nerve in the rat. J Comp Neurol 1982;211(3):248–65.
11. Rhoton AL Jr, O'Leary JL, Ferguson JP. The trigeminal, facial, vagal, and glossopharyngeal nerves in the monkey. Afferent connections. Arch Neurol 1966;14(5): 530–40.
12. Kirchner A, Birklein F, Stefan H, et al. Left vagus nerve stimulation suppresses experimentally induced pain. Neurology 2000;55(8):1167–71.
13. Saper CB. Diffuse cortical projection systems: anatomical organization and role in cortical function. In: Plum F, editor. Handbook of physiology: the nervous system. Bethesda (MD): American Physiological Society; 1987. p. 169–210.
14. Dorr AE, Debonnel G. Effect of vagus nerve stimulation on serotonergic and noradrenergic transmission. J Pharmacol Exp Ther 2006;318(2):890–8.
15. Agostoni E, Chinnock JE, De Daly MB, et al. Functional and histological studies of the vagus nerve and its branches to the heart, lungs and abdominal viscera in the cat. J Physiol 1957;135(1):182–205.
16. Beckstead RM, Morse JR, Norgren R. The nucleus of the solitary tract in the monkey: projections to the thalamus and brain stem nuclei. J Comp Neurol 1980; 190(2):259–82.
17. Saper CB, Loewy AD. Efferent connections of the parabrachial nucleus in the rat. Brain Res 1980;197(2):291–317.
18. Bester H, Bourgeais L, Villanueva L, et al. Differential projections to the intralaminar and gustatory thalamus from the parabrachial area: a PHA-L study in the rat. J Comp Neurol 1999;405(4):421–49.
19. Carmichael ST, Price JL. Sensory and premotor connections of the orbital and medial prefrontal cortex of macaque monkeys. J Comp Neurol 1995;363(4): 642–64.
20. Krout KE, Loewy AD. Parabrachial nucleus projections to midline and intralaminar thalamic nuclei of the rat. J Comp Neurol 2000;428(3):475–94.
21. Saleem KS, Kondo H, Price JL. Complementary circuits connecting the orbital and medial prefrontal networks with the temporal, insular, and opercular cortex in the macaque monkey. J Comp Neurol 2008;506(4):659–93.
22. Ongur D, Price JL. The organization of networks within the orbital and medial prefrontal cortex of rats, monkeys and humans. Cereb Cortex 2000;10(3):206–19.
23. Herbert H, Moga MM, Saper CB. Connections of the parabrachial nucleus with the nucleus of the solitary tract and the medullary reticular formation in the rat. J Comp Neurol 1990;293(4):540–80.

24. Cox CL, Huguenard JR, Prince DA. Nucleus reticularis neurons mediate diverse inhibitory effects in thalamus. Proc Natl Acad Sci U S A 1997;94(16):8854–9.
25. Malow BA, Edwards J, Marzec M, et al. Vagus nerve stimulation reduces daytime sleepiness in epilepsy patients. Neurology 2001;57(5):879–84.
26. Bohning DE, Lomarev MP, Denslow S, et al. Feasibility of vagus nerve stimulation-synchronized blood oxygenation level-dependent functional MRI. Invest Radiol 2001;36(8):470–9.
27. Lomarev M, Denslow S, Nahas Z, et al. Vagus nerve stimulation (VNS) synchronized BOLD fMRI suggests that VNS in depressed adults has frequency/dose dependent effects. J Psychiatr Res 2002;36(4):219–27.
28. Mu Q, Bohning DE, Nahas Z, et al. Acute vagus nerve stimulation using different pulse widths produces varying brain effects. Biol Psychiatry 2004;55(8):816–25.
29. Conway CR, Chibnall JT, Gebara MA, et al. Association of cerebral metabolic activity changes with vagus nerve stimulation antidepressant response in treatment-resistant depression. Brain Stimul 2013;6(5):788–97.
30. Nahas Z, Teneback C, Chae JH, et al. Serial vagus nerve stimulation functional MRI in treatment-resistant depression. Neuropsychopharmacology 2007;32(8):1649–60.
31. Conway CR, Sheline YI, Chibnall JT, et al. Cerebral blood flow changes during vagus nerve stimulation for depression. Psychiatry Res 2006;146(2):179–84.
32. Zobel A, Joe A, Freymann N, et al. Changes in regional cerebral blood flow by therapeutic vagus nerve stimulation in depression: an exploratory approach. Psychiatry Res 2005;139(3):165–79.
33. Kosel M, Brockmann H, Frick C, et al. Chronic vagus nerve stimulation for treatment-resistant depression increases regional cerebral blood flow in the dorsolateral prefrontal cortex. Psychiatry Res 2011;191(3):153–9.
34. Pardo JV, Sheikh SA, Schwindt GC, et al. Chronic vagus nerve stimulation for treatment-resistant depression decreases resting ventromedial prefrontal glucose metabolism. Neuroimage 2008;42(2):879–89.
35. Carpenter LL, Moreno FA, Kling MA, et al. Effect of vagus nerve stimulation on cerebrospinal fluid monoamine metabolites, norepinephrine, and gamma-aminobutyric acid concentrations in depressed patients. Biol Psychiatry 2004;56(6):418–26.
36. Coenen VA, Schlaepfer TE, Maedler B, et al. Cross-species affective functions of the medial forebrain bundle-implications for the treatment of affective pain and depression in humans. Neurosci Biobehav Rev 2011;35(9):1971–81.
37. Baldinger P, Lotan A, Frey R, et al. Neurotransmitters and electroconvulsive therapy. J ECT 2014;30(2):116–21.
38. Saijo T, Takano A, Suhara T, et al. Electroconvulsive therapy decreases dopamine D(2)receptor binding in the anterior cingulate in patients with depression: a controlled study using positron emission tomography with radioligand [(1)(1)C] FLB 457. J Clin Psychiatry 2010;71(6):793–9.
39. Pogarell O, Koch W, Popperl G, et al. Striatal dopamine release after prefrontal repetitive transcranial magnetic stimulation in major depression: preliminary results of a dynamic [123I] IBZM SPECT study. J Psychiatr Res 2006;40(4):307–14.
40. Pogarell O, Koch W, Popperl G, et al. Acute prefrontal rTMS increases striatal dopamine to a similar degree as D-amphetamine. Psychiatry Res 2007;156(3):251–5.
41. Conway CR, Chibnall JT, Gangwani S, et al. Pretreatment cerebral metabolic activity correlates with antidepressant efficacy of vagus nerve stimulation in

treatment-resistant major depression: a potential marker for response? J Affect Disord 2012;139(3):283–90.

42. McGrath CL, Kelley ME, Holtzheimer PE, et al. Toward a neuroimaging treatment selection biomarker for major depressive disorder. JAMA Psychiatry 2013;70(8): 821–9.

43. Roosevelt RW, Smith DC, Clough RW, et al. Increased extracellular concentrations of norepinephrine in cortex and hippocampus following vagus nerve stimulation in the rat. Brain Res 2006;1119(1):124–32.

44. Raedt R, Clinckers R, Mollet L, et al. Increased hippocampal noradrenaline is a biomarker for efficacy of vagus nerve stimulation in a limbic seizure model. J Neurochem 2011;117(3):461–9.

45. Follesa P, Biggio F, Gorini G, et al. Vagus nerve stimulation increases norepinephrine concentration and the gene expression of BDNF and bFGF in the rat brain. Brain Res 2007;1179:28–34.

46. Manta S, El Mansari M, Debonnel G, et al. Electrophysiological and neurochemical effects of long-term vagus nerve stimulation on the rat monoaminergic systems. Int J Neuropsychopharmacol 2013;16(2):459–70.

47. Manta S, Dong J, Debonnel G, et al. Enhancement of the function of rat serotonin and norepinephrine neurons by sustained vagus nerve stimulation. J Psychiatry Neurosci 2009;34(4):272–80.

48. Manta S, El Mansari M, Blier P. Novel attempts to optimize vagus nerve stimulation parameters on serotonin neuronal firing activity in the rat brain. Brain Stimul 2012;5(3):422–9.

49. Aston-Jones G, Zhu Y, Card JP. Numerous GABAergic afferents to locus ceruleus in the pericerulear dendritic zone: possible interneuronal pool. J Neurosci 2004; 24(9):2313–21.

50. Blier P. The pharmacology of putative early-onset antidepressant strategies. Eur Neuropsychopharmacol 2003;13(2):57–66.

51. Nahas Z, Marangell LB, Husain MM, et al. Two-year outcome of vagus nerve stimulation (VNS) for treatment of major depressive episodes. J Clin Psychiatry 2005; 66(9):1097–104.

52. Eriksson PS, Perfilieva E, Bjork-Eriksson T, et al. Neurogenesis in the adult human hippocampus. Nat Med 1998;4(11):1313–7.

53. Biggio F, Gorini G, Utzeri C, et al. Chronic vagus nerve stimulation induces neuronal plasticity in the rat hippocampus. Int J Neuropsychopharmacol 2009; 12(9):1209–21.

54. Revesz D, Tjernstrom M, Ben-Menachem E, et al. Effects of vagus nerve stimulation on rat hippocampal progenitor proliferation. Exp Neurol 2008;214(2):259–65.

55. Gebhardt N, Bar KJ, Boettger MK, et al. Vagus nerve stimulation ameliorated deficits in one-way active avoidance learning and stimulated hippocampal neurogenesis in bulbectomized rats. Brain Stimul 2013;6(1):78–83.

56. Karege F, Perret G, Bondolfi G, et al. Decreased serum brain-derived neurotrophic factor levels in major depressed patients. Psychiatry Res 2002;109(2): 143–8.

57. Karege F, Bondolfi G, Gervasoni N, et al. Low brain-derived neurotrophic factor (BDNF) levels in serum of depressed patients probably results from lowered platelet BDNF release unrelated to platelet reactivity. Biol Psychiatry 2005; 57(9):1068–72.

58. Nibuya M, Morinobu S, Duman RS. Regulation of BDNF and trkB mRNA in rat brain by chronic electroconvulsive seizure and antidepressant drug treatments. J Neurosci 1995;15(11):7539–47.

59. Chen B, Dowlatshahi D, MacQueen GM, et al. Increased hippocampal BDNF immunoreactivity in subjects treated with antidepressant medication. Biol Psychiatry 2001;50(4):260–5.

60. Mallei A, Shi B, Mocchetti I. Antidepressant treatments induce the expression of basic fibroblast growth factor in cortical and hippocampal neurons. Mol Pharmacol 2002;61(5):1017–24.

61. Hanson ND, Owens MJ, Nemeroff CB. Depression, antidepressants, and neurogenesis: a critical reappraisal. Neuropsychopharmacology 2011;36(13): 2589–602.

62. Zhao C, Deng W, Gage FH. Mechanisms and functional implications of adult neurogenesis. Cell 2008;132(4):645–60.

63. Loy R, Koziell DA, Lindsey JD, et al. Noradrenergic innervation of the adult rat hippocampal formation. J Comp Neurol 1980;189(4):699–710.

64. Duman RS. Depression: a case of neuronal life and death? Biol Psychiatry 2004; 56(3):140–5.

65. Chadi G, Tinner B, Agnati LF, et al. Basic fibroblast growth factor (bFGF, FGF-2) immunoreactivity exists in the noradrenaline, adrenaline and 5-HT nerve cells of the rat brain. Neurosci Lett 1993;160(2):171–6.

66. Palmer TD, Markakis EA, Willhoite AR, et al. Fibroblast growth factor-2 activates a latent neurogenic program in neural stem cells from diverse regions of the adult CNS. J Neurosci 1999;19(19):8487–97.

67. Friedman A, Frankel M, Flaumenhaft Y, et al. Programmed acute electrical stimulation of ventral tegmental area alleviates depressive-like behavior. Neuropsychopharmacology 2009;34(4):1057–66.

68. Keck ME, Welt T, Muller MB, et al. Repetitive transcranial magnetic stimulation increases the release of dopamine in the mesolimbic and mesostriatal system. Neuropharmacology 2002;43(1):101–9.

Vagus Nerve Stimulation
Changing the Paradigm for Chronic Severe Depression?

Scott T. Aaronson, MD[a,b,]*, Charles R. Conway, MD[c]

KEYWORDS

- Major depression • Treatment-resistant major depression • Vagus nerve stimulation
- Neurostimulation

KEY POINTS

- Treatment-resistant depression (TRD) affects at least a third of patients with depression and there is scant evidence to guide treatment of those who have failed four or more trials of somatic therapies.
- Vagus nerve stimulation (VNS) was cleared in 2005 by the Food and Drug Administration (FDA) for use in TRD after patients had failed at least four antidepressant trials on the basis of two large clinical trials, although a noncoverage determination (NCD) issued in 2007 by the Centers for Medicare and Medicaid Services has dramatically limited its availability.
- Two large randomized studies failed to reach their primary outcome measure, likely in part because of the 6 to 9 months it takes to achieve response after the device is turned on and because of low, chronic stimulation providing some positive effect.
- A recent open-label, naturalistic study of 795 TRD patients (494 patients receiving VNS and 301 patients receiving treatment as usual) followed over 5 years showed a much great likelihood of achieving response and remission if implanted with VNS.

Epidemiologic evidence suggests that the incidence of major depressive disorder (MDD) is growing with a lifetime prevalence of almost 30% and a yearly prevalence of 9%.[1] Antidepressant medications, the mainstay of somatic therapy for depression, show only a mild to moderate effect size (0.20–0.40) for acute antidepressant response.[2]

Disclosure Statement: Dr C.R. Conway is a research design consultant to LivaNova, the makers of the vagus nerve stimulation device. Dr S.T. Aaronson is a consultant to Neuronetics, Liva-Nova, Alkermes, and Genomind. He serves on the speaker boards for Sunovion, Neurocrine, and Otsuka and has received research support from Neuronetics.

[a] Clinical Research Programs, Sheppard Pratt Health System, 6501 North Charles Street, Towson, MD 21204, USA; [b] Department of Psychiatry, University of Maryland Medical School, 655 West Baltimore Street, Baltimore, MD 21201, USA; [c] Department of Psychiatry, Washington University School of Medicine, 660 South Euclid Avenue, Campus Box 8134, St Louis, MO 63110, USA
* Corresponding author. Sheppard Pratt Health System, 6501 North Charles Street, Towson, MD 21204.
E-mail address: saaronson@sheppardpratt.org

Serial antidepressant treatment trials demonstrate that more than 60% of depressed patients fail to remit after an initial pharmacotherapy trial, and progressively fewer remit with subsequent trials until the fourth antidepressant trial yields a remission rate of 10% to 14%.[3–5] Treatment-resistant depression (TRD) refers to major depression that fails to remit after two antidepressant treatment trials of adequate dose and duration. The Sequenced Treatment Alternatives to Relieve Depression trial (STAR*D) demonstrated that 32% to 41% of depressed patients fail to achieve antidepressant remission after four antidepressant trials, resulting in a large population of symptomatically and functionally impaired individuals with clear TRD.[4] There is scant evidence to guide treatment of TRD patients who have failed more than four trials of somatic therapies.

In 2005, the Food and Drug Administration (FDA) approved vagus nerve stimulation (VNS) for the treatment of MDD (unipolar and bipolar) after failure of at least four adequate trials of antidepressants based on the results of two large clinical trials.[6–8] Despite this, in 2006 the Centers for Medicare and Medicaid Services (CMS) made a noncoverage determination for VNS for MDD. This determination was based on a technology assessment that concluded that the VNS for MDD remained unproven/experimental because the large, randomized trial failed to meet its primary outcome measure of statistically significant antidepressant improvement 12 weeks after implantation. This effect of this decision was that Medicare, Medicaid, and most private insurers have not reimbursed for VNS for this indication. Ongoing efforts, specifically a 5-year, 800-patient naturalistic study comparing VNS with treatment as usual (TAU),[9] may lead to a re-evaluation of this policy, potentially increasing the availability of VNS for those with the most severe forms of TRD.

This article reviews the clinical development of VNS starting with the first recognition of its potential for treating depression, parses the results several large clinical trials, and suggests a future path for optimal clinical development and use.

EARLY DEVELOPMENT OF VAGUS NERVE STIMULATION

VNS was first developed and FDA-approved in 1997 for use in treatment-refractory epilepsy. Anecdotal reports of mood improvement seen in VNS-implanted epilepsy patients led to two open-label pilot studies tracking changes in mood. The first compared outcomes in 20 VNS-implanted epilepsy patients and 20 epilepsy patients who were not implanted with VNS but received stable anticonvulsant medication.[10] This study showed a significant reduction in depression scores within the VNS-implanted subjects ($P = .017$) but not a between-groups difference. Two potential significant limitations for this study were that on average, the two groups were not depressed; and the VNS group had significantly more baseline seizures per month compared with the control group. The second study reported on 11 patients implanted with VNS for medication-refractory partial complex seizures, who had at least a mild depression. These patients were then randomized to low- or high-dose stimulation.[11] Depression rating scores were done at baseline, 3 months, and 6 months. This group found statistically significant differences in several depression scores at both postimplant time points; however, only a trend toward significance between high- and low-dose stimulation ($P = .1$). Both studies also demonstrated that the decrease in depression scores was independent of the VNS antiseizure benefit.

THE VAGUS NERVE STIMULATION DEVICE

The primary VNS device used in the US and European clinical trials described next is the Neurocybernetic Prosthesis system now marketed by LivaNova (Houston, TX) (**Fig. 1**). The stimulus generator consists of a titanium-encased lithium battery that is

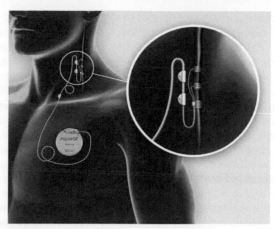

Fig. 1. Illustration of the attachment of the VNS lead to the mid-cervical region of the left vagus nerve. The bipolar lead is coiled around the vagus in two adjacent regions with a tether attached to the surrounding fascia to prevent lead movement under tension. (*Courtesy of* LivaNova USA, Inc, Houston, TX.)

implanted under the skin in the upper chest wall. Pig-tailed electrodes emerge from the device, are tunneled under the skin, and are then wrapped around the left cervical vagus nerve. The device is implanted under general or local anesthesia typically in 1 to 2 hours. Two weeks following the surgery the device is activated and set by a wand connected to a handheld programming device. The telemetric programming wand sets the four stimulation parameters for the device: current (from 0.25 to 3.0 mA), stimulation frequency (from 20 to 50 Hz), pulse width (from 130 to 500 ms), and duty cycle (adjustable from the usual settings of 30 seconds on and 5 minutes off). The initial settings are gradually titrated up, usually over the first 2 weeks of treatment as tolerated by the patient. Although the mechanism of action of VNS in TRD is not fully established, several animal studies and human neuroimaging studies demonstrate significant changes in regions known to be associated with depression (prefrontal and cingulate cortex, and brainstem) following chronic treatment.[12] Both clinical and neuroimaging studies support that the effects of VNS in TRD occur gradually. Statistically significant improvement may take 6 months to develop and continue to improve beyond that time up to about 2 years. The proposed mechanisms of action are discussed elsewhere in this issue.

CLINICAL TRIALS OF VAGUS NERVE STIMULATION IN TREATMENT-RESISTANT DEPRESSION

After seeing support for mood improvement in epilepsy patients receiving VNS, the first experience in a primarily depressed population was a 30-patient open-label study.[6] As with most VNS trials, the study population included patients with either unipolar or bipolar MDD. Subjects had to have failed at least two antidepressants from two different classes and be depressed in the current episode for at least 2 years or have had more than four episodes of depression. After implantation, the device was turned on after 2 weeks, and then titrated to maximum tolerated dose for 2 weeks. For this study, the primary antidepressant outcome measure was at 12 weeks postimplantation or 8 weeks postimplantation at full stimulation dose. Forty percent (12 of 30) of subjects met response criteria, which was a 50% reduction from baseline on the 28-item Hamilton Depression Rating Scale and 17% met remission criteria.

This cohort was followed and reported on after 1 year[13] and 2 years.[14] At 1 year, the response rate was sustained going from 40% to 46% and the remission rate increased significantly from 17% to 29% (P = .045). The 2-year data included an expanded cohort of 59 patients and showed a response rate of 42% and a remission rate of 22%.

The initial response and remission rates were promising given the chronicity, disability, and severity of TRD. These sustained response and remission rates are even more striking given the evidence of extremely high relapse rates in longer term TRD treatment studies including one involving electroconvulsive therapy (ECT).[15,16] Also, the VNS was exceptionally well tolerated. These early studies were limited by the absence of a control group but supported the need for a prospective, double-blind, controlled trial of VNS in TRD.

In the first randomized clinical trial studying VNS for TRD, 235 TRD patients who had failed between two and six adequate trials of antidepressant treatment were implanted with VNS devices, but only half had active treatment for the first 12 weeks, whereas the other half had the device implanted but not activated.[7] This trial defined treatment response as a 50% drop from baseline in the 24-item Hamilton Depression Rating Scale. Following 10 weeks of stimulation (including 2 weeks of gradual increase in output current) there was no significant difference (P = .251) in response rate between active VNS (15.2%) and sham VNS (10%). A secondary depression measurement scale, the 30-item Inventory of Depression Symptomatology—Self Report did show a significant difference at 8 weeks of stimulation (P = .032).

It is unclear why there was such a large difference between the open-label pilot study (response rate of 40%) and the double-blinded trial (15.2%). In addition to the most obvious reason, that is, observer bias, the open-label study was conducted at only four sites, which may have allowed for more careful patient selection, likely critical given the tremendous heterogeneity of TRD.

A subsequent report on the open-label extension arm of this initially double-blind study demonstrated a growing response and remission rate over the subsequent months of VNS treatment.[8] A cumulative increase in response rate was observed over time: 15% at 3 months, 18% at 6 months, 25% at 9 months, and 30% at 12 months. The 12-month remission rate was 15.8%. This gradually increasing response rate was duplicated in a European open-label study[17] that showed increasing response and remission rates at 3, 6, 9, and 12 months with the median time to response at 9 months. Curiously, the European study had a much higher response rate at 12 months (53% with a remission rate of 33%). This is likely because the European patients being markedly less ill than the American subjects: fewer episodes, fewer failed medication trials, less ECT exposure, and less severe baseline depression scores.

To compare 1-year outcomes for TRD patients with and without VNS (VNS + TAU vs TAU), a naturalistic nonrandomized comparator group was identified and followed at the same centers doing the randomized trial.[18] Patients in this cohort could receive any treatment, including ECT, to manage their TRD. The patients selected were equally treatment resistant (same number of failed trials, severity of illness, and so forth) as those in the VNS randomized controlled trial (RCT).[7,8] This study found a significantly higher response rate at 1 year (21.1% for VNS + TAU vs 11.6% for TAU alone; P = .029) and a significantly better remission rate (15.0% for VNS + TAU vs 3.6% for TAU; P = .006). Although compelling, using an equivalent population in a separate study has not been the gold standard for demonstrating significant efficacy in psychiatric trials. The special difficulties of studying a severely ill population with a treatment that takes months to demonstrated effectiveness is discussed later.

The only other large randomized trial of VNS in TRD was a dose-finding study that although not repeating the error of placing the primary outcome measure too soon in the course of treatment, found another hurdle in the path toward acceptance of VNS for TRD.[19] There are four programmable parameters with implantable VNS: (1) output current (milliampere), (2) pulse width of each individual stimulation (microsecond), (3) frequency (Hertz), and (4) duty cycle (how much stimulation time in seconds and how much off time in minutes). For this study amount of stimulation varied by three randomization groups: (1) low, (2) medium, and (3) high. Across all groups frequency was kept at 20 Hz and duty cycle was kept at 30 seconds on and 5 minutes off. The pulse width was 250 μs for the medium- and high-dose groups and 125 μs for the low-dose group. The main variable was the current, programmed at 0.25 mA for low, 1.0 mA for medium, and 1.5 mA for high. In the study 331 patients were randomized. The patient population had failed at least four antidepressant treatments and 97% failed six or more treatments. The acute treatment phase lasted 22 weeks and had a longer term, still blinded phase that allowed upward dosing titration. All treatment groups showed significant improvement in the acute phase; however, there was no significant difference identified between dosing groups. Other findings from this study included significantly better durability of response at 52 weeks in the medium- and high-dose acute-phase responders than the low-dose responders and a post hoc analysis that demonstrated higher total charge delivered per day was associated with greater improvement in depressive symptoms. An important lesson from this study is that even low-current treatment over months (intended to be a sham equivalent) has considerable antidepressant activity; that is, it is difficult to determine if it is possible to have a low-dose "sham" control in future studies.

More recently, results from the largest and longest observational study of TRD were published, which compared the 5-year outcomes for patients implanted with VNS with a similar population getting TAU alone in a TRD registry.[9] The study included 795 patients, 494 received VNS (including 159 patients rolled over from the dose-finding study) and 301 patient got TAU. More than 97% of patients had failed at least six antidepressant treatments. At baseline the VNS patients had slightly greater depressive illness history than TAU comparison group; that is, they had higher depression rating scale scores, more failed treatments, and a higher likelihood of past ECT treatment than the TAU group. The registry results indicated that the adjunctive VNS group had better clinical outcomes than the TAU group, including a significantly higher 5-year cumulative response rate (67.6% compared with 40.9%; $P<.001$) and a significantly higher remission rate (cumulative first-time remitters, 43.3% compared with 25.7%; $P<.001$).

Compelling evidence of the severity of depressive illness under investigation in this registry study was the finding that 58.7% of the VNS group and 36.2% of the TAU had previous exposure to ECT to manage their illness. A subanalysis demonstrated that among patients with a history of response to ECT by history, those in the adjunctive VNS group had a significantly higher 5-year cumulative response rate than those in the TAU group (71.3% compared with 56.9%; $P = .006$). A similar significant response differential was observed among ECT nonresponders (59.6% compared with 34.1%; $P<.001$). This last finding is particularly noteworthy, because failure of TRD to respond to ECT is often considered a bad prognostic sign.

INTERPRETATION OF STUDY RESULTS

Because there is no existing evidence base for the effective management of TRD once it passes the threshold of more than four treatment failures, one needs to be thoughtful as to how to parse the existing data for VNS. A meta-analysis of six trials (including randomized and nonrandomized cohorts) of VNS and TAU for TRD using a Bayesian hierarchical model found that the response and remission rates increased over the duration of stimulation and VNS patients were more likely to respond than those receiving TAU alone.[20] The odds ratio for response based on the Montgomery Asberg Depression Rating Scale was 3.19 (confidence interval [CI], 2.12–4.66) and the Clinical Global Inventory-Improvement scale demonstrated an odds ratio of 7.00 (CI, 4.63–10.83) both favoring VNS over TAU.

Although compelling, these data do not fit the standard paradigm of evaluating antidepressant efficacy by presence of statistical separation between outcomes of a treated group versus placebo or sham control. In the two RCT of VNS for TRD unforeseen complications prevented the achievement of statistical separation. In the first study[7] the primary outcome measure was measured many weeks before optimal VNS benefit could be expected to occur. In the dose-finding study,[19] the cumulative low dose provided sufficient antidepressant neurostimulation over 6 months to not provide a sham control; hence, lowering the chance of statistical separation.

In summary, the totality of the extensive data collected on VNS in TRD supports that there is strong evidence of the antidepressant efficacy of VNS for a population of TRD patients for whom there are no obvious somatic options. The response rate ranges from 30% to 53% and seems to be decidedly higher than comparable TAU cohorts. The absence of clear separation in the two RCTs has limited the acceptability of VNS for third-party payers but the large, positive albeit naturalistic data set released in 2017[9] may provoke re-evaluation of this position.

SIDE EFFECTS AND SAFETY

With at least 80,000 individuals (4000 for TRD, remainder for refractory epilepsy) in 70 countries implanted with VNS as of 2015 (data provided by LivaNova) there is a considerable safety and tolerability database. As reported in 1999 from the experience with VNS for refractory epilepsy[21] and confirmed by the subsequent experience from multiple TRD studies, most side effects are related to the stimulation from the device or an extremely low risk of surgical complication. The electrodes attach to the left vagus nerve just below/distal to where the recurrent laryngeal nerve comes off the vagus. Leakage of the afferent signal to the recurrent laryngeal frequently causes hoarseness or voice alteration while the device is delivering stimulation. At 3 months the frequency of hoarseness/voice alteration varies by study from 25% to 68%; however, the incidence drops at 12 to 24 months.[8,14,17] There is a dose effect, higher stimulation parameters having a higher incidence of voice alteration.[19] Other side effects seen in more than 10% of VNS patients include shortness of breath, increased cough, difficulty swallowing, and general pain. Several adverse events are related to complications from surgical implantation including pain or infection at the incision site or incision site reaction. Typically, when these were reported the symptoms would dissipate after 2 weeks.

In the TRD Registry, both the VNS and TAU groups had a decrease in suicidal ideation, although on two of three scales used the VNS group had a statistically greater improvement. All-cause mortality was markedly lower in the VNS arm than in the TAU arm (3.53 per 1000 person-years [95% CI, 1.41–7.27] and 8.63 per 1000 person-years [95% CI, 3.72–17.01], respectively). The rate of completed suicides was also lower in the VNS arm than in the TAU arm (1.01 per 1000 person-years [95% CI, 0.11–3.64] and 2.20 per 1000 person-years [95% CI, 0.24–7.79]).

Serious adverse events related to either VNS implantation or stimulation occurred at a low rate in all the studies cited. A concern about increased risk of cardiac serious adverse events was in part addressed in a recent paper looking at more than 40,000 epilepsy patients implanted with VNS in the United States between 1988 and 2012 and covering 277,661 patient-years of treatment.[22] The incidence of sudden unexpected death in these medication-resistant epilepsy patients was significantly reduced after VNS implantation.

Perhaps the best indication of tolerability is in the original RCT for VNS. In this trial 98% of the active VNS treatment arm completed the acute phase of the study.[7]

CONTRAINDICATIONS

VNS is contraindicated for patients with a left or bilateral cervical vagotomy and it is not recommended for patients with severe cardiac or pulmonary disease.[23] Because stimulation can lead to an onset of sleep apnea, there is an increased risk for apneic events for those with obstructive sleep apnea. Patients implanted with a VNS device should not receive shortwave, microwave, or therapeutic ultrasound diathermy. There are important limitations to the use of whole-body MRI with VNS and this should be taken into account before implanting the device. Concurrent ECT treatment showed no complications when the VNS device was turned off.[14]

CLINICAL USE

The target population for VNS is patients with unipolar or bipolar MDD who have failed at least four adequate trials of antidepressant medication and/or ECT. Consideration for its use should also take into account that response may take 6 to 12 months. Hence, patients who are actively suicidal or unable to care for themselves because of depression or otherwise requiring a rapid response would not be good candidates.

Conversely, patients who have required multiple medication adjustments, multiple courses of ECT or maintenance ECT, or who typically have only transient responses to therapies may be ideal candidates. VNS provides ongoing, well-tolerated, persistent neurostimulation (unique among the current neurostimulation treatments for depression), which is delivered as long as the battery life lasts. Although ECT is a superb treatment for TRD, its effects in TRD are not sustained: afterward, even with aggressive psychopharmacologic support, the positive antidepressant response is lost.[24] VNS has been found to often be helpful in patients with a past history of ECT response and nonresponse.[9] Perhaps VNS could be a chronic neurostimulation delivery system for patients responding to an acute course of stimulation from ECT. There is suggestive evidence that even in patients for who ECT has not been effective VNS may provide a possible option.

COURSE OF TREATMENT

The device is surgically implanted under general or local anesthesia as an out-patient procedure. Two incisions are made, one on the left side of the neck over the vagus nerve, the other in the left upper chest where a subdermal pocket is made for the device. The leads attached to the VNS device are tunneled under the skin and wrapped around the vagus nerve. The entire operation takes about 90 minutes.

A waiting period of 2 weeks after surgery is typical to allow healing before the device is turned on. The device is programmed externally via a wand attached to a handheld device or electronic tablet. For the management of depression, four parameters are adjusted: (1) the output current, (2) the pulse width, (3) the frequency of pulses, and

(4) the duty cycle (how much time the device is on). Typically, the pulse width is held constant at 250 µs and the frequency at 20 Hz (cycles per second). The duty cycle at the start of titration is 30 seconds on and 5 minutes off. At the start of dose titration current is 0.25 mA and is gradually titrated up often over 2 weeks to a goal of 1.0 to 1.5 mA. Although most patients can tolerate these settings, for those patients who cannot the current and/or pulse width are downward adjusted. Usually after the first series of dose titrations to best-tolerated settings, the device parameters are held constant for several months. The existing data support waiting 6 to 12 months before further upward titrations.

Should response be inadequate after 12 months, one strategy is to increase the duty cycle to a longer on time and/or a shorter off time. It is not recommended to exceed a duty cycle of 50% on time (vs the initial setting, which is a 10% on time). Alternatively, the current is set to a higher level as tolerated. Some clinicians find that increases in pulse width or frequency tend to be less well tolerated.

WHAT CONSTITUTES A GOOD VAGUS NERVE STIMULATION RESPONSE?

There is a wide range of responses to VNS. The evidence from clinical trials suggests that in addition to the third of patients who meet the typical threshold of antidepressant response of a 50% drop in a depression rating scale, another third may have a 25% to 50% response. For TRD patients with severe, chronic depression this decrease in depressive symptoms may well represent a meaningful change. The remaining third seems to have little to no response. This seems to be wise counsel to prospective VNS patients: about one-third have an excellent response, one-third a more limited but meaningful response, and one-third have minimal/no response.

Clinical experience has demonstrated that some patients with only minimal antidepressant response have requested to keep receiving VNS, because they report no longer being suicidal and are better able to enjoy some activities. Some may report that the worst they get is less severe than it once was, that is, VNS seems to "raise the floor" on the severity of MDD. Conversely, some patients who feel they have not benefitted from VNS have the device turned off only to experience a worsening depression and request the device be turned back on. Many clinicians have learned to wait a full year after maximal dose titration before attempting to turn off the device for nonresponse and to wait 6 months after turning off the device before considering explantation.

FUTURE OF VAGUS NERVE STIMULATION AND EXTERNAL STIMULATION

The current availability of VNS for TRD in the United States is extremely limited. Despite the FDA approval of VNS for depression in July of 2005, the CMS made a noncoverage determination for VNS for TRD in May of 2007. The report issued at that time cited a lack of clear definition of what determines treatment-resistance in MDD. Furthermore, the report concluded that, in the opinion of CMS, in 2007 the available clinical evidence did not support the clinical efficacy of VNS in TRD, primarily because of the pivotal trial not meeting its primary end point.[7] This decision has had a decidedly negative effect because most private medical insurance has followed the CMS determination, essentially limiting the access of VNS to only the wealthy. Of note, CMS and several private insurers have funded reimplantations of the VNS in TRD device after the battery life had expired.

Since the time of this decision several subsequent clinical trials (described previously), a meta-analysis,[20] and a medical economic study[25] have supported the use of VNS for TRD on a broader scale. In particular the large TRD Registry, although not a randomized or blinded study, offered results that may compel reconsideration of the noncoverage determination.

On a final note, preliminary research into a transcutaneous stimulation of the vagus nerve through its auricular branch in the tragus of the ear may provide another clinical tool. A nonblinded study from China on an external noninvasive VNS device demonstrated some efficacy albeit in mild to moderate, non-treatment-refractory depression.[26]

REFERENCES

1. Kessler RC, Petukhova M, Sampson NA, et al. Twelve-month and lifetime prevalence and lifetime morbid risk of anxiety and mood disorders in the United States. Int J Methods Psychiatr Res 2012;21(3):169–84.
2. Leucht S, Hierl S, Kissling W, et al. Putting the efficacy of psychiatric and general medicine medication into perspective: review of meta-analyses. Br J Psychiatry 2012;200(2):97–106.
3. Fava M, Rush AJ, Wisniewski SR, et al. A comparison of mirtazapine and nortriptyline following two consecutive failed medication treatments for depressed outpatients: a STAR*D report. Am J Psychiatry 2006;163(7):1161–72.
4. Rush AJ, Trivedi MH, Wisniewski SR, et al. Acute and longer-term outcomes in depressed outpatients requiring one or several treatment steps: a STAR*D report. Am J Psychiatry 2006;163(11):1905–17.
5. McGrath PJ, Stewart JW, Fava M, et al. Tranylcypromine versus venlafaxine plus mirtazapine following three failed antidepressant medication trials for depression: a STAR*D report. Am J Psychiatry 2006;163(9):1531–41 [quiz: 1666].
6. Rush AJ, George MS, Sackeim HA, et al. Vagus nerve stimulation (VNS) for treatment-resistant depressions: a multicenter study. Biol Psychiatry 2000;47(4):276–86.
7. Rush AJ, Marangell LB, Sackeim HA, et al. Vagus nerve stimulation for treatment-resistant depression: a randomized, controlled acute phase trial. Biol Psychiatry 2005;58(5):347–54.
8. Rush AJ, Sackeim HA, Marangell LB, et al. Effects of 12 months of vagus nerve stimulation in treatment-resistant depression: a naturalistic study. Biol Psychiatry 2005;58(5):355–63.
9. Aaronson ST, Sears P, Ruvuna F, et al. A 5-year observational study of patients with treatment-resistant depression treated with vagus nerve stimulation or treatment as usual: comparison of response, remission, and suicidality. Am J Psychiatry 2017;174(7):640–8.
10. Harden CL, Pulver MC, Ravdin LD, et al. A pilot study of mood in epilepsy patients treated with vagus nerve stimulation. Epilepsy Behav 2000;1(2):93–9.
11. Elger G, Hoppe C, Falkai P, et al. Vagus nerve stimulation is associated with mood improvements in epilepsy patients. Epilepsy Res 2000;42(2–3):203–10.
12. Carreno FR, Frazer A. Vagal nerve stimulation for treatment-resistant depression. Neurotherapeutics 2017;14(3):716–27.
13. Marangell LB, Rush AJ, George MS, et al. Vagus nerve stimulation (VNS) for major depressive episodes: one year outcomes. Biol Psychiatry 2002;51(4):280–7.
14. Nahas Z, Marangell LB, Husain MM, et al. Two-year outcome of vagus nerve stimulation (VNS) for treatment of major depressive episodes. J Clin Psychiatry 2005; 66(9):1097–104.
15. Dunner DL, Rush AJ, Russell JM, et al. Prospective, long-term, multicenter study of the naturalistic outcomes of patients with treatment-resistant depression. J Clin Psychiatry 2006;67(5):688–95.

16. Sackeim HA, Prudic J, Devanand DP, et al. The impact of medication resistance and continuation pharmacotherapy on relapse following response to electroconvulsive therapy in major depression. J Clin Psychopharmacol 1990;10(2):96–104.
17. Schlaepfer TE, Frick C, Zobel A, et al. Vagus nerve stimulation for depression: efficacy and safety in a European study. Psychol Med 2008;38(5):651–61.
18. George MS, Rush AJ, Marangell LB, et al. A one-year comparison of vagus nerve stimulation with treatment as usual for treatment-resistant depression. Biol Psychiatry 2005;58(5):364–73.
19. Aaronson ST, Carpenter LL, Conway CR, et al. Vagus nerve stimulation therapy randomized to different amounts of electrical charge for treatment-resistant depression: acute and chronic effects. Brain Stimul 2013;6(4):631–40.
20. Berry SM, Broglio K, Bunker M, et al. A patient-level meta-analysis of studies evaluating vagus nerve stimulation therapy for treatment-resistant depression. Med Devices (Auckl) 2013;6:17–35.
21. Morris GL 3rd, Mueller WM. Long-term treatment with vagus nerve stimulation in patients with refractory epilepsy. The Vagus Nerve Stimulation Study Group E01-E05. Neurology 1999;53(8):1731–5.
22. Ryvlin P, So EL, Gordon CM, et al. Long-term surveillance of SUDEP in drug-resistant epilepsy patients treated with VNS therapy. Epilepsia 2018;59(3):562–72.
23. VNS therapy physician's manual. Houston (TX): LivaNova PLC; 2017. Available at: https://us.livanova.cyberonics.com/.
24. Prudic J, Haskett RF, McCall WV, et al. Pharmacological strategies in the prevention of relapse after electroconvulsive therapy. J ECT 2013;29(1):3–12.
25. Feldman RL, Dunner DL, Muller JS, et al. Medicare patient experience with vagus nerve stimulation for treatment-resistant depression. J Med Econ 2013;16(1):62–74.
26. Rong P, Liu J, Wang L, et al. Effect of transcutaneous auricular vagus nerve stimulation on major depressive disorder: a nonrandomized controlled pilot study. J Affect Disord 2016;195:172–9.

Updates on Transcranial Magnetic Stimulation Therapy for Major Depressive Disorder

Sarah L. Garnaat, PhD[a,b], Shiwen Yuan, MD[a],
Haizhi Wang, MD, PhD[a], Noah S. Philip, MD[a,b,c],
Linda L. Carpenter, MD[a,b],*

KEYWORDS

- Noninvasive neuromodulation • Depression • Treatment-resistant depression
- Transcranial magnetic stimulation

KEY POINTS

- Transcranial magnetic stimulation is a noninvasive brain stimulation therapy developed for use in treatment-resistant depression.
- Metaanalyses and large, randomized, controlled trials largely support efficacy of transcranial magnetic stimulation targeting the dorsolateral prefrontal cortex for major depressive disorder.
- Transcranial magnetic stimulation for depression continues to advance, with studies focusing on refining parameters for treatment optimization, and identification of biomarkers related to treatment response.

INTRODUCTION

Major depression is a leading cause of disability; however, a subset of patients do not experience sufficient relief from existing first-line treatments[1] or have trouble tolerating the side effects of antidepressant medications. Thus, identifying alternative treatments

Disclosure Statement: Dr L.L. Carpenter has received consulting income from Magstim, LTD, and Drs N.S. Philip and L.L. Carpenter have received clinical trials/research support from Neuronetics, Neosync, and Janssen. Dr N.S. Philip has been an unpaid scientific advisory board member for Neuronetics. None of the other authors has any relevant commercial or financial disclosures to report.
This work was supported in part by grants from the National Institute of Mental Health (NIMH) (R25MH101076; S. Yuan & H. Wang) and the US Department of Veterans Affairs (IK2CX000724 and I01RX002450; N.S. Philip). The views expressed in this article are those of the authors and do not necessarily reflect the position or policy of NIMH or Department of Veterans Affairs.
[a] Department of Psychiatry and Human Behavior, Alpert Medical School of Brown University, Box G-BH, Providence, RI 02912, USA; [b] Butler Hospital, 345 Blackstone Boulevard, Providence, RI 02906, USA; [c] Center for Neurorestoration and Neurotechnology, Providence VA Medical Center, 830 Chalkstone Avenue, Providence, RI 02908, USA
* Corresponding author.
E-mail address: linda_carpenter_md@brown.edu

Psychiatr Clin N Am 41 (2018) 419–431
https://doi.org/10.1016/j.psc.2018.04.006
0193-953X/18/© 2018 Elsevier Inc. All rights reserved.

Abbreviations	
DLPFC	Dorsolateral prefrontal cortex
DMN	Default model network
DMPFC	Dorsomedial prefrontal cortex
EEG	Electroencephalography
MDD	Major depressive disorder
MT	Motor threshold
rCBF	Regional cerebral blood flow
RCT	Randomized, controlled trial
sgACC	Subgenual anterior cingulate cortex
TMS	Transcranial magnetic stimulation
VMPFC	Ventromedial prefrontal cortex

has been an area of significant interest. Transcranial magnetic stimulation (TMS) has emerged over the last few decades as one such potential option for treatment-resistant depression.

TMS involves application of a strong, pulsed magnetic field to a targeted brain region. A coil generating an electromagnetic field is placed on the scalp, such that strong magnetic pulses are delivered to a relatively focal area of cerebral cortex, resulting in regional neuronal depolarization and generation of action potentials. In treatment protocols, TMS is typically delivered in bundles or "trains" of pulses, separated by periods of rest; this is called repetitive TMS (hereafter referred to as "TMS"). In 2008, the US Food and Drug Administration cleared the first TMS device to treat major depressive disorder (MDD); now multiple devices have regulatory approval in the United States and internationally.

The most common target for TMS for depression is the dorsolateral prefrontal cortex (DLPFC). Both high-frequency (eg, pulses delivered at 10 Hz)[2,3] TMS to the left DLPFC and low-frequency (1 Hz) TMS to the right DLPFC[4] have shown efficacy for pharmacoresistant depression, as well as bilateral TMS (a combination of these approaches).[5] Antidepressant efficacy has also been suggested for high-frequency TMS targeting broader prefrontal cortex.[6] In addition, open trial results show preliminary support for TMS to the dorsomedial prefrontal cortex (DMPFC)[7] for depression. Recent research has examined efficacy of TMS delivered using a pulse pattern called theta-burst,[8] a form of stimulation that has shown ability to promote synaptic plasticity in motor cortex; preliminary evidence suggests theta-burst TMS is as effective as a standard stimulation for MDD, but sessions are much shorter. Additionally, a small number of studies have investigated accelerated TMS protocols, delivering 2 or more TMS sessions per day, potentially shortening the number of weeks that comprise a course of TMS therapy. Preliminary findings suggest accelerated approaches may be efficacious,[9,10] although definitive trials have yet to be conducted.

The TMS for depression field depression is growing quickly, with new studies seeking to optimize parameters for delivery and to identify biomarkers of treatment response. Hereafter, we review efficacy data from controlled TMS trials for depression and discuss ongoing areas of research aimed at further improving this treatment, including research identifying neuroimaging and neurophysiologic biomarkers.

EVIDENCE FOR THE EFFICACY OF TRANSCRANIAL MAGNETIC STIMULATION FOR DEPRESSION

Over the past 20 to 30 years, studies of TMS for depression have shifted from small trials focused on safety, tolerability, and preliminary efficacy to larger multicenter trials and refinement of treatment parameters. Thus, many randomized, controlled trials

(RCTs) of TMS for depression in the literature are underpowered. Additionally, studies have varied in target population (ie, unipolar vs bipolar depression), patient medication status, quality of sham procedures, and total sessions in a course of treatment (with studies generally increasing the number of sessions over time, from 5–10 in early studies, to 20–30 sessions in more recent trials, now comprising the standard of care). Accordingly, metaanalyses have been conducted to clarify findings across studies.

Metaanalytic Findings

Metaanalyses of TMS for depression have largely supported statistically significant differences favoring active TMS over sham in terms of symptom improvement,[11–14] as well as clinical response.[12,15] Most metaanalyses have focused on high-frequency TMS, although metaanalyses examining antidepressant efficacy of low-frequency TMS also found it superior to sham in terms of effect size[16] and rates of response and remission.[15] One metaanalysis found better outcomes with bilateral TMS versus sham.[17] A recent metaanalysis by Brunoni and colleagues[14] used a network-based approach to compare multiple TMS approaches and sham. This analysis, including 81 studies, found low-frequency, high-frequency, and bilateral TMS all to be more effective than sham.

Findings from Large Multisite, Sham-Controlled, Randomized, Controlled Trials

To date, 3 large multisite, sham-controlled trials have been conducted to more definitively evaluate efficacy of TMS as a monotherapy for depression.[2,3,6] The first study[3] randomized 325 medication-free patients with treatment-resistant depression to undergo 5 sessions per week of high-frequency TMS to left DLPFC or sham over 4 to 6 weeks.[18] In this pivotal trial, TMS was delivered at 120% resting motor threshold (MT) in a series of 4-second trains of 10 Hz, separated by 26-second intervals of no stimulation, totaling 3000 pulses per session. After 4 weeks, change in the primary outcome (Montgomery-Asberg Depression Rating Scale score) fell short of the threshold for statistical significance (p = .057). However, change in secondary measures of depression severity (Hamilton Depression Rating Scale-17 and -24) showed significant improvement for active TMS versus sham, and post hoc analyses aiming to correct for baseline differences between conditions in Montgomery-Asberg Depression Rating Scale scores also suggested significant differences in outcomes between conditions. Additionally, response rates on all 3 depression measures were significantly higher following 4 weeks of active TMS (18.1%–20.6%), relative to sham (11.0%–11.6%). Data from this trial supported US Food and Drug Administration clearance of the first TMS device for depression.

A second large multisite RCT for TMS for depression was reported by George and colleagues.[2] TMS was delivered using the same devices and parameters described, but with 5 sessions per week for 3 weeks. After 3 weeks, participants showing improvement continued for up to 3 additional weeks. Those not showing improvement were crossed over to open treatment. In total, 199 patients were randomized, with 190 comprising the intent-to-treat sample used for primary analyses. Primary findings indicated a significant difference in remission rates for active TMS (14.1%) versus sham (5.1%) in the blinded phase. Response rates also differed between conditions, favoring active stimulation (15% vs 5%). Secondary analyses showed significant differences between conditions at the end of the blinded phase in Montgomery-Asberg Depression Rating Scale score, global severity ratings, and self-reported depressive symptoms.

A third multicenter trial sought to evaluate efficacy of TMS using an H-coil.[6] Patients with treatment-resistant depression received 4 weeks of high-frequency TMS delivered to a broad prefrontal cortex area (left > right). During the acute treatment phase (4 weeks), participants received 5 daily sessions per week at 18 Hz before transitioning to a twice a week treatment schedule in weeks 5 to 12. Stimulation was delivered at 120% MT, with 2-second stimulation trains separated by 20-second rest intervals, totaling 1980 pulses per session. Intent-to-treat analyses failed to reach statistical significance for the primary outcome (change in Hamilton Depression Rating Scale-21 after 22 sessions; p = .0578), although secondary analyses investigating response and remission rates showed significant group differences at week 5, favoring active TMS. Analyses using a per-protocol sample, excluding participants who did not receive stimulation at the specified intensity (120% MT), showed significant group differences in HDRS change from baseline to week 5, as well as significant differences between conditions in both response and remission rates at week 5.

A recent multisite, RCT investigated a 2-coil TMS array for treatment-resistant or -intolerant depression[19] in patients (n = 92) allowed to remain on stable (ineffective) pharmacotherapy regimens. The 2-coil array was designed to stimulate deeper into the cortex through placement of center-folded double coils over the DMPFC and the DLPFC. Participants were randomized to 20 sessions of active or sham 10-Hz TMS over 4 weeks, with pulse trains delivered from both coils (3000 pulses per session, 120% MT). The per-protocol sample, but not the intent-to-treat sample, showed significantly greater change in Hamilton Depression Rating Scale for active versus sham. No significant differences were found in response or remission rates. A future, fully powered trial may be warranted to more definitely determine the efficacy of this approach.

Naturalistic Findings

After US Food and Drug Administration approval and launch of the first US TMS device, a study was published describing real-life outcomes from TMS delivered by non-research psychiatrists at 42 real-world clinics.[20] Patients with MDD (n = 307) paid for TMS therapy out of pocket or through insurance. Parameters and course were determined by treating physicians. Results confirmed that positive TMS outcomes were achievable in a variety of psychiatry clinical practice settings, with naturalistic data showing significant improvement in depression severity from baseline to end of treatment, and response (58.0%) and remission (37.1%) rates consistent with those in research populations. A subset of this naturalistically treated sample (n = 257) completed long-term follow-up assessments over 1 year to examine durability outcomes.[21] These data revealed that acute TMS benefits were generally sustained throughout the follow-up period, with the majority (62.5%) of acute TMS responders maintaining their status over a year; approximately one-third of patients received some "reintroduction" TMS sessions during the year-long follow-up period. Statistically significant improvement was also found in functional status on a broad range of mental health and physical health domains after acute TMS.[22]

OPTIMIZING TRANSCRANIAL MAGNETIC STIMULATION THERAPY FOR MAJOR DEPRESSIVE DISORDER

Pressing clinical questions surrounding TMS therapy today concern the selection of optimal stimulation parameters, treatment schedules, and other variables in protocols used for treating depression, with increasing interest in individually customizing stimulation. Data from RCTs have underscored the safety and potential efficacy of TMS, even with protocols expanding well beyond those used in predecessor trials, with regard to magnetic stimuli exposure.[23] Outcomes from both blinded[24] and open-label[25] continuation phase studies suggest there is not a one-size-fits-all dosing strategy, and that some patients will require more treatments than others to experience maximal symptom relief.[26] A metaanalysis of RCTs using high-frequency stimulation confirmed greater number of daily sessions (within a single TMS course) was associated more favorable outcomes.[13] Positive effects of TMS may only last a few weeks in some patients,[27] and although open-label data[28] support a plan for offering "booster" treatments,[21,29] the best approach for achieving durable positive effect with TMS remains unknown. It is, however, fairly clear that, after positive response is achieved with TMS therapy, about one-third of patients will need a reintroduction of stimulation within 1 year to avoid relapse or to recapture prior level of benefits in the face of depressive symptom reemergence.[21,30] The ideal schedule or protocol for maintenance of effect has yet to be identified and confirmed in a prospective trial.[31]

The questions of ideal treatment target site[32] and laterality for TMS stimulation also remain critical, with some studies yielding preliminary suggestions that TMS sequential delivery to both hemispheres is better than one-sided stimulation,[14] and others suggesting that right-sided stimulation is better for cognition,[33] and that benefits may still be derived from left-sided stimulation after a patient has failed a TMS course over the right DLPFC.[34] Stimulation protocols for MDD using the theta-burst pulse pattern appear to be effective when compared with sham treatments,[8] but have not yet demonstrated superiority over standard TMS parameters with regard to symptom improvement or response rates in RCTs. Retrospective analyses of a large open-label Canadian database recently suggested that TMS sessions delivered twice daily, rather than once, may bring about earlier clinical response,[35] but again, prospective controlled trials are needed to properly test this notion.

IMAGING BIOMARKERS

The development of biomarkers for guiding TMS application for depression is in its infancy, in part owing to great voids in our understanding of neurobiological underpinnings of MDD and only nascent insights about how stimulation impacts the brain. Nevertheless, findings emerging from metabolic imaging and functional connectivity studies have begun to identify specific regional and network abnormalities, and their alterations after TMS.

RESTING STATE SINGLE PHOTON EMISSION COMPUTED TOMOGRAPHY/PET (METABOLIC IMAGING)

Regional cerebral blood flow (rCBF) and metabolic activity of brain areas can be evaluated with either single photon emission computed tomography or PET by evaluating the regional uptake of a tagged metabolic substrate, (eg, 18-fluordeoxyglucose).[36] Findings of hypofrontality in the left DLPFC observed in MDD[37,38] provided some rationale for application of high-frequency TMS to that region in early treatment studies. This approach was reinforced by PET studies observing that high-frequency (20 Hz) stimulation increased prefrontal rCBF (including amygdala, hippocampus, insula, parahippocampus, thalamus, and cerebellum), whereas low-frequency (1 Hz) stimulation was associated with distal rCBF reductions in the right prefrontal cortex, left medial temporal cortex, and amygdala.[38–40]

However, the directionality of rCBF changes under different stimulation frequencies correlate modestly with clinical improvement. For instance, high-frequency stimulation studies (20 Hz)[41] found that higher baseline subgenual anterior cingulate cortex (sgACC) activity predicted superior clinical outcomes, and clinical response corresponded to reduced sgACC activity. Clinical efficacy is correlated with changes in numerous regions related to mood regulation, including DLPFC; basal ganglia, orbitofrontal cortex, and ventromedial prefrontal cortex (VMPFC; which have direct anatomic connections with the DLPFC); and the sgACC and posterior cingulate cortex[41–43] (which have polysynaptic relationships to the DLPFC). Contrarily, Kito and colleagues[44–46] found that an increased rCBF in the VMPFC predicted treatment response to 1 Hz TMS. Treatment efficacy was also associated with decreased rCBF in prefrontal cortex, orbitofrontal cortex, putamen, anterior insula, and sgACC. Reduced sgACC activity after stimulation has been consistently shown in single photon emission computed tomography/positron emission tomography studies to associate with positive treatment effect.[41,45] However, these studies have been limited by lower stimulation intensity, fewer sessions, and modest sample sizes.

RESTING STATE FUNCTIONAL CONNECTIVITY AND NEURAL NETWORKS

The 3 principle networks in mood regulation are the default model network (DMN), frontoparietal executive control network, and the attention/limbic or salience network.[47] These are often measured via fluctuations in resting state blood oxygenation levels with functional MRI (ie, functional connectivity). In MDD, sgACC/DMN activity is considered a core component of pathologic network dysfunction, which compromises the ability for dynamic network change of an otherwise healthy brain in response to changing demands.[48] Fox and colleagues[32,49] conducted several studies linking MDD treatment response and reduced sgACC connectivity, and suggesting that suppression of sgACC connectivity leads to clinical improvement.

Transcranial Magnetic Stimulation to the Dorsolateral Prefrontal Cortex

Connectivity changes associated with TMS can also be interpreted in the context of the primary stimulation site. An ACC-centered network was shown to be the only mediator of TMS effects in an experiment with healthy individuals, and only with TMS delivered to the DLPFC.[50] After TMS treatment targeting the DLPFC, sgACC-to-DMN connectivity was attenuated, and reduced connectivity was observed between the DLPFC and the medial prefrontal cortex/VMPFC.[51] Reducing sgACC-to-DMN connectivity and inducing negative connectivity between DLPFC and DMN have been considered possible putative mechanisms of TMS therapy.

Considering clinical response, patients who experience significant symptom reduction with TMS have demonstrated, at baseline, greater negative connectivity between the sgACC and superior medial prefrontal cortex, including portions of the DMPFC,[52] greater connectivity between the sgACC and orbitofrontal cortex,[53] stronger DMN-to-salience network connectivity,[54] and higher left DLPFC-to-striatum connectivity.[55] Greater pretreatment sgACC connectivity generally predicts superior clinical outcomes.[51] In contrast, greater baseline connectivity between the posterior cingulate and insula has predicted TMS nonresponse.[56] After a course of TMS, sgACC connectivity was reduced in all responders, whereas no sgACC changes were observed in nonresponders.[52] TMS responders have also shown reduced negative connectivity between sgACC and medial prefrontal cortex, reduced sgACC connectivity with the middle frontal gyrus and motor cortex, increased sgACC connectivity with VMPFC,[57] and reduced DLFPC-to-caudate connectivity.[58]

Transcranial Magnetic Stimulation to the Dorsomedial Prefrontal Cortex

Clinical responders to TMS targeting DMPFC have been found to have intact reward circuit function[7,59] while nonresponders displayed lower connectivity in reward pathways comprised of VMPFC, ventral tegmental area, and striatum. Examination of clinical response predictors revealed that superior antidepressant outcomes were associated with positive midcingulate-to-sgACC/medial prefrontal cortex connectivity; negative midcingulate-to-thalamus, -hippocampus, and -amygdala connectivity; higher sgACC-to-DLPFC connectivity; and lower sgACC-to-insula, -putamen, and -parahippocampus/amygdala connectivity.[60] Coinciding with DLPFC-based studies, better clinical responses were associated with more negative DMPFC-sgACC connectivity.

Seeking to characterize global neurobiological changes in depression, a multisite study[61] provided evidence of 4 discrete biotypes within depression, according to frontostriatal and limbic connectivity. For a subset of patients with MDD (n = 124) who received TMS to DMPFC, one specific imaging biotype, characterized by reduced connectivity in frontoamygdala networks and in anterior cingulate and orbitofrontal areas, showed the best treatment response.

Findings arising from TMS imaging studies should be interpreted with the caveat of the considerable heterogeneity of variables in these neuroimaging studies, including treatment parameters, imaging modalities, and analytical approaches. Although these preliminary findings do not yet lend themselves to clinical application, a convergence of evidence to date underscores the sgACC as a critically important target for TMS to treat depression. With further investigation and refinement, imaging biomarkers might someday be useful for clinical decision making in delivering TMS for depression.

Electroencephalographic biomarkers
Electroencephalography (EEG) is a noninvasive method for measuring brain activity using superficial recording electrodes on the scalp to detect rhythmic electrical events generated by large populations of neurons. EEG recordings reflect regional oscillatory brain activity defined by key anatomic landmarks according to a standardized topographic method, capturing signals in discrete frequency "bands" based on periodicity of the waveform, for example, delta (0.5–3 Hz), theta (3–7 Hz), alpha (7–13 Hz), beta (13–30 Hz), and gamma (>30 Hz). Quantitative EEG analyses can locate the source, strength, and orientation of brain activity; provide its spatial representation; compare temporal relationships of signals from different recording sites (coherence analysis); and capture event-related potentials (small voltage changes in EEG in response to certain events in real time). Because spatially discrete neuronal groups can interact effectively only when they are oscillating at a coherent (synchronized) rhythm, an analysis of phase synchronization or coherence of change in EEG data can reveal functional connectivity among multiple cortical and deeper brain regions, representing functional circuits or hubs in a coordinated network. For example, a combined EEG–functional MRI experiment found that frontal theta activity correlated significantly with activation of the DMN.[62] Owing to the relative ease of application in clinical settings, EEG holds significant promise for elucidating biomarkers to guide customization of TMS treatments, or for predicting negative outcomes before investing substantial time, and resources in a course of TMS.

Studies comparing EEG pre-TMS and post-TMS treatment have identified changes induced by stimulation and/or by resolution of depressive symptoms and provide preliminary insights regarding possible therapeutic mechanisms of TMS for depression. Llinas and colleagues[63] proposed that perturbation in thalamocortical neural oscillations may be central to MDD pathogenesis, with abnormal increases in theta activity and coherence of low-frequency oscillations. In a study of 44 healthy subjects, resting EEG showed that TMS induces short-term effects in the thalamocortical interplay of low-frequency brain oscillatory activities: 10-Hz stimulation induced transient synchronization of delta and theta rhythms, whereas low-frequency (1 Hz, 5 Hz) stimulation induced desynchronization of these slow waves.[64] The transient desynchronizing effects of TMS at thalamocortical neural circuits in healthy subjects (inferred by decreased power of delta and theta rhythms) resembles the opposite of patterns observed in depression,[65] raising the possibility that TMS effects on oscillatory neural rhythms are related to its therapeutic mechanism of action. Furthermore, TMS transiently induces oscillations that synchronize with the stimulating frequency (ie, entrainment),[66–68] followed by a reemergence of intrinsic natural local cortical oscillations.[69] Transient entrainment of brain oscillations by TMS has, thus, been hypothesized to promote normal intrinsic rhythm and plasticity to bring about therapeutic effects in MDD.[70,71]

Activity in the gamma frequency band has produced several potential EEG biomarkers relevant to TMS for depression. In an open label study comparing pretreatment and posttreatment EEGs in 31 patients with depression, TMS targeting the left DLPFC induced significant increases in resting gamma power at the F3 electrode, corresponding with symptom improvement.[72] TMS treatment has also been shown to alter functional connectivity within gamma band in resting EEG, with increased gamma activity in the left DLPFC and decreased gamma activity in the precuneus after TMS.[73]

Cordance is an EEG measure using various algorithms to yield indicators corresponding to cerebral perfusion/metabolism. In a retrospective study of patients with MDD or dysthymia (n = 90) treated with TMS, several pretreatment EEG variables were shown to distinguish nonresponders from responders. Before treatment, TMS nonresponders had slower anterior individual alpha peak frequency, increased frontocentral theta power, and decreased prefrontal delta and theta cordance.[74] Another study of 25 patients with MDD treated with TMS showed that decreases in prefrontal theta cordance at week 1, compared with pretreatment baseline, successfully predicted week 4 response.[75] A study analyzing nonlinear metrics in baseline EEG identified a measure of alpha signal complexity that significantly predicted TMS response.[76] Here, slower anterior alpha peak frequency was also found in nonresponders. Another study with 18 clinically stable depressed outpatients receiving open-label TMS found change in theta cordance in left DLPFC at week 1 was a significant predictor of outcome at week 6.[77] Finally, using machine learning, an artificial neural network was developed using pretreatment frontal EEG cordance to identify TMS responder status in MDD subjects (n = 55); responders were identified with a sensitivity of 93% and an overall accuracy of 89%.[78]

Some EEG researchers have posited that optimal clinical outcomes may be achieved with individually customized stimulation protocols matching pulse frequency to the patient's individual alpha frequency. Pilot studies[79,80] have begun investigating this approach using a low-field TMS device with promising preliminary results that require further testing with standard intensity TMS protocols. With continued research, the refinement of EEG biomarkers may someday enhance TMS treatment outcomes. However, at present, data are insufficient to suggest individual EEG could be used to guide treatment decisions in standard TMS care settings.

SUMMARY

Overall, these findings continue to support efficacy of TMS for treatment-resistant depression. Work continues on the development of alternative treatment regimens and optimization of protocols, including stimulation parameters, treatment targets, and TMS delivery schedules. Ongoing research using neuroimaging and EEG is laying the foundation for a deeper understanding of treatment-resistant depression and therapeutic mechanisms of TMS. Although these findings are still in their infancy, these efforts may someday provide valuable insights for optimizing TMS for treatment-resistant depression.

REFERENCES

1. McIntyre RS, Filteau MJ, Martin L, et al. Treatment-resistant depression: definitions, review of the evidence, and algorithmic approach. J Affect Disord 2014; 156:1–7.
2. George MS, Lisanby SH, Avery D, et al. Daily left prefrontal transcranial magnetic stimulation therapy for major depressive disorder: a sham-controlled randomized trial. Arch Gen Psychiatry 2010;67(5):507–16.
3. O'Reardon JP, Solvason HB, Janicak PG, et al. Efficacy and safety of transcranial magnetic stimulation in the acute treatment of major depression: a multisite randomized controlled trial. Biol Psychiatry 2007;62(11):1208–16.
4. Berlim MT, Van den Eynde F, Jeff Daskalakis Z. Clinically meaningful efficacy and acceptability of low-frequency repetitive transcranial magnetic stimulation (rTMS) for treating primary major depression: a meta-analysis of randomized, double-blind and sham-controlled trials. Neuropsychopharmacology 2013;38(4):543–51.
5. Zhang YQ, Zhu D, Zhou XY, et al. Bilateral repetitive transcranial magnetic stimulation for treatment-resistant depression: a systematic review and meta-analysis of randomized controlled trials. Braz J Med Biol Res 2015;48(3):198–206.
6. Levkovitz Y, Isserles M, Padberg F, et al. Efficacy and safety of deep transcranial magnetic stimulation for major depression: a prospective multicenter randomized controlled trial. World Psychiatry 2015;14(1):64–73.
7. Downar J, Daskalakis ZJ. New targets for rTMS in depression: a review of convergent evidence. Brain Stimul 2013;6(3):231–40.
8. Berlim MT, McGirr A, Rodrigues Dos Santos N, et al. Efficacy of theta burst stimulation (TBS) for major depression: an exploratory meta-analysis of randomized and sham-controlled trials. J Psychiatr Res 2017;90:102–9.
9. Holtzheimer PE 3rd, McDonald WM, Mufti M, et al. Accelerated repetitive transcranial magnetic stimulation for treatment-resistant depression. Depress Anxiety 2010;27(10):960–3.
10. McGirr A, Van den Eynde F, Tovar-Perdomo S, et al. Effectiveness and acceptability of accelerated repetitive transcranial magnetic stimulation (rTMS) for treatment-resistant major depressive disorder: an open label trial. J Affect Disord 2015;173:216–20.
11. McNamara B, Ray JL, Arthurs OJ, et al. Transcranial magnetic stimulation for depression and other psychiatric disorders. Psychol Med 2001;31(7):1141–6.
12. Gaynes BN, Lloyd SW, Lux L, et al. Repetitive transcranial magnetic stimulation for treatment-resistant depression: a systematic review and meta-analysis. J Clin Psychiatry 2014;75(5):477–89 [quiz: 489].
13. Teng S, Guo Z, Peng H, et al. High-frequency repetitive transcranial magnetic stimulation over the left DLPFC for major depression: session-dependent efficacy: a meta-analysis. Eur Psychiatry 2017;41:75–84.
14. Brunoni AR, Chaimani A, Moffa AH, et al. Repetitive transcranial magnetic stimulation for the acute treatment of major depressive episodes: a systematic review with network meta-analysis. JAMA Psychiatry 2017;74(2):143–52.
15. Berlim MT, van den Eynde F, Tovar-Perdomo S, et al. Response, remission and drop-out rates following high-frequency repetitive transcranial magnetic stimulation (rTMS) for treating major depression: a systematic review and meta-analysis

of randomized, double-blind and sham-controlled trials. Psychol Med 2014;44(2): 225–39.

16. Schutter DJ. Quantitative review of the efficacy of slow-frequency magnetic brain stimulation in major depressive disorder. Psychol Med 2010;40(11):1789–95.

17. Berlim MT, Van den Eynde F, Daskalakis ZJ. A systematic review and meta-analysis on the efficacy and acceptability of bilateral repetitive transcranial magnetic stimulation (rTMS) for treating major depression. Psychol Med 2013;43(11): 2245–54.

18. Horvath JC, Mathews J, Demitrack MA, et al. The NeuroStar TMS device: conducting the FDA approved protocol for treatment of depression. J Vis Exp 2010;(45) [pii:2345].

19. Carpenter LL, Aaronson ST, Clarke GN, et al. rTMS with a two-coil array: safety and efficacy for treatment resistant major depressive disorder. Brain Stimul 2017;10(5):926–33.

20. Carpenter LL, Janicak PG, Aaronson ST, et al. Transcranial magnetic stimulation (TMS) for major depression: a multisite, naturalistic, observational study of acute treatment outcomes in clinical practice. Depress Anxiety 2012;29(7):587–96.

21. Dunner DL, Aaronson ST, Sackeim HA, et al. A multisite, naturalistic, observational study of transcranial magnetic stimulation for patients with pharmacoresistant major depressive disorder: durability of benefit over a 1-year follow-up period. J Clin Psychiatry 2014;75(12):1394–401.

22. Janicak PG, Dunner DL, Aaronson ST, et al. Transcranial magnetic stimulation (TMS) for major depression: a multisite, naturalistic, observational study of quality of life outcome measures in clinical practice. CNS Spectr 2013;18(6):322–32.

23. Hadley D, Anderson BS, Borckardt JJ, et al. Safety, tolerability, and effectiveness of high doses of adjunctive daily left prefrontal repetitive transcranial magnetic stimulation for treatment-resistant depression in a clinical setting. J ECT 2011; 27(1):18–25.

24. Yip AG, George MS, Tendler A, et al. 61% of unmedicated treatment resistant depression patients who did not respond to acute TMS treatment responded after four weeks of twice weekly deep TMS in the Brainsway pivotal trial. Brain Stimul 2017;10(4):847–9.

25. Avery DH, Isenberg KE, Sampson SM, et al. Transcranial magnetic stimulation in the acute treatment of major depressive disorder: clinical response in an open-label extension trial. J Clin Psychiatry 2008;69(3):441–51.

26. McDonald WM, Durkalski V, Ball ER, et al. Improving the antidepressant efficacy of transcranial magnetic stimulation: maximizing the number of stimulations and treatment location in treatment-resistant depression. Depress Anxiety 2011; 28(11):973–80.

27. Kedzior KK, Reitz SK, Azorina V, et al. Durability of the antidepressant effect of the high-frequency repetitive transcranial magnetic stimulation (rTMS) In the absence of maintenance treatment in major depression: a systematic review and meta-analysis of 16 double-blind, randomized, sham-controlled trials. Depress Anxiety 2015;32(3):193–203.

28. Rapinesi C, Bersani FS, Kotzalidis GD, et al. Maintenance deep transcranial magnetic stimulation sessions are associated with reduced depressive relapses in patients with unipolar or bipolar depression. Front Neurol 2015;6:16.

29. Harel EV, Rabany L, Deutsch L, et al. H-coil repetitive transcranial magnetic stimulation for treatment resistant major depressive disorder: an 18-week continuation safety and feasibility study. World J Biol Psychiatry 2014;15(4): 298–306.

30. Janicak PG, Nahas Z, Lisanby SH, et al. Durability of clinical benefit with transcranial magnetic stimulation (TMS) in the treatment of pharmacoresistant major depression: assessment of relapse during a 6-month, multisite, open-label study. Brain Stimul 2010;3(4):187–99.

31. Philip NS, Dunner DL, Dowd SM, et al. Can medication free, treatment-resistant, depressed patients who initially respond to TMS be maintained off medications? A prospective, 12-month multisite randomized pilot study. Brain Stimul 2016;9(2):251–7.

32. Fox MD, Liu H, Pascual-Leone A. Identification of reproducible individualized targets for treatment of depression with TMS based on intrinsic connectivity. Neuroimage 2013;66:151–60.

33. Nadeau SE, Bowers D, Jones TL, et al. Cognitive effects of treatment of depression with repetitive transcranial magnetic stimulation. Cogn Behav Neurol 2014; 27(2):77–87.

34. Fitzgerald PB, McQueen S, Herring S, et al. A study of the effectiveness of high-frequency left prefrontal cortex transcranial magnetic stimulation in major depression in patients who have not responded to right-sided stimulation. Psychiatry Res 2009;169(1):12–5.

35. Schulze L, Feffer K, Lozano C, et al. Number of pulses or number of sessions? An open-label study of trajectories of improvement for once-vs. twice-daily dorsomedial prefrontal rTMS in major depression. Brain Stimul 2018;11(2):327–36.

36. Chi KF, Korgaonkar M, Grieve SM. Imaging predictors of remission to anti-depressant medications in major depressive disorder. J Affect Disord 2015; 186:134–44.

37. Buchsbaum MS, Wu J, DeLisi LE, et al. Frontal cortex and basal ganglia metabolic rates assessed by positron emission tomography with [18F]2-deoxyglucose in affective illness. J Affect Disord 1986;10(2):137–52.

38. Martinot JL, Hardy P, Feline A, et al. Left prefrontal glucose hypometabolism in the depressed state: a confirmation. Am J Psychiatry 1990;147(10):1313–7.

39. Nahas Z, Teneback CC, Kozel A, et al. Brain effects of TMS delivered over prefrontal cortex in depressed adults: role of stimulation frequency and coil-cortex distance. J Neuropsychiatry Clin Neurosci 2001;13(4):459–70.

40. Speer AM, Kimbrell TA, Wassermann EM, et al. Opposite effects of high and low frequency rTMS on regional brain activity in depressed patients. Biol Psychiatry 2000;48(12):1133–41.

41. Baeken C, Marinazzo D, Everaert H, et al. The impact of accelerated HF-rTMS on the subgenual anterior cingulate cortex in refractory unipolar major depression: insights from 18FDG PET brain imaging. Brain Stimul 2015;8(4):808–15.

42. Klein JC, Rushworth MF, Behrens TE, et al. Topography of connections between human prefrontal cortex and mediodorsal thalamus studied with diffusion tractography. Neuroimage 2010;51(2):555–64.

43. Padberg F, George MS. Repetitive transcranial magnetic stimulation of the prefrontal cortex in depression. Exp Neurol 2009;219(1):2–13.

44. Kito S, Fujita K, Koga Y. Regional cerebral blood flow changes after low-frequency transcranial magnetic stimulation of the right dorsolateral prefrontal cortex in treatment-resistant depression. Neuropsychobiology 2008;58(1):29–36.

45. Kito S, Hasegawa T, Koga Y. Neuroanatomical correlates of therapeutic efficacy of low-frequency right prefrontal transcranial magnetic stimulation in treatment-resistant depression. Psychiatry Clin Neurosci 2011;65(2):175–82.

46. Kito S, Hasegawa T, Koga Y. Cerebral blood flow in the ventromedial prefrontal cortex correlates with treatment response to low-frequency right prefrontal

repetitive transcranial magnetic stimulation in the treatment of depression. Psychiatry Clin Neurosci 2012;66(2):138–45.

47. Hamilton JP, Farmer M, Fogelman P, et al. Depressive rumination, the default-mode network, and the dark matter of clinical neuroscience. Biol Psychiatry 2015;78(4):224–30.

48. Buckner RL, Andrews-Hanna JR, Schacter DL. The brain's default network: anatomy, function, and relevance to disease. Ann N Y Acad Sci 2008;1124:1–38.

49. Fox MD, Buckner RL, White MP, et al. Efficacy of transcranial magnetic stimulation targets for depression is related to intrinsic functional connectivity with the subgenual cingulate. Biol Psychiatry 2012;72(7):595–603.

50. Tik M, Hoffmann A, Sladky R, et al. Towards understanding rTMS mechanism of action: stimulation of the DLPFC causes network-specific increase in functional connectivity. Neuroimage 2017;162:289–96.

51. Liston C, Chen AC, Zebley BD, et al. Default mode network mechanisms of transcranial magnetic stimulation in depression. Biol Psychiatry 2014;76(7): 517–26.

52. Baeken C, Marinazzo D, Wu GR, et al. Accelerated HF-rTMS in treatment-resistant unipolar depression: insights from subgenual anterior cingulate functional connectivity. World J Biol Psychiatry 2014;15(4):286–97.

53. Cooney RE, Joormann J, Eugene F, et al. Neural correlates of rumination in depression. Cogn Affect Behav Neurosci 2010;10(4):470–8.

54. Ge R, Blumberger DM, Downar J, et al. Abnormal functional connectivity within resting-state networks is related to rTMS-based therapy effects of treatment resistant depression: a pilot study. J Affect Disord 2017;218:75–81.

55. Avissar M, Powell F, Ilieva I, et al. Functional connectivity of the left DLPFC to striatum predicts treatment response of depression to TMS. Brain Stimul 2017;10(5): 919–25.

56. Taylor SF, Ho SS, Abagis T, et al. Changes in brain connectivity during a sham-controlled, transcranial magnetic stimulation trial for depression. J Affect Disord 2018;232:143–51.

57. Duprat R, Desmyter S, Rudi de R, et al. Accelerated intermittent theta burst stimulation treatment in medication-resistant major depression: a fast road to remission? J Affect Disord 2016;200:6–14.

58. Kang JI, Lee H, Jhung K, et al. Frontostriatal connectivity changes in major depressive disorder after repetitive transcranial magnetic stimulation: a randomized sham-controlled study. J Clin Psychiatry 2016;77(9):e1137–43.

59. Sheline YI, Price JL, Yan Z, et al. Resting-state functional MRI in depression unmasks increased connectivity between networks via the dorsal nexus. Proc Natl Acad Sci U S A 2010;107(24):11020–5.

60. Salomons TV, Dunlop K, Kennedy SH, et al. Resting-state cortico-thalamic-striatal connectivity predicts response to dorsomedial prefrontal rTMS in major depressive disorder. Neuropsychopharmacology 2014;39(2):488–98.

61. Drysdale AT, Grosenick L, Downar J, et al. Resting-state connectivity biomarkers define neurophysiological subtypes of depression. Nat Med 2017; 23(1):28–38.

62. Scheeringa R, Bastiaansen MC, Petersson KM, et al. Frontal theta EEG activity correlates negatively with the default mode network in resting state. Int J Psychophysiol 2008;67(3):242–51.

63. Llinas RR, Ribary U, Jeanmonod D, et al. Thalamocortical dysrhythmia: a neurological and neuropsychiatric syndrome characterized by magnetoencephalography. Proc Natl Acad Sci U S A 1999;96(26):15222–7.

64. Fuggetta G, Noh NA. A neurophysiological insight into the potential link between transcranial magnetic stimulation, thalamocortical dysrhythmia and neuropsychiatric disorders. Exp Neurol 2013;245:87–95.
65. Schulman JJ, Cancro R, Lowe S, et al. Imaging of thalamocortical dysrhythmia in neuropsychiatry. Front Hum Neurosci 2011;5:69.
66. Brignani D, Manganotti P, Rossini PM, et al. Modulation of cortical oscillatory activity during transcranial magnetic stimulation. Hum Brain Mapp 2008;29(5): 603–12.
67. Hamidi M, Slagter HA, Tononi G, et al. Repetitive transcranial magnetic stimulation affects behavior by biasing endogenous cortical oscillations. Front Integr Neurosci 2009;3:14.
68. Johnson JS, Hamidi M, Postle BR. Using EEG to explore how rTMS produces its effects on behavior. Brain Topogr 2010;22(4):281–93.
69. Rosanova M, Casali A, Bellina V, et al. Natural frequencies of human corticothalamic circuits. J Neurosci 2009;29(24):7679–85.
70. Leuchter AF, Cook IA, Jin Y, et al. The relationship between brain oscillatory activity and therapeutic effectiveness of transcranial magnetic stimulation in the treatment of major depressive disorder. Front Hum Neurosci 2013;7:37.
71. Leuchter AF, Hunter AM, Krantz DE, et al. Rhythms and blues: modulation of oscillatory synchrony and the mechanism of action of antidepressant treatments. Ann N Y Acad Sci 2015;1344:78–91.
72. Noda Y, Zomorrodi R, Saeki T, et al. Resting-state EEG gamma power and theta-gamma coupling enhancement following high-frequency left dorsolateral prefrontal rTMS in patients with depression. Clin Neurophysiol 2017;128(3):424–32.
73. Kito S, Hasegawa T, Fujita K, et al. Changes in hypothalamic-pituitary-thyroid axis following successful treatment with low-frequency right prefrontal transcranial magnetic stimulation in treatment-resistant depression. Psychiatry Res 2010; 175(1–2):74–7.
74. Arns M, Drinkenburg WH, Fitzgerald PB, et al. Neurophysiological predictors of non-response to rTMS in depression. Brain Stimul 2012;5(4):569–76.
75. Bares M, Brunovsky M, Novak T, et al. QEEG theta cordance in the prediction of treatment outcome to prefrontal repetitive transcranial magnetic stimulation or venlafaxine ER in patients with major depressive disorder. Clin EEG Neurosci 2015;46(2):73–80.
76. Arns M, Cerquera A, Gutierrez RM, et al. Non-linear EEG analyses predict non-response to rTMS treatment in major depressive disorder. Clin Neurophysiol 2014;125(7):1392–9.
77. Hunter AM, Nghiem TX, Cook IA, et al. Change in quantitative EEG theta cordance as a potential predictor of repetitive transcranial magnetic stimulation clinical outcome in major depressive disorder. Clin EEG Neurosci 2017. [Epub ahead of print].
78. Erguzel TT, Ozekes S, Gultekin S, et al. Neural network based response prediction of rTMS in major depressive disorder using QEEG cordance. Psychiatry Investig 2015;12(1):61–5.
79. Jin Y, Phillips B. A pilot study of the use of EEG-based synchronized Transcranial Magnetic Stimulation (sTMS) for treatment of major depression. BMC Psychiatry 2014;14:13.
80. Louchtor AF, Cook IA, Feifel D, et al. Efficacy and safety of low-field synchronized transcranial magnetic stimulation (sTMS) for treatment of major depression. Brain Stimul 2015;8(4):787–94.

Clinical Repetitive Transcranial Magnetic Stimulation for Posttraumatic Stress Disorder, Generalized Anxiety Disorder, and Bipolar Disorder

F. Andrew Kozel, MD, MSCR[a,b,*]

KEYWORDS

- Transcranial magnetic stimulation • TMS • Posttraumatic stress disorder • PTSD
- Generalized anxiety disorder • GAD • Bipolar disorder

KEY POINTS

- A growing body of literature is demonstrating the possibility of using repetitive transcranial magnetic stimulation (rTMS) to treat posttraumatic stress disorder (PTSD), generalized anxiety disorder (GAD), and bipolar disorder.
- These findings are still preliminary and require well-designed and adequately powered studies before rTMS can be recommended for use clinically in PTSD, GAD, or bipolar disorder.
- More studies are required to determine optimal treatment parameters with the caveat that the results may suggest that choice of certain parameters are not critical to efficacy.
- A better understanding of the neuropathology of these disorders as well as how the mechanism of action of rTMS interacts with that pathology could help with optimizing treatment parameters.

INTRODUCTION

Transcranial magnetic stimulation (TMS) is a noninvasive brain stimulation technology that has been investigated as both a clinical and neurophysiology research tool. When the stimulation is given repetitively, it is commonly referred to as repetitive transcranial

Disclosure Statement. See last page of article.
[a] Mental Health and Behavioral Sciences & HSR&D Center of Innovation on Disability and Rehabilitation Research (CINDRR), James A. Haley Veterans' Administration Hospital and Clinics, 116A, 13000 Bruce B. Downs Boulevard, Tampa, FL 33612, USA; [b] Department of Psychiatry and Behavioral Neurosciences, University of South Florida, 3515 E Fletcher Avenue, Tampa, FL 33613, USA
* James A. Haley Veterans' Hospital and Clinics, 116A, 13000 Bruce B. Downs Boulevard, Tampa, FL 33612.
E-mail address: Frank.Kozel@va.gov

Psychiatr Clin N Am 41 (2018) 433–446
https://doi.org/10.1016/j.psc.2018.04.007
0193-953X/18/Published by Elsevier Inc.

magnetic stimulation (rTMS).[1] An acute course of rTMS for major depressive disorder (MDD) generally consists of daily visits (Monday through Friday) for about 6 weeks.[2] The treatment dose is individualized for each patient and reported as a percentage of the motor threshold (MT). The MT is typically defined as the intensity of stimulation that moves the contralateral abductor pollicis brevis 50% of the time determined by either visual observation or electromyography measures. Several large trials and meta-analyses have demonstrated its antidepressant effect in MDD.[3–6] In 2008, the Food and Drug Administration (FDA) in the United States cleared the first rTMS device for the treatment of MDD targeting the left dorsolateral prefrontal cortex (DLPFC) using 10 Hz stimulation at 120% MT. Subsequently, the FDA has cleared 5 additional rTMS devices as well as expanded the initial rTMS device's indication to a broader range of treatment resistance in patients with MDD. Beyond efficacy studies for MDD, other studies have supported the effectiveness of rTMS across a variety of settings outside randomized trials.[7–11] Given its effectiveness in MDD and excellent safety profile, rTMS is being investigated in several other neuropsychiatric disorders, including posttraumatic stress disorder (PTSD), generalized anxiety disorder (GAD), and both phases of bipolar disorder.[12]

REPETITIVE TRANSCRANIAL MAGNETIC STIMULATION AND POSTTRAUMATIC STRESS DISORDER

PTSD is a significant public health problem. The National Co-morbidity Survey (NCS) reported a lifetime prevalence rate of 7.8% for PTSD in a national sample,[13,14] whereas the data from the Wave 2 National Epidemiologic Survey on Alcohol and Related Conditions found the lifetime prevalence of PTSD to be 6.4%.[15] Current clinical guidelines support evidence-based psychotherapies such as prolonged exposure and cognitive processing therapy as first-line treatments for PTSD.[16] However, a recent review of randomized clinical trials for military-related PTSD demonstrated that although these therapies do result in meaningful improvement in patients with PTSD, approximately two-thirds of patients continued to meet full criteria for PTSD.[17] Thus, new treatment approaches are critically needed to improve treatment outcomes.

Early in clinical development, rTMS was considered for PTSD, and the research has progressed through increasing levels of evidence for its clinical utility. In 1998, Grisaru and colleagues[18] (n = 10) were among the first to report some benefit for treating PTSD using 1-Hz rTMS stimulation to the right and left motor cortex. They, however, used only 15 pulses on each side and the improvement lasted only a short time. McCann and colleagues,[19] also in 1998, administered 1 Hz rTMS at 80% MT over the right DLPFC to 2 patients with PTSD and demonstrated temporary reduction in several core symptoms in both patients. Rosenberg and colleagues[20] in 2002 found (n = 12) that 1 Hz and 5 Hz over the left DLPFC for 10 days demonstrated improvement in depressive symptoms but did not lead to a significant change in PTSD symptoms, although the treatment dose was small, with only 6000 pulses over the 10 days. Taghva and colleagues[21] in 2015 studied (n = 16) whether rTMS frequencies determined by electroencephalography (EEG) and electrocardiography at 80% MT for 30 trains of 6 second stimulation and 30 second intertrain intervals were effective for PTSD symptoms. The location of stimulation was determined by the area in the prefrontal cortex with the highest EEG irregularity. After 5 times a week for 2 weeks, the participants who completed the treatment demonstrated positive clinical as well as EEG changes.

Several studies have investigated rTMS for PTSD in patients specifically with co-morbid conditions. Nakama and colleagues[22] in 2014 reported on the successful treatment of an active duty soldier with both MDD and PTSD using standard rTMS treatment parameters for MDD. Also in 2014, Oznur and colleagues[23] reported on a case series of 20 combat veterans with comorbid PTSD and MDD treated with right prefrontal rTMS using 1 Hz for 20 daily treatments but only at 80% of the resting MT. Although there was no significant change in the depression rating or total PTSD scale, there was a significant change in the hyperarousal subscale. Given that the patients were only treated at 80% of MT, it was unclear if the lack of response was simply related to the low-intensity dose. Philip and colleagues[24] reported in 2016 on a case series of 10 patients with comorbid PTSD and MDD treated with left prefrontal cortex stimulation at 5 Hz using 120% MT. The patients were offered up to 36 treatments, with significant improvement found when baseline compared with endpoint PTSD and MDD symptoms. Woodside and colleagues[25] in 2017 reported on a case series of 14 female patients with comorbid PTSD and eating disorders, who received around 20 to 30 treatment sessions using various treatment parameters. Patients demonstrated a significant improvement in both trauma symptoms and eating disorder symptoms. These reports demonstrate that rTMS could possibly be an effective treatment of PTSD including those with various comorbidities. Given the nature of the reports, however, they are only a starting point from which to support the use of rTMS for PTSD.

Adding to the evidence provided by noncontrolled studies, there have been several small randomized controlled trials that do support the use of rTMS for PTSD. Cohen and colleagues[26] in 2004 (n = 24) used 10 Hz stimulation over the right DLPFC to demonstrate that rTMS significantly improved PTSD symptoms compared with sham and 1 Hz stimulation. The stimulation dose, however, was only 80% of MT, and the number of 1 Hz pulses (100 per treatment × 10 days) and 10 Hz pulses (200 per treatment × 10 days) were quite small, thus making any firm conclusion difficult except that it was well tolerated and that the 10 Hz demonstrated an effect. In 2010, Boggio and colleagues[27] (n = 30) compared right versus left DLPFC with sham stimulation using 20 Hz at 80% of MT for 10 treatments. They found that although both active protocols achieved better results than sham, the right prefrontal cortex stimulation produced a larger effect on PTSD symptoms. Watts and colleagues[28] in 2012 (n = 20) demonstrated that 10 sessions of right DLPFC 1-Hz rTMS at 90% of MT could significantly improve the symptoms of PTSD compared with what was achieved using sham stimulation. Similarly, Nam and colleagues[29] in 2013 (n = 18) also used a sham-controlled design to determine that 1-Hz right DLPFC rTMS at 100% MT for 15 treatments significantly improved PTSD symptoms in patients with various types of trauma. Although preliminary because of the small sample sizes and multiple parameters chosen, most of the results did support the use of rTMS for PTSD.[30–32] In addition, there was some support for the more effective location of stimulation being over the right versus left DLPFC, but larger studies are required to confirm these findings. Another unanswered question is regarding the optimal frequency for treating PTSD. Given the findings discussed earlier, there is some evidence for both high frequency (>1 Hz) and low frequency (1 Hz) as being effective. Given the limited data, especially of direct comparisons with equal pulses per treatment, however, the available results do not provide a clear optimal frequency choice for rTMS to treat PTSD.[33]

In addition to randomized controlled trials using rTMS alone to treat PTSD, there are several trials that have combined rTMS with psychotherapy or script-driven imagery to determine if the combination has an additive or synergistic effect. Osuch and colleagues[34] in 2009 (n = 9) explored combining exposure therapy (traumatic recall) with either 1 Hz or sham rTMS delivered for 30 minutes to the right DLPFC for 20 sessions in a cross-over, double-blind study. Moderate improvement in hyperarousal symptoms on the Clinician-Administered PTSD Scale (CAPS) with exposure plus active rTMS was found but no effect with exposure plus sham rTMS; however, the difference between active and sham groups was not statistically significant. Isserles and colleagues[35] in 2013 (n = 30) reported on testing an H-coil with script-driven imagery from a traumatic event to relieve the symptoms of PTSD. The H-coil (H-coil TMS [H-TMS]) was thought to provide deeper penetration into the brain compared with the standard figure-8 coils. The participants were randomized to 1 of 3 groups: H-TMS after imagery of traumatic experience; H-TMS after imagery of positive experience; and sham H-TMS after imagery of traumatic experience. Treatment sessions were 3 times a week for 4 weeks, stimulating over the medial prefrontal cortex using 20 Hz at 120% MT for 1680 pulses per session. The group of H-TMS after imagery of traumatic experience demonstrated a significant improvement in the intrusive component of the CAPS score and a trend for improvement in the total CAPS score, but the other groups demonstrated no significant improvements. One of the largest studies of rTMS for PTSD to date involved randomizing 103 combat veterans to either active or sham 1-Hz right DLPFC rTMS just prior to weekly cognitive processing therapy (CPT). Although CPT was effective in both groups, the active rTMS group had significantly greater improvements than the sham rTMS group in clinician (CAPS) and patient (PTSD symptom checklist) rated scales of PTSD that were maintained for 6 months. Although both groups had significant improvement in depressive symptoms and function, the active TMS plus CPT group was not significantly improved on either depression or function scales compared with the sham plus CPT group. Thus, the significant improvements in PTSD symptoms from active rTMS versus sham rTMS were not solely attributed to the improvement in depression symptoms.[36] If these results can be replicated, rTMS with CPT would serve as a much-needed treatment for a very disabling illness.

Several questions would be important to address in order to optimize the outcome of rTMS augmenting exposure-based or other psychotherapy interventions for PTSD. An important question is the timing of rTMS with respect to the psychotherapy. The 3 studies discussed earlier used rTMS during, after, and before the indicated intervention. As the timing of rTMS with respect to intervention was stable within the studies as well as differing interventions across studies, no assessment of which timing is the most effective can be made. A second important question is if particular types of psychotherapy interventions are more likely to be augmented by rTMS than others. All 3 of these interventions had an exposure component; whether this is critical to the benefit from adding rTMS should be investigated in future studies.

PTSD is a significant cause of suffering and disability for many patients. For those patients who do not respond to current therapies or are unable to tolerate them, other treatment options are critically needed. A growing body of evidence is supporting the use of rTMS with and without psychotherapy/exposure for PTSD; however, the level of evidence is not sufficient to currently recommend rTMS specifically for PTSD. Future work involving randomized controlled trials of rTMS for PTSD with adequate sample sizes will be required to demonstrate its effectiveness. In addition to demonstrating clinical effectiveness, studies should also investigate ways to optimize treatment with respect to location of stimulation (eg, left vs right, DLPFC vs dorsomedial prefrontal cortex), treatment parameters (eg, frequency, number of pulses, number of treatments), and timing of rTMS with respect to psychotherapy intervention to achieve optimal augmenting results. Understanding the mechanism of action of rTMS for PTSD would dramatically help with investigating these treatment factors. Unfortunately, the information on mechanism of action of rTMS to treat PTSD is limited. Philip and colleagues[37] investigated resting state connectivity measures in patients treated with left DLPFC 5 Hz rTMS for PTSD comorbid with PTSD. The study demonstrated circuit-based changes that predicted treatment outcome as well as those associated with treatment improvement. Future work will be required to determine how consistently these changes occur and whether they can be clinically informative.

REPETITIVE TRANSCRANIAL MAGNETIC STIMULATION FOR GENERALIZED ANXIETY DISORDER

GAD is a common psychiatric illness that has a 12-month prevalence of approximately 3.1% of the population with high rates of comorbidity with depression.[14] In addition to being common, GAD causes considerable morbidity in patients especially in combination with depression.[38] Although there are several effective psychotherapy and medication treatments, these treatments do not work for a significant percentage of patients.[39,40]

Given that rTMS has been shown to be effective for MDD and that there is a significant overlap with MDD and GAD, investigators have been examining the role that rTMS could play in treating GAD. One of the first studies on GAD by Bystritsky and colleagues[41] used an open design to see if 1-Hz right prefrontal rTMS for 6 sessions could improve the anxiety symptoms of 10 patients with only GAD and no other psychiatric comorbidities. They used a gambling task during functional MRI acquisition to determine the target location within the right prefrontal cortex for each individual. Participants were treated 2 times a week for 3 weeks at 90% MT with 900 pulses per day. A significant reduction was found on the anxiety scales as well as 6 of the 10 participants achieving criteria for remission. Given the potential for effectiveness on GAD symptoms alone, several studies have assessed impact of generalized anxiety symptoms with respect to rTMS treatment of MDD. Diefenbach and colleagues[42] in 2013 examined a case series of 32 patients treated with 10-Hz left DLPFC rTMS who were titrated up to 130% MT for approximately 31 treatments. They found that patients with and without anxious depression demonstrated significant improvement in both depression and anxiety symptoms and to a similar degree. Similarly, White and colleagues[43] (n = 13) and Kozel and colleagues[8] (n = 40) found significant improvement in both anxiety and depressive measures in patients treated with rTMS using various treatment locations. Given the open nature of these reports, the role of rTMS versus other factors associated with rTMS could not be assessed.

Randomized sham-controlled trials of GAD with limited depressive symptoms, however, have begun to address whether rTMS can be effective specifically for GAD. Diefenbach and colleagues[44] randomized participants to an active coil or a sham coil in participants with principal or co-principal diagnosis of GAD with a 17-item Hamilton Rating Scale[45] for depression score less than or equal to 17. Subjects were treated with 900 pulses per day using 1 Hz stimulation at 90% MT over the right DLPFC. Treatments occurred on weekdays for 30 treatments. Stimulation location was determined individually based on the MNI coordinates generated in the Bystritsky study discussed earlier and targeted using participants' structural MRIs. Posttreatment and at 3-months follow-up, the active group (n = 13) had a significantly greater response than the sham group (n = 12) on anxiety rating scales.[44] In addition, a secondary analysis demonstrated that self-reported emotional regulation difficulties were statistically improved for only the active rTMS group at posttreatment and 3-month follow-up visits.[46] Dilkov and colleagues also investigated using right DLPFC rTMS in a randomized control trial of GAD but used high-frequency (20 HZ) stimulation as opposed to low-frequency (1 Hz) stimulation. Participants randomized to active treatment were treated at 110% MT for 9 seconds of stimulation and 51 seconds intertrain interval for 3600 pulses per day. Treatments were 5 days a week for 4 weeks and then tapered for a total of 25 treatments. The participants randomized to the sham group had the same procedures except that the coil was held 90° from the skull. The location of right prefrontal stimulation was determined by moving the coil 5 cm anteriorly from the location of the site for determining the MT. The active stimulation group (n = 15) experienced a significant decrease in anxiety symptoms, whereas the sham group (n = 25) demonstrated very little improvement. One of the participants in the active group, however, experienced a generalized tonic–clonic seizure. Importantly, the treatment parameters in this study were outside the safety guidelines provided by the treatment safety parameter tables.[47,48]

The available information for rTMS for GAD is limited but growing. There are open trials and case reports that point to the effectiveness of rTMS for GAD but mostly in the context of treating MDD. These reports demonstrated various treatment locations (eg, right DLPFC, left DLPFC, and sequential right then left DLPFC) as well as treatment parameters including high- versus low-frequency stimulation and treatment schedules (eg, treating only twice a week for multiple weeks vs 5 days a week for multiple weeks). The 2 randomized controlled trials provide more convincing support but have small samples. Future studies are needed with adequate power and sham-controlled designs before rTMS can be clinically recommended for GAD. Also, the Dilkov study highlights the importance of using treatment parameters within the safety guidelines to prevent seizures from occurring.

REPETITIVE TRANSCRANIAL MAGNETIC STIMULATION FOR BIPOLAR DISORDER

Bipolar disorder is a serious condition that causes significant morbidity and mortality that affects approximately 2.5% of the population.[49] Bipolar disorder is generally classified as either bipolar I disorder or bipolar II disorder. Bipolar I disorder requires the history of a manic episode but is often accompanied by depressive episodes. Conversely, bipolar II disorder requires the presence of both a hypomanic episode and a major depressive episode.[50] Treatment with rTMS has been investigated for manic/hypomanic episodes, depressive episodes, and mixed episodes in bipolar disorder.

Repetitive Transcranial Magnetic Stimulation to Treat Mania in Bipolar Disorder

Early in the development of rTMS as a clinical tool, Grisaru and colleagues[51] in 1998 published a manuscript comparing left versus right DLPFC 20 Hz rTMS for mania. They found that 10 rTMS treatments resulted in a significantly greater improvement in mania symptoms when rTMS was positioned over the right (n = 7) versus the left DLPFC (n = 9). A follow-up study by this group in 2003 compared right DLPFC 20-Hz rTMS with sham rTMS in 19 participants. Compared with sham, however, right-sided stimulation did not provide any benefit in mania symptoms. Subsequently in 2004, there were 2 small case series using 10-Hz and 20-Hz rTMS over the right DLPFC that reported significant improvements in mania symptoms.[52,53] Providing conflicting evidence regarding the usefulness of rTMS to treat mania, there have been 2 subsequent randomized controlled trials of high-frequency rTMS over the right DLPFC. Praharaj and colleagues[54] in 2009 reported that 20-Hz rTMS (n = 21) versus sham rTMS (n = 20) over the right DLPFC for 10 days in adults resulted in a significantly greater improvement in mania symptoms. The treatments were well tolerated, but one of the patients treated with active stimulation developed mild depression during the study period whereas none in the sham group developed depression. Conversely, using a similar design in adolescent participants, Pathak and colleagues[55] reported in 2015 that active stimulation did not result in a greater reduction in mania scores in participants aged 12 to 17 years. Because of the small sample sizes, determining whether the differences observed were because of the differences in age groups or some other factor is not possible. The results of rTMS in treating mania are clearly mixed. Currently, there is no compelling evidence for the use of rTMS in mania. Adequately powered randomized controlled trials demonstrating benefit are required before rTMS can be recommended for mania in a clinical setting.

Repetitive Transcranial Magnetic Stimulation to Treat Depression in Bipolar Disorder

Several studies investigating rTMS for depression included patients with bipolar disorder as well as MDD. Especially in early trials, the number of participants was too small to adequately assess for differences in response or safety between the conditions, but rTMS seemed to work similarly in both conditions.[56–58] One of the first randomized trials for rTMS, specifically for depressive episodes in patients with bipolar disorder (ie, bipolar depression), was reported by Dolberg and colleagues[59] in 2002. Their pilot study of rTMS (n = 10) versus sham (n = 10) demonstrated significant improvement for rTMS versus sham at 2 weeks but not 4 weeks. Several key rTMS treatment parameters were not reported. Similarly, Nahas and colleagues[60] in 2003 reported on a randomized controlled trial of 5-Hz left DLPFC rTMS (n = 11) versus sham (n = 12) at 110% MT for 2 weeks that failed to show a significant difference in outcome between the 2 groups but was well tolerated with no appearance of hypomanic symptoms. Both studies, however, were underpowered from the standpoint of number of treatments and number of participants. Taking a different approach, Tamas and colleagues[61] in 2007 reported on using 1-Hz right DLPFC rTMS at 95% MT for 100 stimuli twice a week for 4 weeks. The 5 participants randomized to active versus the 1 participant assigned to sham rTMS demonstrated improvement but the number of subjects was too small for any meaningful statistical analysis. Combining 1-Hz right DLPFC rTMS followed by left 10-Hz DLPFC rTMS (ie, sequential bilateral rTMS) both at 110% MT, Fitzgerald and colleagues[62] reported in 2016 on a well-designed trial of active (n = 23) versus sham (n = 23) rTMS for 20 sessions over 4 weeks in the treatment of bipolar depression. At 4 weeks, both groups demonstrated significant improvement but there was no difference in clinical outcome between the 2 groups. In an attempt to augment the effect of quetiapine in bipolar depression, Hu and colleagues[63] in 2016 reported on a trial of randomizing participants being started on quetiapine to augmentation with 3 rTMS groups: 10-Hz left DLPFC rTMS; 1-Hz right DLPFC rTMS; and sham rTMS. The rTMS was performed for 20 sessions at 80% MT with 1200 pulses per session. The sham condition involved positioning the coil vertical to the scalp and using the left 10 Hz parameters. Although there was a significant improvement over the course of the trial for all groups, there was no significant difference between the groups, which may have been the result of using a low-dose (80% MT) stimulation. An encouraging randomized controlled study for rTMS over the left DLPFC in bipolar depression was published by Tavares and colleagues[64] in 2017. They used an H1-coil with capability for active and sham stimulation using the parameters of 18 Hz stimulation at 120% MT for 1980 pulses per day. Participants were randomized to active (n = 25) or sham (n = 25) stimulation for 20 daily treatments. The active group demonstrated significant improvement in depression rating scales compared with the sham group at the completion of treatments at 4 weeks, but that significant difference in improvement was lost after 4 additional weeks of follow-up. There were no reported episodes of mania observed in the trial.

Because bipolar disorder is a chronic illness, several investigators have reported on small case series supporting the safety and long-term effects of rTMS for bipolar depression.[65-68] To more formally test the potential long-term impact of rTMS in depression, Rapinesi and colleagues[69] reported in 2015 on the benefits of a protracted taper period of 3 months resulting in better outcomes at 6 and 12 months for participants who were diagnosed with bipolar disorder and MDD.

Treatment with rTMS for bipolar depression seems to be safe and well tolerated. Although there are case reports of inducing mania/hypomania with rTMS in bipolar depression, the actual incidence is small and similar to rates seen with traditional mood stabilizers.[70] Importantly, inducing mania/hypomania may be more common in patients with bipolar disorder, but it has also been reported in healthy controls and participants with psychiatric disorders other than mood disorders.[71] Although rTMS for bipolar depression is generally accepted as a safe treatment, the question of whether it is clinically useful is still unclear. Although there is some support for rTMS being useful for bipolar depression acutely and in the long term, most of the evidence is not in randomized controlled studies. The randomized controlled studies to date have actually failed to demonstrate a benefit or only provided a fleeting benefit. This may be related to methodological problems in the design, such as being underpowered or using an inadequate duration of therapy. Regardless, randomized controlled trials with adequate power are required before rTMS can be recommended for bipolar depression.

Repetitive Transcranial Magnetic Stimulation to Treat Mixed State in Bipolar Disorder

In addition to trials of rTMS in bipolar disorder for the episodes of mania or depression, Pallanti and colleagues[72] in 2014 reported on an open trial using 1-Hz right DLPFC rTMS in patients in a mixed state. Forty participants were treated initially with valproate for 4 weeks. Subsequently, rTMS was started at 110% MT for 420 stimuli per session for 15 treatments over 3 weeks. There was evidence of benefit for both the depressive and manic symptoms, but this was an open trial. Further positive studies using a randomized controlled design are required before rTMS can be recommended for mixed states of bipolar disorder.

SUMMARY

As rTMS has demonstrated clinical efficacy,[4] effectiveness,[8,10] and cost-effectiveness[73,74] in treating MDD, treatment of other indications has been explored. Although the data supporting treating other indications are not nearly as strong, the data for using rTMS in PTSD, GAD, and bipolar disorder is growing. The level of support, however, has not currently reached a point that rTMS is clinically indicated for use with PTSD, GAD, or bipolar disorder.

This technology has some unique aspects that promise both great potential and significant hurdles, specifically the multiple treatment parameters that can be prescribed. The promise is that treatment parameters might be tailored to a particular illness and/or person, and the hurdle is that the broad parameter space offers an almost infinite number of treatment combinations to test. Theories are important to provide a framework for testing, but the final assessment of clinical utility must be based on clinical trial data in specified populations using detailed reports of treatment parameters. Several key questions remain. Does targeting of treatment based on a neuroanatomic functional/structural location improve outcome over a probabilistic target? There is no convincing evidence, even in MDD, that neuroanatomic targeting improves outcome. Determining the benefit of this technology is critical for clinical use because the cost in time and money is significantly greater for neuroanatomic targeting. Does frequency affect long-term outcome? We have rather convincing evidence that different frequencies can have diverging effects on brain circuitry; however, whether that translates into differences in treatment outcome is still unknown. Another important question is whether rTMS should be coupled with psychotherapy or other intervention to maximize clinical utility? These and several other concerns will need to be addressed in future studies in order for this exciting technology to provide critically needed evidence-based treatment.

DISCLOSURE STATEMENT

I do not believe that I have any financial conflicts of interest but have included my full disclosure for transparency. Current Research and/or Salary Support: 04/2015 to Present (PI - Kozel), VA Office of Research and Development—"Targeting Disability from PTSD with Transcranial Magnetic Stimulation", Role: Principal Investigator 30% (No salary support per VA rules). Past Research and/or Salary Support: 10/14/2014 to 9/30/2016 RX 14-009, (PI - Chapman), VA Office of Research and Development—RRD SPiRE— "Pre treatment Physiological Reactivity and Treatment Outcome", Role: Co-investigator 10% (No salary support per VA rules); 02/2011 to 04/2014 DM090122, (PI - Hart), Department of Defense—"Novel Treatment of Emotional Dysfunction in PTSD", Role: Co-investigator 10% (No Salary Support after Apr 2014); 09/30/10 to 06/30/14 1 U01MH092221-01, (PI - Trivedi), NIMH—"Establishing Moderators and Biosignatures of Antidepressant Response for Clinical Care (EMBARC)", Role: Co-investigator (No Salary Support after July 2011); Neuronetics (Kozel Site PI) 2013 "An open-label study to evaluate the efficacy and safety of the Neuronetics Neurostar TMS therapy system in patients with major depressive disorder (MDD) with postpartum onset." No support other than research funds for regulatory submission but then discontinued due to change in personnel. More than 3 years ago: The National Institute of Mental Health K23 NIMH 5 K23 MH070897-02, Role: PI 2005 to 2009; NIH, NCRR 5 UL1 RR024982-02 Packer (PI) Role: Pilot Study PI; Neuronetics Grant-in-kind support for supplies and use of equipment; the Defense Academy for Credibility Assessment (formerly the Department of Defense Polygraph Institute), Cephos Corp., Stanley Medical Research Institute, Cyberonics (Treatment studies D01, D02, D04, AN01) 2001 to 2005; Glaxo Smith Kline (Interleaved TMS-fMRI) 2002 to 2003. Paid Advisory/Consulting: None. Speaking: None. Equity Holdings (exclude mutual funds): None. Royalty/patent, other income: patents as an inventor through the Medical University of South Carolina on fMRI Detection of Deception, patents pending for Guided rTMS Inhibition of Deception, Optimizing VNS dose with rTMS. Other: 2004 Monthly Case Discussion Group Leader x1 Sponsored by Astra Zeneca; Unpaid scientific consultant to Neuronetics and Cephos Corp. (none in > 5 years).

ACKNOWLEDGMENTS

The author alone is responsible for the content and writing of the article. The views expressed in this article are those of the author and do not necessarily reflect the official policy or position of the Department of Veteran Affairs or the United States Government.

REFERENCES

1. George MS, Belmaker RH. Transcranial magnetic stimulation in clinical psychiatry. Washington, DC: American Psychiatric Publishing, Inc; 2007.

2. Van Trees K, Rustad JK, Weisman M, et al. Comprehensive guide for the safe administration of rTMS while providing for patient comfort. Issues Ment Health Nurs 2017;38(2):182–7.

3. O'Reardon JP, Solvason HB, Janicak PG, et al. Efficacy and safety of transcranial magnetic stimulation in the acute treatment of major depression: a multisite randomized controlled trial. Biol Psychiatry 2007;62(11):1208–16.

4. Gaynes BN, Lloyd SW, Lux L, et al. Repetitive transcranial magnetic stimulation for treatment-resistant depression: a systematic review and meta-analysis. J Clin Psychiatry 2014;75(5):477–89.

5. George MS, Lisanby SH, Avery D, et al. Daily left prefrontal transcranial magnetic stimulation therapy for major depressive disorder: a sham-controlled randomized trial. Arch Gen Psychiatry 2010;67(5):507–16.

6. Kozel FA, George MS. Meta-analysis of left prefrontal repetitive transcranial magnetic stimulation (rTMS) to treat depression. J Psychiatr Pract 2002;8(5):270–5.

7. Taylor SF, Bhati MT, Dubin MJ, et al. A naturalistic, multi-site study of repetitive transcranial magnetic stimulation therapy for depression. J Affect Disord 2017; 208:284–90.

8. Kozel FA, Hernandez M, Van Trees K, et al. Clinical repetitive transcranial magnetic stimulation for veterans with major depressive disorder. Ann Clin Psychiatry 2017;29(4):242–8.

9. Connolly KR, Helmer A, Cristancho MA, et al. Effectiveness of transcranial magnetic stimulation in clinical practice post-FDA approval in the United States: results observed with the first 100 consecutive cases of depression at an academic medical center. J Clin Psychiatry 2012;73(4):e567–73.

10. Carpenter LL, Janicak PG, Aaronson ST, et al. Transcranial magnetic stimulation (TMS) for major depression: a multisite, naturalistic, observational study of acute treatment outcomes in clinical practice. Depress Anxiety 2012;29(7):587–96.

11. Janicak PG, Dunner DL, Aaronson ST, et al. Transcranial magnetic stimulation (TMS) for major depression: a multisite, naturalistic, observational study of quality of life outcome measures in clinical practice. CNS Spectr 2013;18(6): 322–32.

12. Lefaucheur JP, Andre-Obadia N, Antal A, et al. Evidence-based guidelines on the therapeutic use of repetitive transcranial magnetic stimulation (rTMS). Clin Neurophysiol 2014;125(11):2150–206.

13. Kessler RC, Sonnega A, Bromet E, et al. Posttraumatic stress disorder in the National Comorbidity Survey. Arch Gen Psychiatry 1995;52(12):1048–60.

14. Kessler RC, Chiu WT, Demler O, et al. Prevalence, severity, and comorbidity of 12-month DSM-IV disorders in the National Comorbidity Survey Replication. Arch Gen Psychiatry 2005;62(6):617–27.

15. Pietrzak RH, Goldstein RB, Southwick SM, et al. Prevalence and Axis I comorbidity of full and partial posttraumatic stress disorder in the United States: results from Wave 2 of the National Epidemiologic Survey on Alcohol and Related Conditions. J Anxiety Disord 2011;25(3):456–65.

16. IOM (Institute of Medicine). Treatment for posttraumatic stress disorder in military and veteran populations: final assessment. Washington, DC: The National Academies Press; 2014.

17. Steenkamp MM, Litz BT, Hoge CW, et al. Psychotherapy for military-related PTSD: a review of randomized clinical trials. JAMA 2015;314(5):489–500.

18. Grisaru N, Amir M, Cohen H, et al. Effect of transcranial magnetic stimulation in posttraumatic stress disorder: a preliminary study. Biol Psychiatry 1998;44(1): 52–5.

19. McCann UD, Kimbrell TA, Morgan CM, et al. Repetitive transcranial magnetic stimulation for posttraumatic stress disorder (letter). Arch Gen Psychiatry 1998;55:276–9.

20. Rosenberg PB, Mehndiratta RB, Mehndiratta YP, et al. Repetitive transcranial magnetic stimulation treatment of comorbid posttraumatic stress disorder and major depression. J Neuropsychiatry Clin Neurosci 2002;14(3):270–6.

21. Taghva A, Silvetz R, Ring A, et al. Magnetic resonance therapy improves clinical phenotype and EEG alpha power in posttraumatic stress disorder. Trauma Mon 2015;20(4):e27360.

22. Nakama H, Garcia A, O'Brien K, et al. Case report of a 24-year-old man with resolution of treatment-resistant major depressive disorder and comorbid PTSD using rTMS. J ECT 2014;30(1):e9–10.

23. Oznur T, Akarsu S, Celik C, et al. Is transcranial magnetic stimulation effective in treatment-resistant combat related posttraumatic stress disorder? Neurosciences (Riyadh) 2014;19(1):29–32.

24. Philip NS, Ridout SJ, Albright SE, et al. 5-Hz transcranial magnetic stimulation for comorbid posttraumatic stress disorder and major depression. J Trauma Stress 2016;29(1):93–6.

25. Woodside DB, Colton P, Lam E, et al. Dorsomedial prefrontal cortex repetitive transcranial magnetic stimulation treatment of posttraumatic stress disorder in eating disorders: an open-label case series. Int J Eat Disord 2017;50(10):1231–4.

26. Cohen H, Kaplan Z, Kotler M, et al. Repetitive transcranial magnetic stimulation of the right dorsolateral prefrontal cortex in posttraumatic stress disorder: a double-blind, placebo-controlled study. Am J Psychiatry 2004;161(3):515–24.

27. Boggio PS, Rocha M, Oliveira MO, et al. Noninvasive brain stimulation with high-frequency and low-intensity repetitive transcranial magnetic stimulation treatment for posttraumatic stress disorder. J Clin Psychiatry 2010;71(8):992–9.

28. Watts BV, Landon B, Groft A, et al. A sham controlled study of repetitive transcranial magnetic stimulation for posttraumatic stress disorder. Brain Stimul 2012; 5(1):38–43.

29. Nam DH, Pae CU, Chae JH. Low-frequency, repetitive transcranial magnetic stimulation for the treatment of patients with posttraumatic stress disorder: a double-blind, sham-controlled study. Clin Psychopharmacol Neurosci 2013; 11(2):96–102.

30. Karsen EF, Watts BV, Holtzheimer PE. Review of the effectiveness of transcranial magnetic stimulation for post-traumatic stress disorder. Brain Stimul 2014;7(2): 151–7.

31. Berlim MT, Van Den Eynde F. Repetitive transcranial magnetic stimulation over the dorsolateral prefrontal cortex for treating posttraumatic stress disorder: an exploratory meta-analysis of randomized, double-blind and sham-controlled trials. Can J Psychiatry 2014;59(9):487–96.

32. Clark C, Cole J, Winter C, et al. A review of transcranial magnetic stimulation as a treatment for post-traumatic stress disorder. Curr Psychiatry Rep 2015;17(10):83.

33. Yan T, Xie Q, Zheng Z, et al. Different frequency repetitive transcranial magnetic stimulation (rTMS) for posttraumatic stress disorder (PTSD): a systematic review and meta-analysis. J Psychiatr Res 2017;89:125–35.

34. Osuch EA, Benson BE, Luckenbaugh DA, et al. Repetitive TMS combined with exposure therapy for PTSD: a preliminary study. J Anxiety Disord 2009;23(1): 54–9.

35. Isserles M, Shalev AY, Roth Y, et al. Effectiveness of deep transcranial magnetic stimulation combined with a brief exposure procedure in post-traumatic stress disorder–a pilot study. Brain Stimul 2013;6(3):377–83.

36. Kozel FA, Motes MA, Didehbani N, et al. Repetitive TMS to augment cognitive processing therapy in combat veterans of recent conflicts with PTSD: a randomized clinical trial. J Affect Disord 2017;229:506–14.
37. Philip NS, Barredo J, van 't Wout-Frank M, et al. Network mechanisms of clinical response to transcranial magnetic stimulation in posttraumatic stress disorder and major depressive disorder. Biol Psychiatry 2018;83(3): 263–72.
38. Revicki DA, Travers K, Wyrwich KW, et al. Humanistic and economic burden of generalized anxiety disorder in North America and Europe. J Affect Disord 2012;140(2):103–12.
39. Gersh E, Hallford DJ, Rice SM, et al. Systematic review and meta-analysis of dropout rates in individual psychotherapy for generalized anxiety disorder. J Anxiety Disord 2017;52:25–33.
40. Reinhold JA, Mandos LA, Rickels K, et al. Pharmacological treatment of generalized anxiety disorder. Expert Opin Pharmacother 2011;12(16):2457–67.
41. Bystritsky A, Kaplan JT, Feusner JD, et al. A preliminary study of fMRI-guided rTMS in the treatment of generalized anxiety disorder. J Clin Psychiatry 2008; 69(7):1092–8.
42. Diefenbach GJ, Bragdon L, Goethe JW. Treating anxious depression using repetitive transcranial magnetic stimulation. J Affect Disord 2013;151(1):365–8.
43. White D, Tavakoli S. Repetitive transcranial magnetic stimulation for treatment of major depressive disorder with comorbid generalized anxiety disorder. Ann Clin Psychiatry 2015;27(3):192–6.
44. Diefenbach GJ, Bragdon LB, Zertuche L, et al. Repetitive transcranial magnetic stimulation for generalised anxiety disorder: a pilot randomised, double-blind, sham-controlled trial. Br J Psychiatry 2016;209(3):222–8.
45. Hamilton M. A rating scale for depression. J Neurol Neurosurg Psychiatry 1960; 12:56–62.
46. Diefenbach GJ, Assaf M, Goethe JW, et al. Improvements in emotion regulation following repetitive transcranial magnetic stimulation for generalized anxiety disorder. J Anxiety Disord 2016;43:1–7.
47. Rossi S, Hallett M, Rossini PM, et al. Safety, ethical considerations, and application guidelines for the use of transcranial magnetic stimulation in clinical practice and research. Clin Neurophysiol 2009;120(12):2008–39.
48. Wassermann EM. Risk and safety of repetitive transcranial magnetic stimulation: report and suggested guidelines from the International Workshop on the Safety of Repetitive Transcranial Magnetic Stimulation, June 5-7, 1996. Electroencephalogr Clin Neurophysiol 1998;108(1):1–16.
49. Kessler RC, Petukhova M, Sampson NA, et al. Twelve-month and lifetime prevalence and lifetime morbid risk of anxiety and mood disorders in the United States. Int J Methods Psychiatr Res 2012;21(3):169–84.
50. American Psychiatric Association. Diagnostic and statistical manual of mental health disorders: DSM-5. 5th edition. Washington, DC: American Psychiatric Publishing; 2013.
51. Grisaru N, Chudakov B, Yaroslavsky Y, et al. Transcranial magnetic stimulation in mania: a controlled study. Am J Psychiatry 1998;155(11):1608–10.
52. Saba G, Rocamora JF, Kalalou K, et al. Repetitive transcranial magnetic stimulation as an add-on therapy in the treatment of mania: a case series of eight patients. Psychiatry Res 2004;128(2):199–202.
53. Michael N, Erfurth A. Treatment of bipolar mania with right prefrontal rapid transcranial magnetic stimulation. J Affect Disord 2004;78(3):253–7.

54. Praharaj SK, Ram D, Arora M. Efficacy of high frequency (rapid) suprathreshold repetitive transcranial magnetic stimulation of right prefrontal cortex in bipolar mania: a randomized sham controlled study. J Affect Disord 2009;117(3): 146–50.

55. Pathak V, Sinha VK, Praharaj SK. Efficacy of adjunctive high frequency repetitive transcranial magnetic stimulation of right prefrontal cortex in adolescent mania: a randomized sham-controlled study. Clin Psychopharmacol Neurosci 2015;13(3): 245–9.

56. McGirr A, Karmani S, Arsappa R, et al. Clinical efficacy and safety of repetitive transcranial magnetic stimulation in acute bipolar depression. World Psychiatry 2016;15(1):85–6.

57. Rachid F, Moeglin C, Sentissi O. Repetitive transcranial magnetic stimulation (5 and 10 Hz) with modified parameters in the treatment of resistant unipolar and bipolar depression in a private practice setting. J Psychiatr Pract 2017; 23(2):92–100.

58. Carnell BL, Clarke P, Gill S, et al. How effective is repetitive transcranial magnetic stimulation for bipolar depression? J Affect Disord 2017;209:270–2.

59. Dolberg OT, Dannon PN, Schreiber S, et al. Transcranial magnetic stimulation in patients with bipolar depression: a double blind, controlled study. Bipolar Disord 2002;4(Suppl 1):94–5.

60. Nahas Z, Kozel FA, Li X, et al. Left prefrontal transcranial magnetic stimulation (TMS) treatment of depression in bipolar affective disorder: a pilot study of acute safety and efficacy. Bipolar Disord 2003;5(1):40–7.

61. Tamas RL, Menkes D, El-Mallakh RS. Stimulating research: a prospective, randomized, double-blind, sham-controlled study of slow transcranial magnetic stimulation in depressed bipolar patients. J Neuropsychiatry Clin Neurosci 2007;19(2):198–9.

62. Fitzgerald PB, Hoy KE, Elliot D, et al. A negative double-blind controlled trial of sequential bilateral rTMS in the treatment of bipolar depression. J Affect Disord 2016;198:158–62.

63. Hu SH, Lai JB, Xu DR, et al. Efficacy of repetitive transcranial magnetic stimulation with quetiapine in treating bipolar II depression: a randomized, double-blinded, control study. Sci Rep 2016;6:30537.

64. Tavares DF, Myczkowski ML, Alberto RL, et al. Treatment of bipolar depression with deep TMS: results from a double-blind, randomized, parallel group, sham-controlled clinical trial. Neuropsychopharmacology 2017;42(13):2593–601.

65. Li X, Nahas Z, Anderson B, et al. Can left prefrontal rTMS be used as a maintenance treatment for bipolar depression? Depress Anxiety 2004;20(2):98–100.

66. Li X, Fryml L, Rodriguez JJ, et al. Safe management of a bipolar depressed patient with prefrontal repetitive transcranial magnetic stimulation (rTMS) Over 7 years and >2 million stimuli. Brain Stimul 2014;7(6):919–21.

67. Dell'osso B, D'Urso N, Castellano F, et al. Long-term efficacy after acute augmentative repetitive transcranial magnetic stimulation in bipolar depression: a 1-year follow-up study. J ECT 2011;27(2):141–4.

68. Kito S, Matsuda Y, Sewaki Y, et al. A 6-month follow-up case study of low-frequency right prefrontal repetitive transcranial magnetic stimulation in treatment-resistant bipolar depression. J ECT 2017;33(4):o43 4.

69. Rapinesi C, Bersani FS, Kotzalidis GD, et al. Maintenance deep transcranial magnetic stimulation sessions are associated with reduced depressive relapses in patients with unipolar or bipolar depression. Front Neurol 2015;6:16.

70. Xia G, Gajwani P, Muzina DJ, et al. Treatment-emergent mania in unipolar and bipolar depression: focus on repetitive transcranial magnetic stimulation. Int J Neuropsychopharmacol 2008;11(1):119–30.
71. Rachid F. Repetitive transcranial magnetic stimulation and treatment-emergent mania and hypomania: a review of the literature. J Psychiatr Pract 2017;23(2): 150–9.
72. Pallanti S, Grassi G, Antonini S, et al. rTMS in resistant mixed states: an exploratory study. J Affect Disord 2014;157:66–71.
73. Kozel FA, George MS, Simpson KN. Decision analysis of the cost-effectiveness of repetitive transcranial magnetic stimulation versus electroconvulsive therapy for treatment of nonpsychotic severe depression. CNS Spectr 2004;9(6):476–82.
74. Simpson KN, Welch MJ, Kozel FA, et al. Cost-effectiveness of transcranial magnetic stimulation in the treatment of major depression: a health economics analysis. Adv Ther 2009;26(3):346–68.

Transcranial Direct Current Stimulation in Psychiatric Disorders: A Comprehensive Review

Adriano H. Moffa, PsyD, Mphil[a],*, Andre R. Brunoni, MD, PhD[b,c],
Stevan Nikolin, BSc, MCom[a], Colleen K. Loo, MB BS, FRANZCP, MD[a]

KEYWORDS

- Transcranial direct current stimulation • tDCS • NIBS • Psychiatric disorders
- Major depression • Schizophrenia • Obsessive-compulsive disorder

KEY POINTS

- Transcranial direct current stimulation (tDCS) is a noninvasive brain stimulation modality increasingly used for psychiatric disorders treatment.
- Because of the mixed results regarding efficacy, the authors performed a review exploring the current evidence in relation to major depression, schizophrenia, and obsessive-compulsive disorder (OCD).
- Current findings indicate that tDCS is probably effective in non-treatment-resistant depressive patients.
- Regarding schizophrenia and OCD, present evidence is promising but not robust enough.

INTRODUCTION

Transcranial direct current stimulation (tDCS) is a form of noninvasive brain stimulation (NIBS), and arguably one of humanity's earliest attempts at neuromodulation, predating electroconvulsive therapy (ECT). Its use as a therapeutic intervention can be traced as far back as the first century, with the application of torpedo fish to the scalp as a cure for

A.H. Moffa is the recipient of a Scientia PhD Scholarship from the University of New South Wales, Sydney, Australia. A.R. Brunoni is the recipient of a Capes/Alexander von Humboldt fellowship award for experienced researchers and a consultant of the Neurocare group GmbH (Munich, Germany). C.K. Loo received equipment support from the Soterix Company for an investigator-initiated trial of tDCS.
[a] School of Psychiatry, University of New South Wales, Black Dog Institute, Prince of Wales Hospital, Hospital Road, Randwick, Sydney, New South Wales 2031, Australia; [b] Service of Interdisciplinary Neuromodulation, Laboratory of Neurosciences (LIM-27) and National Institute of Biomarkers in Psychiatry (INBioN), Department and Institute of Psychiatry, Hospital das Clinicas HCFMUSP, Faculdade de Medicina, Universidade de Sao Paulo, R. Dr. Ovídio Pires de Campos 785, Sao Paulo, Sao Paulo 01060-970, Brazil; [c] Department of Psychiatry and Psychotherapy, Ludwig-Maximilians-University, Leopoldstr. 13, Munich 80802, Germany
* Corresponding author.
E-mail address: adriano.moffa@student.unsw.edu.au

Psychiatr Clin N Am 41 (2018) 447–463
https://doi.org/10.1016/j.psc.2018.05.002
0193-953X/18/© 2018 Elsevier Inc. All rights reserved.

headaches,[1] as well as to manage epilepsy.[2] A more refined and contemporary form of tDCS, known as "brain polarization," was trialed in the middle of the twentieth century for the treatment of psychiatric disorders with promising results.[3,4] Unfortunately, further research into the technique languished, with greater efforts instead devoted to ECT and pharmacologic interventions. This brief period of stagnation ended in the early 2000s following a short, but influential report detailing the antidepressant effects of tDCS,[5] heralding the return of tDCS as a treatment of psychiatric illnesses.

In-depth understandings of the workings of the central nervous system, and its electrical underpinnings, in combination with advances in technology, have led to the development and growing application of tDCS, which has been steadily gaining favor as a viable tool in the psychiatric toolbox. The appeal of tDCS as a therapeutic intervention is multifactorial: it is safe and tolerable, producing only mild side effects, such as localized paresthesia and erythema at the site of stimulation.[6,7] The device itself is portable and relatively inexpensive, and application of tDCS electrodes to the scalp is a simple process that can even be done by the patients on themselves while in the comfort of their own homes.[8]

As such, the field of brain stimulation has grown exponentially, with research currently underway examining the efficacy of tDCS across a variety of conditions, including dementia, schizophrenia, sensorineural tinnitus, chronic pain, depression, and many more. The purpose of this review is to summarize the evidence for tDCS as a treatment of psychiatric disorders.

To this end, 3 separate PubMed searches were performed including the terms "transcranial direct current stimulation" or "tDCS" and the following psychiatric disorders: major depressive disorder/depression, schizophrenia, and obsessive-compulsive disorder (verbatim and in abbreviated forms). The search was conducted from the year 2000 until November 15, 2017. Also, the authors examined recent reviews and meta-analyses for potentially relevant references.

MECHANISM OF ACTION

In tDCS, a continuous electric current of low intensity (typically between 1 and 2.5 mA) is passed between 2 electrodes placed over the scalp, for 10 to 30 minutes, to stimulate the underlying brain tissue. The stimulation results in partial depolarization of neuronal cell membranes in regions near the anode, and hyperpolarization near the cathode, causing a shift in the spontaneous rate of neuronal firing,[9] thereby modulating cortical excitability.[10,11]

Anodal stimulation lowers the firing threshold for propagation of action potentials, facilitating activity,[12] whereas cathodal stimulation inhibits activity.[13] The after effects of tDCS, which can persist up to an hour beyond the cessation of stimulation, are due to changes in synaptic neuroplasticity,[14] whereby increases in postsynaptic potentials, and decreases in synaptic efficacy, result in long-term potentiation and long-term depression, respectively.[15–17]

Interestingly, the effect of tDCS is dependent on the direction of current flow (ie, parallel or perpendicular to the orientation of underlying pyramidal neurons).[17] Because of the folding of the neocortex, the dominant flow of current is perpendicular to the neuronal columns, such that the mechanism of action of tDCS is mostly driven by polarization of synaptic terminals.[18] The influence of current direction and the importance of electrode polarity with regards to facilitation or inhibition of cortical activity highlight the relevance of electrode placement ("montages") to achieve desired tDCS outcomes.

Commonly used tDCS montages produce widespread, diffuse activation of the brain.[19] As such, on the macro scale, tDCS modulates network dynamics within functionally connected areas beyond the cortical regions located beneath the electrodes.[20,21] This mechanism of action has been demonstrated to produce lasting changes in populations of neurons with ongoing brain activity.[22] As a result, tDCS is not as spatially specific and targeted as other forms of NIBS, but rather is functionally specific in that it is capable of modulating task-relevant brain networks.[23,24] The therapeutic application of tDCS relies precisely on these effects, with the potential to normalize dysfunctional activity specific to the psychiatric disorder being treated.

DEPRESSION

Depression is a common, debilitating, severe, and often recurrent psychiatric disorder, associated with significant morbidity and substantial functional impairment.[25] Depression has been associated with pathologic interhemispheric cortical asymmetry.[26,27] Neuroimaging and electroencephalography (EEG) studies suggest relative hypoactivity of the left dorsolateral prefrontal cortex (DLPFC/F3 in 10–20 EEG system) and hyperactivity of this same region on the right side when compared with healthy subjects.[28] Furthermore, neuroimaging studies suggest that the patients with depression exhibit abnormalities in the relative functioning of cortical and subcortical regions.[29] It has been proposed that the increased activity of regions, such as the amygdala, insula, and ventral striatum, and the decrease in areas such as the DLPFC and dorsomedial prefrontal cortex can result in impairment in the identification of negative emotions, among other cognitive and vegetative symptoms of the depressive disorder.[30] tDCS stimulates large areas of the brain and has been shown to alter activity in deeper limbic structures such as the anterior cingulate.[31] These aspects provide the theoretic rationale for the most common tDCS montages in depression. The anode is most commonly placed over F3, to facilitate the activity of this region, whereas the cathode can be placed on either another cephalic location like the right DLPFC/F4 (**Fig. 1**B), the right supraorbital/Fp2 (**Fig. 1**A) or frontotemporal area/F8 (**Fig. 1**C), or in an extracephalic position, usually the shoulder or upper arm (eg, deltoid muscle).[32,33]

The first randomized sham-controlled clinical trial (RCT) of the "modern era" of tDCS was published in 2006, when Fregni and colleagues[5] recruited 10 antidepressant (AD)-free participants and verified that there was a significant reduction in the Hamilton Depression Rating Scale (HDRS) and Beck Depression Inventory in the active group between posttreatment and baseline. Since then, several RCTs explored the efficacy of tDCS in depression (**Table 1**). Results were mixed, which can be partly attributed to heterogeneity of the parameters of stimulation, the clinical and demographic characteristics of the patients, and low sample size of the initial pilot studies. The largest single trial to date, the ELECT-tDCS, was designed with the primary objective of comparing the efficacy of tDCS with the maximally effective dose of a commonly used AD (escitalopram 20 mg/d).[34] It was designed as a noninferiority trial to verify if the difference in HDRS scores between the tDCS and escitalopram groups would be ≥50% of the difference between escitalopram and the placebo group. There were 245 patients divided into 3 groups: active tDCS and placebo pill; sham tDCS and escitalopram; and sham tDCS and placebo pill. Because the lower limit of the confidence interval (CI) for the difference in decrease between tDCS and escitalopram (−4.3) was lower than the noninferiority mark (−2.75), tDCS was superior to placebo but not as effective as escitalopram. Consequently, based on these results, tDCS should not be used as a first-line monotherapy in depression, although could be considered for specific populations that cannot tolerate AD drugs.

A randomized, sham-controlled, and factorial clinical trial called SELECT-tDCS[35] was performed to evaluate the combined efficacy of tDCS and sertraline compared

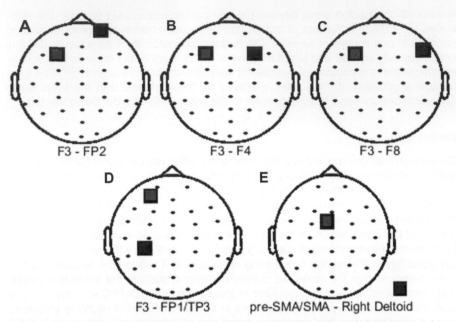

Fig. 1. tDCS montages. Montages commonly used in tDCS studies of depression, schizophrenia, and OCD (anode: *red*; cathode: *blue*) with locations specified according to the International 10-20 EEG system. (*A*) Anode: F3, Cathode: Fp2. (*B*) Anode: F3, Cathode: F4. (*C*) Anode: F3, Cathode: F8. (*D*) Anode: F3-FP1, Cathode: TP3. (*E*) Anode: pre-SMA/SMA (between presupplementary motor area and supplementary motor area), Cathode: right deltoid muscle.

with tDCS, AD, or sham alone. The results showed that tDCS accelerated and enhanced sertraline response and that the association of sertraline with active tDCS was superior for the treatment of depression over sham and sertraline or tDCS alone.

In 2016, to better clarify the efficacy of the technique and to identify predictors of response, a meta-analysis[36] was performed using individual patient data (IPD) from 289 patients from 6 RCTs[35,37–41] comparing active tDCS with sham. Active tDCS was statistically superior to sham for all outcomes: response (34% vs 19% odds ratio [OR] = 2.44, 95% CI [1.4–4.3]), remission (23% vs 13% OR = 2.38 [1.2–4.6]), and depression improvement (β = 0.347[0.12–0.57]) with all *P*s<.01. These effect sizes were small to moderate but comparable to those reported for ADs in primary care[42] and from a recent transcranial magnetic stimulation meta-analysis.[43] Regarding predictors of response, treatment-resistant patients had lower responses to tDCS, and higher "dose" of tDCS was positively associated with efficacy. Because there is no consensus on how to measure tDCS "dose," the authors used charge density, a measurement that included the variables of session duration, current intensity, electrode size, and number of sessions to run the multivariate analyses. Whereas charge density was an independent predictor for both continuous and categorical outcomes, it was not possible to identify whether current intensity or number of sessions was more important, although a longer session duration (30 vs 20 minutes) was directly associated with depression improvement.

The most recent study to examine the efficacy of tDCS in depression was an international RCT[44] with 130 unipolar and bipolar participants treated for 20 sessions over 4 weeks. This trial was the first multicenter study and assessed a longer period of tDCS treatment than prior trials. It also investigated whether the brain-derived

Table 1
Randomized controlled trials of transcranial direct current stimulation for the treatment of depression

Author, Year	Sample	Anode	Cathode	Current Intensity (mA)	Current Density (mA/cm²)	Sessions	Duration (min)	Effects
Bennabi et al,[41] 2015	24	F3	Fp2	2	0.06	10 (twice a day)	30	tDCS did not induce clinically relevant AD effect
Blumberger et al,[40] 2012	24	F3	F4	2	0.06	15 (once a day)	20	No significant difference in remission rates between active and sham
Boggio et al,[52] 2008	40	F3	F4	2	0.06	10 (once a day)	20	The DLPFC group accomplished a significantly greater improvement in HDRS (40% vs 21% occipital and 10% sham) persisting for 30 d
Brunoni et al,[35] 2013	120	F3	F4	2	0.08	12 (10 daily + 2 weekly)	30	tDCS accelerated and enhanced sertraline response; this association was superior for the treatment of depression than AD or tDCS alone
Brunoni et al,[51] 2014	37	F3	F4	2	0.08	10 (once a day)	30	CCT did not enhance the effects of tDCS
Brunoni et al,[34] 2017	245	F3	F4	2	0.08	15 daily + 7 weekly	30	tDCS was superior to placebo but not as effective as Escitalopram
Fregni et al,[5] 2006	10	F3	Fp2	1	0.03	5 (every other day)	20	Mean reduction of 60% in HDRS and BDI in the active group vs 12% in the sham group
Fregni et al,[53] 2006	18	F3	Fp2	1	0.03	5 (every other day)	20	Significant mood improvement in the active group of 58.5% vs 13.1% in sham (HDRS)
Loo et al,[38] 2010	40	F3	Fp2	1	0.03	5 (every other day)	20	No difference between active and sham tDCS

(continued on next page)

Table 1
(continued)

Author, Year	Sample	Anode	Cathode	Current Intensity (mA)	Current Density (mA/cm²)	Sessions	Duration (min)	Effects
Loo et al,[39] 2012	64	F3	F8	2	0.06	15 (once a day)	20	Active treatment improved mood compared with sham, although no difference in responder rates (13% in both groups)
Loo et al,[44] 2017	130	F3	F8	2.5	0.07	20 (once a day)	30	A significant improvement in mood was observed in the unipolar and bipolar groups; both active and sham treatments improved mood
Palm et al,[37] 2012	22	F3	Fp2	1/2	0.03/0.06	10 (once a day)	20	No difference between active and sham tDCS
Rigonatti et al,[54] 2008	42	F3	Fp2	2	—	10 (once a day)	20	The AD response of tDCS is similar to a 6-wk course of fluoxetine (20 mg/d), however, with faster time to response
Sampaio-Junior et al,[46] 2018	59[a]	F3	F4	2	0.08	12 (10 daily + 2 weekly)	30	Cumulative response rates, but not remission rates, were higher in the active group compared with sham
Salehinejad et al,[55] 2017	24	F3	F4	2	0.06	10 (once a day)	20	tDCS improves cognitive control
Segrave et al,[56] 2014	27	F3	Fp2	2	0.06	5 (once a day)	24	CCT enhanced the effects of tDCS
Valiengo et al,[57] 2017	48	F3	F4	2	0.08	12 (10 daily + 2 weekly)	30	Active tDCS was significantly superior to sham at end (response: 37.5% vs 4.1%; remission: 20.8% vs 0%, respectively).
Vanderhasselt et al,[58] 2015	33	F3	F4	2	0.08	10 (once a day)	30	tDCS did not moderate the association between changes in working memory and changes in depressive brooding

Abbreviations: BDI, Beck Depression Inventory; CCT, cognitive control therapy.
[a] RCT restricted to patients with bipolar disorder only.

neurotrophic factor (BDNF) genotype, a marker of neuroplasticity, would be associated with the AD response of these patients. At the end of the treatment, a significant improvement in mood was observed in the unipolar ($P = .001$) and bipolar groups ($P<.001$), but both active and sham treatments led to mood improvement, prompting the authors to speculate that the "sham" method, which involved a low (microampere) level of stimulation, may have had positive neuromodulatory effects. A subsequent study of the "sham" stimulation method used supported this interpretation.[45] No relation was found between BDNF genotype and the AD effect, although the study was not specifically powered for this aim.

A recent RCT investigated the efficacy of tDCS in a pure sample of 59 patients with bipolar depression that received active or sham tDCS. The main findings in the intention-to-treat analyses were that patients in the active tDCS group effected significantly superior improvement ($\beta = -1.68$; number needed to treat [NNT] = 5.8; 95% CI, 3.3–25.8; $P = .01$) and cumulative response rates (67.6% vs 30.4%; NNT = 2.69; 95% CI, 1.84–4.99; $P = 0.01$) but not remission rates ($P = .18$) compared with the ones receiving sham.[46]

Regarding the safety and acceptability of tDCS for the treatment of depression, 289 IPD from 6 RCTs were meta-analyzed and showed that there were no significant differences between active and sham groups regarding dropout ($P = .38$) and adverse event rates ($P = .23$),[47] an indication that the most commonly used tDCS parameters in depression RCTs are safe and well tolerated. The most common adverse events were equally observed in both arms and included tingling, itching, redness, headache, and discomfort.

The consensus from the European Expert Group[48] suggests that for depression, tDCS given with the anode over F3 and the cathode at Fp2 (see **Fig. 1**A) is probably effective in non-treatment-resistant patient cohorts. Guidelines from the UK National Institute of Clinical Excellence permit the use of tDCS in treating depression, given its good safety profile, although specifying that further data should be collected to assess outcomes.[49] tDCS devices are now gaining approval from governing bodies such as the Therapeutic Goods Administration (Australia), including registration of devices allowing for home-administered tDCS. The home-administered tDCS will increase treatment access, particularly in remote areas, an approach that is currently being researched for depression. Another area of interest is the combination of exogenous stimulation via tDCS with task-related endogenous activation of cognitive control regions, such as the DLPFC (for example, by using a computer task, meditation, or CBT).[50,51]

SCHIZOPHRENIA

Schizophrenia is a chronic and debilitating psychiatric disorder that affects approximately 1% of the world population.[59] Patients with schizophrenia have low functionality in daily living activities, lower quality of life, and a higher incidence of comorbidities, such as depressive symptoms, substance-related disorders, suicidal behavior, and cardiovascular risk.[60] Despite the advances in pharmacotherapy, up to 30% of patients treated with 2 or more antipsychotic drugs still present significantly disabling symptoms.[61]

The disorder is characterized by the variable presentation of "positive" and "negative" symptoms. The positive (or psychotic) symptoms like hallucinations, delusions, and disturbance of thoughts[62] affect approximately 70% of schizophrenic patients.[63] Negative symptoms comprise avolition, alogia, emotional withdrawal,[48] and anhedonia[62] and seem to be related to a decrease in DLPFC activity and disturbances in dopaminergic functioning.[64]

Considering positive symptoms, the left temporoparietal junction (TP3), an area associated with the speech perception, has been identified as an essential structural factor in the topography of auditory verbal hallucination (AVH) symptoms.[65] Neuroimaging studies in patients with schizophrenia show pathologically increased activity in TP3 in addition to frontotemporal dysconnectivity.[66]

These abnormalities observed during AVH and negative symptoms guide the most common tDCS montages, with the anode over F3 and the cathode over TP3 (**Fig. 1D**).[67] If the focus of treatment is to ease negative symptoms, the anode is placed over F3 and the cathode over Fp2, F4 (see **Fig. 1A**, B, respectively) or extracephalically.[68]

The first RCT in this field was published only 5 years ago by Brunelin and colleagues[69] in which the cathode was placed over TP3 and the anode over F3-Fp1 (see **Fig. 1D**), to relieve the severity of the AVH as well as improve negative symptoms, respectively (**Table 2**). The primary outcome was the change in AVH severity after 5 days of tDCS. Regarding the acute effects, there was a mean improvement of 31% in the active tDCS compared with 8% in sham. In respect to the follow-up, the improvements in the Auditory Hallucination Rating Scale (AHRS) scores were 36% and 38% in active and 3% and 5% in the sham groups, respectively, in first and third months. In relation to negative symptoms (evaluated with the Positive and Negative Syndrome Scale [PANSS]), there was a significant improvement with tDCS treatment in comparison to sham.

In 2014, Fitzgerald and colleagues[70] examined 2 tDCS montages for the treatment of AVH and negative symptoms. In the "unilateral" montage, the anode was placed over F3, while the cathode was on TP3. In the "bilateral" montage, the anodes were over F3 and F4 and the cathodes on TP3 and TP4. No differences in severity of AVH or negative symptoms were observed after treatment in any of the montages. The main difference relative to the Brunelin and colleagues[69] study, apart from the montage, was the number of sessions and its application scheme: 2 daily sessions for 5 days in the former while the present study stimulated once a day for 3 weeks. This result draws attention to the issue of the dose as an important factor. Indeed, a subset of participants from a previous trial[69] received twice daily tDCS instead of once daily, with all other tDCS parameters held constant.[71] The twice daily regime resulted in a significant reduction in AVH frequency. The most recent RCT from Bose and colleagues[72] replicated the Brunelin protocol, exploring the efficacy of the frontotemporal montage (see **Fig. 1D**), twice daily sessions for 5 days to improve refractory AVH symptoms. The reduction in AVH (measured by AHRS scores) was significantly higher in comparison with sham. Thus, evidence suggests improved efficacy using an increased frequency of stimulation (ie, twice daily).

Mondino and colleagues[73] evaluated the effects of tDCS on the resting-state functional connectivity (rs-FC) of TP3 in 23 subjects with AVH. After 10 sessions, there was a significant decrease in rs-FC ($P<.005$) between TP3 and the inferior frontal areas (left anterior insula and right inferior frontal gyrus) in the active tDCS group compared with sham; the AHRS scores of the active group also significantly decreased from 27.2 (SD = ±4.1) to 19.1 (±7.1), corresponding to a 28% (±26) reduction ($P<.01$), whereas the decline in scores for sham participants between baseline and endpoint was nonsignificant ($P = .09$).

Contrary to the previous findings, Smith and colleagues[74] showed no differences in PANSS or AVH scores between active and sham stimulation (anode over F3 and cathode on Fp2; see **Fig. 1A**).

Fröhlich and colleagues[75] assessed the effects of tDCS on AVH severity in 26 schizophrenic/schizoaffective subjects. No difference was observed in AVH reduction between the active and sham.

Table 2
Randomized controlled trials of transcranial direct current stimulation for the treatment of schizophrenia

Author, Year	Sample	Anode	Cathode	Current Intensity (mA)	Current Density (mA/cm²)	Sessions	Duration (min)	Effects
Bose et al,[72] 2018	25	F3-Fp1	TP3	2	0.06	10 (twice a day)	20	Reduction in AVH (AHRS) was significantly greater in tDCS compared with the sham (t = 5.01; P<.001; effect size Cohen's d = 1.98)
Brunelin et al,[69] 2012	30	F3-Fp1	TP3 (T3-P3)	2	0.06	10 (twice a day)	20	Mean improvement of 31%/36% (acute/follow-up) in AHRS in active tDCS. Significant improvement in negative symptoms
Fitzgerald et al,[70] 2014	11	F3	TP3	2	0.06	15 (once a day)	20	No differences in severity of auditory hallucinations or negative symptoms were observed in any of the montages
Fröhlich et al,[75] 2016	26	F3-Fp1	TP3	2	0.06	5 (once a day)	20	No differences in AVH reduction between active and sham
Gomes et al,[78] 2015	15	F3	F4	2	N/A	10 (once a day)	20	Active stimulation showed reduced PANSS negative, general, and total scores. No effects were observed for depression scores, functional outcomes, or for positive symptoms
Mondino et al,[71] 2015	28	F3-Fp1	TP3	2	0.06	10 (twice a day)	20	Reduction in AVH frequency (46% AHRS)
Mondino et al,[73] 2015	23	F3-Fp1	TP3	2	0.06	10 (twice a day)	20	AHRS scores decreased significantly by 28% (P<.01) in active group
Palm et al,[76] 2016	20	F3	Fp2	2	0.06	10 (once a day)	20	Significant results were found at SANS and PANSS (P<.01) at weeks 2 (endpoint) and 4 (follow-up)
Shiozawa et al,[79] 2016	9	F3	F4	2	0.06	5 (twice a day)	20	tDCS and cognitive training was not effective to improve clinical outcomes
Smith et al,[74] 2015	33	F3	Fp2	2	0.39	10 (twice a day)	20	No differences in PANSS or AVH scores between active and sham

In 2016 Palm and colleagues[76] conducted a study with 20 schizophrenic patients with predominately negative symptoms that were randomized to 10 sessions of active or sham tDCS with the anode at F3 and cathode at Fp2 (see **Fig. 1**A). Significant results were found at both primary and secondary outcomes: Scale for the Assessment of Negative Symptoms (SANS) and PANSS at weeks 2 (endpoint) and 4 (follow-up).

Regarding efficacy, present evidence is not robust enough, although preliminary results[77] indicate that tDCS is a promising technique as an add-on treatment of persistent symptoms of schizophrenia. There is a need for further RCTs with larger and more homogeneous sampling before using it in a clinical setting.

OBSESSIVE COMPULSIVE DISORDER

OCD is a common and debilitating disease with a transcultural lifetime prevalence of about 2.5%.[80,81] It is characterized by the presence of obsessions and compulsions. Obsessions are recurring, intrusive, and unwanted thoughts or needs. Compulsions are repetitive behaviors or mental acts that the individual feels compelled to perform according to specific rules to alleviate the stress and anxiety caused by the obsessions.[82]

Treatment options include pharmacologic interventions, such as selective serotonin reuptake inhibitors, clomipramine, and antipsychotics. This approach presents limited efficacy with up to 40% to 60% of patients showing no satisfactory response.[83]

Based on neuroimaging findings, it has been proposed that OCD results from dysfunctions in the cortico-striatal-thalamic-cortical circuit, including the prefrontal cortex (orbitofrontal cortex [OFC]), dorsal anterior cingulate cortex, the basal ganglia, and the thalamus.[84] It has additionally been suggested that there is increased recruitment of pre–supplementary motor area (pre-SMA) during response inhibition and action control.[85] The increased activity of the OFC is also associated with the severity of OCD symptoms.[86] Three areas have been mostly used as a target for tDCS: F3, OFC, and the pre-SMA/SMA.

A common montage is an active electrode (anode or cathode) placed over the pre-SMA and the reference electrode placed in an extracephalic position (eg, the arm)[87] (**Fig. 1**E). The SMA has usually been chosen because of its superficial location and extensive connections with the thalamus, which is much involved in cognitive processes and motor control.

The first clinical use of tDCS in OCD was a case report[88] in which the cathode was placed over F3 and the anode on the posterior neck base (**Table 3**). After the course of treatment, a beneficial effect was observed in symptoms of anxiety and depression, but not in obsessive-compulsive symptoms. In 2 case reports,[89] the anode was placed over the left pre-SMA/SMA and the cathode over Fp2. Both patients had a significant improvement with 40% to 46% Yale-Brown Obsessive-Compulsive Scale (Y-BOCS) reduction. Using the same montage, Hazari and colleagues[90] also reported positive results with remission of obsessive-compulsive symptoms. D'Urso and colleagues[87] initially treated a resistant OCD patient with 10 sessions of anodal tDCS placed on the pre-SMA and the cathode on the right deltoid (see **Fig. 1**E). In the last 10 sessions, the montage was inverted. After the initial 10 sessions, there was a worsening of OCD symptoms. With the inverted montage, there was a significant clinical improvement (Y-BOCS decrease of 30%).

Using the previous montages, D'Urso and colleagues[91] conducted the first randomized controlled, partial crossover trial with 12 patients and confirmed that cathodal but not anodal tDCS over pre-SMA significantly improved OCD symptoms.

Exploring another promising target area in OCD (OFC), Mondino and colleagues[92] stimulated a patient with the cathode on the left OFC and the anode on right occipital

Table 3
Studies of transcranial direct current stimulation for the treatment of obsessive compulsive disorder

Author, Year	Sample	Anode	Cathode	Current Intensity (mA)	Current Density (mA/cm²)	Sessions	Duration (min)	Effects
Bation et al,[93] 2016	8[a,b]	Right cerebellum	Left OFC	2	0.06	5 (once a day)	20	Significant beneficial effect on obsessive and compulsive symptoms (25.4% decrease in Y-BOCS, SD = 15.8; $P = .002$)
Dinn et al,[94] 2016	5[a,b]	F3	Fp2	2	0.06	15 (once a day)	20	Significant OCD symptom reduction; however, gains were not maintained at 1-mo follow-up
D'Urso et al,[87] 2016	1[b,c]	Pre-SMA	Right deltoid	2	0.08	10 (once a day)	20	Significant clinical improvement with cathode in SMA (30% decrease in Y-BOCS)
D'Urso et al,[91] 2016	12[a,c]	Active pre-SMA[d]	Right deltoid[d]	2	0.08	10 (once a day)	20	Cathodal but not anodal tDCS over pre-SMA significantly improved OCD symptoms
Hazari et al,[90] 2016	1[b,c]	Pre-SMA/SMA	Fp2	2	N/A write author	20 (twice a day)	20	Remission of obsessive-compulsive symptoms
Mondino et al,[92] 2015	1[b,c]	Right occipital area	OFC	2	0.02	10 (twice a day)	20	26% decrease in Y-BOCS
Narayanaswamy et al,[89] 2015	2[b,c]	Pre-SMA/SMA	Fp2	2	0.06	20 (twice a day)	20	Both patients with significant improvement with 40%–46% decrease in Y-BOCS
Volpato et al,[88] 2013	1[b,c]	Posterior neck base	F3	2	0.06	10 (once a day)	20	Beneficial effect in relation to symptoms of anxiety and depression, but not on obsessive-compulsive symptoms

[a] Open label.
[b] Case report.
[c] RCT; Randomized Clinical Trial.
[d] Switched polarity in case of symptom worsening following 10 sessions of tDCS.

region. One month after the end of the tDCS sessions, there was a 26% reduction in the severity of obsessive and compulsive symptoms. Bation and colleagues[93] also placed the cathode over the left OFC (anode over the right cerebellum) in an open-label pilot study with 8 treatment-resistant patients. A significant beneficial effect on obsessive and compulsive symptoms was observed immediately after 10 sessions.

The case reports and RCT presented so far suggest that tDCS is a safe intervention and has possible efficacy in OCD that must be confirmed by RCTs. The most promising montages appear to involve a cathode over the left OFC or pre-SMA. On the other hand, anodal DLPFC stimulation seems to have effects mainly on depression,[88] and less on obsessive-compulsive symptoms.

SUMMARY

The goal of this review was to highlight the main evidence base on the efficacy of tDCS in major psychiatric disorders and to clarify important questions regarding the most commonly used stimulation parameters and montages.

The main advantages of tDCS among all forms of NIBS are its low cost, portability, and potential for home-administered use, ease of use, and absence of severe adverse effects, which may increase the adherence of psychiatric patients to the treatment. Nonetheless, the evidence base is preliminary with some promising results in depression, and mixed results in other disorders. Heterogeneity in efficacy outcomes may mainly relate to small study sample sizes, variability between individuals and clinical conditions, and the use of different devices and stimulus parameters.

In the face of the current findings, a level A (definite efficacy) recommendation has not been achieved for any clinical indication according to a guideline published by a group of European experts.[48] The most promising clinical results were obtained when treating depression, with a level B of evidence (probable efficacy).

Therefore, future larger controlled tDCS studies should aim to better understand tDCS mechanisms of action and the neurobiological effects of tDCS. In addition, identification of biomarkers and clinical predictors of response, and ideally, individualization of the treatment parameters (current, montage, density, duration, number of sessions), are fundamental to improving tDCS delivery. Finally, if the efficacy of tDCS is proven, further studies should explore long-term effects of tDCS treatment and its role as monotherapy or add-on with medications and/or other therapies.

REFERENCES

1. Largus S. De compositionibus medicamentorum. Paris: liber unus; 1529.
2. Kellayway P. The part played by the electric fish in the early history of bioelectricity and electrotherapy. Bull Hist Med 1946;20:112–37.
3. Redfearn J, Lippold O, Costain R. Preliminary account of the clinical effects of polarizing the brain in certain psychiatric disorders. Br J Psychiatry 1964; 110(469):773–85.
4. Costain R, Redfearn J, Lippold O. A controlled trial of the therapeutic effect of polarization of the brain in depressive illness. Br J Psychiatry 1964;110:786–99.
5. Fregni F, Boggio PS, Nitsche MA, et al. Treatment of major depression with transcranial direct current stimulation. Bipolar Disord 2006;8(2):203–4.
6. Nikolin S, Huggins C, Martin D, et al. Safety of repeated sessions of transcranial direct current stimulation: a systematic review. Brain Stimul 2018;11(2): 278–88.
7. Bikson M, Grossman P, Thomas C, et al. Safety of transcranial direct current stimulation: evidence based update 2016. Brain Stimul 2016;9(5):641–61.

8. Charvet LE, Kasschau M, Datta A, et al. Remotely-supervised transcranial direct current stimulation (tDCS) for clinical trials: guidelines for technology and protocols. Front Syst Neurosci 2015;9:26.

9. Nitsche MA, Cohen LG, Wassermann EM, et al. Transcranial direct current stimulation: state of the art 2008. Brain Stimul 2008;1(3):206–23.

10. Bindman LJ, Lippold O, Redfearn J. Long-lasting changes in the level of the electrical activity of the cerebral cortex produced by polarizing currents. Nature 1962; 196(4854):584–5.

11. Purpura DP, McMurtry JG. Intracellular activities and evoked potential changes during polarization of motor cortex. J Neurophysiol Jan 1965;28:166–85.

12. Nitsche MA, Paulus W. Sustained excitability elevations induced by transcranial DC motor cortex stimulation in humans. Neurology 2001;57(10):1899–901.

13. Nitsche MA, Nitsche MS, Klein CC, et al. Level of action of cathodal DC polarisation induced inhibition of the human motor cortex. Clin Neurophysiol 2003;114(4): 600–4.

14. Nitsche MA, Liebetanz D, Antal A, et al. Modulation of cortical excitability by weak direct current stimulation–technical, safety and functional aspects. Suppl Clin Neurophysiol 2003;56:255–76.

15. George MS, Aston-Jones G. Noninvasive techniques for probing neurocircuitry and treating illness: vagus nerve stimulation (VNS), transcranial magnetic stimulation (TMS) and transcranial direct current stimulation (tDCS). Neuropsychopharmacology 2010;35(1):301–16.

16. Pascual-Leone A, Tormos JM, Keenan J, et al. Study and modulation of human cortical excitability with transcranial magnetic stimulation. J Clin Neurophysiol 1998;15(4):333–43.

17. Bikson M, Inoue M, Akiyama H, et al. Effects of uniform extracellular DC electric fields on excitability in rat hippocampal slices in vitro. J Physiol 2004;557(1): 175–90.

18. Rahman A, Reato D, Arlotti M, et al. Cellular effects of acute direct current stimulation: somatic and synaptic terminal effects. J Physiol 2013;591(10):2563–78.

19. Bai S, Dokos S, Ho K-A, et al. A computational modelling study of transcranial direct current stimulation montages used in depression. Neuroimage 2014;87:332–44.

20. Hunter MA, Coffman BA, Gasparovic C, et al. Baseline effects of transcranial direct current stimulation on glutamatergic neurotransmission and large-scale network connectivity. Brain Res 2015;1594:92–107.

21. Peña-Gómez C, Sala-Lonch R, Junqué C, et al. Modulation of large-scale brain networks by transcranial direct current stimulation evidenced by resting-state functional MRI. Brain Stimul 2012;5(3):252–63.

22. Reato D, Bikson M, Parra LC. Lasting modulation of in vitro oscillatory activity with weak direct current stimulation. J Neurophysiol 2015;113(5):1334–41.

23. Pereira JB, Junqué C, Bartrés-Faz D, et al. Modulation of verbal fluency networks by transcranial direct current stimulation (tDCS) in Parkinson's disease. Brain Stimul 2013;6(1):16–24.

24. Bikson M. Origins of specificity during tDCS: anatomical, activity-selective, and input-bias mechanisms. Front Hum Neurosci 2013;7:668.

25. McKenna SP, Doward LC. The translation and cultural adaptation of patient-reported outcome measures. Value Health 2005;8(2):89–91.

26. Bench C, Frackowiak R, Dolan R. Changes in regional cerebral blood flow on recovery from depression. Psychol Med 1995;25(2):247–61.

27. Grimm S, Beck J, Schuepbach D, et al. Imbalance between left and right dorsolateral prefrontal cortex in major depression is linked to negative emotional

judgment: an fMRI study in severe major depressive disorder. Biol Psychiatry 2008;63(4):369–76.

28. Vanderhasselt M-A, De Raedt R, Baeken C. Dorsolateral prefrontal cortex and Stroop performance: tackling the lateralization. Psychon Bull Rev 2009;16(3):609–12.

29. Koenigs M, Grafman J. The functional neuroanatomy of depression: distinct roles for ventromedial and dorsolateral prefrontal cortex. Behav Brain Res 2009;201(2): 239–43.

30. Grimm S, Ernst J, Boesiger P, et al. Increased self-focus in major depressive disorder is related to neural abnormalities in subcortical-cortical midline structures. Hum Brain Mapp 2009;30(8):2617–27.

31. Keeser D, Meindl T, Bor J, et al. Prefrontal transcranial direct current stimulation changes connectivity of resting-state networks during fMRI. J Neurosci 2011; 31(43):15284–93.

32. Arul-Anandam AP, Loo C. Transcranial direct current stimulation: a new tool for the treatment of depression? J Affect Disord 2009;117(3):137–45.

33. Martin DM, Alonzo A, Mitchell PB, et al. Fronto-extracephalic transcranial direct current stimulation as a treatment for major depression: an open-label pilot study. J Affect Disord 2011;134(1):459–63.

34. Brunoni AR, Moffa AH, Sampaio-Junior B, et al. Trial of electrical direct-current therapy versus escitalopram for depression. N Engl J Med 2017;376(26):2523–33.

35. Brunoni AR, Valiengo L, Baccaro A, et al. The sertraline vs electrical current therapy for treating depression clinical study: results from a factorial, randomized, controlled trial. JAMA Psychiatry 2013;70(4):383–91.

36. Brunoni AR, Moffa AH, Fregni F, et al. Transcranial direct current stimulation for acute major depressive episodes: meta-analysis of individual patient data. Br J Psychiatry 2016;208(6):522–31.

37. Palm U, Schiller C, Fintescu Z, et al. Transcranial direct current stimulation in treatment resistant depression: a randomized double-blind, placebo-controlled study. Brain Stimul 2012;5(3):242–51.

38. Loo CK, Sachdev P, Martin D, et al. A double-blind, sham-controlled trial of transcranial direct current stimulation for the treatment of depression. Int J Neuropsychopharmacol 2010;13(1):61–9.

39. Loo CK, Alonzo A, Martin D, et al. Transcranial direct current stimulation for depression: 3-week, randomised, sham-controlled trial. Br J Psychiatry 2012; 200(1):52–9.

40. Blumberger DM, Tran LC, Fitzgerald PB, et al. A randomized double-blind shamcontrolled study of transcranial direct current stimulation for treatment-resistant major depression. Front Psychiatry 2012;3:74.

41. Bennabi D, Nicolier M, Monnin J, et al. Pilot study of feasibility of the effect of treatment with tDCS in patients suffering from treatment-resistant depression treated with escitalopram. Clin Neurophysiol 2015;126(6):1185–9.

42. Arroll B, Elley CR, Fishman T, et al. Antidepressants versus placebo for depression in primary care. Cochrane Database Syst Rev 2009;(3):CD007954.

43. Berlim M, Van den Eynde F, Tovar-Perdomo S, et al. Response, remission and drop-out rates following high-frequency repetitive transcranial magnetic stimulation (rTMS) for treating major depression: a systematic review and meta-analysis of randomized, double-blind and sham-controlled trials. Psychol Med 2014;44(2): 225–39.

44. Loo CK, Husain MM, McDonald WM, et al. International randomized-controlled trial of transcranial direct current stimulation in depression. Brain Stimul 2018; 11(1):125–33.

45. Nikolin S, Martin D, Loo CK, et al. Effects of TDCS dosage on working memory in healthy participants. Brain Stimul 2018;11(3):518–27.
46. Sampaio-Junior B, Tortella G, Borrione L, et al. Efficacy and safety of transcranial direct current stimulation as an add-on treatment for bipolar depression: a randomized clinical trial. JAMA Psychiatry 2018;75(2):158–66.
47. Moffa AH, Brunoni AR, Fregni F, et al. Safety and acceptability of transcranial direct current stimulation for the acute treatment of major depressive episodes: analysis of individual patient data. J Affect Disord 2017;221:1–5.
48. Lefaucheur J-P, Antal A, Ayache SS, et al. Evidence-based guidelines on the therapeutic use of transcranial direct current stimulation (tDCS). Clin Neurophysiol 2017;128(1):56–92.
49. National Institute for Health and Care Excellence. Transcranial direct current stimulation (tDCS) for depression. Interventional procedures guidance [IPG530]. 2015. Available at: https://www.nice.org.uk/guidance/ipg530. Accessed March 9, 2018.
50. D'Urso G, Mantovani A, Micillo M, et al. Transcranial direct current stimulation and cognitive-behavioral therapy: evidence of a synergistic effect in treatment-resistant depression. Brain Stimul 2013;6(3):465–7.
51. Brunoni A, Boggio P, De Raedt R, et al. Cognitive control therapy and transcranial direct current stimulation for depression: a randomized, double-blinded, controlled trial. J Affect Disord 2014;162:43–9.
52. Boggio PS, Rigonatti SP, Ribeiro RB, et al. A randomized, double-blind clinical trial on the efficacy of cortical direct current stimulation for the treatment of major depression. Int J Neuropsychopharmacol 2008;11(2):249–54.
53. Fregni F, Boggio PS, Nitsche MA, et al. Cognitive effects of repeated sessions of transcranial direct current stimulation in patients with depression. Depress Anxiety 2006;23(8):482–4.
54. Rigonatti SP, Boggio PS, Myczkowski ML, et al. Transcranial direct stimulation and fluoxetine for the treatment of depression. Eur Psychiatry 2008;23(1):74–6.
55. Salehinejad MA, Ghanavai E, Rostami R, et al. Cognitive control dysfunction in emotion dysregulation and psychopathology of major depression (MD): evidence from transcranial brain stimulation of the dorsolateral prefrontal cortex (DLPFC). J Affect Disord 2017;210:241–8.
56. Segrave R, Arnold S, Hoy K, et al. Concurrent cognitive control training augments the antidepressant efficacy of tDCS: a pilot study. Brain Stimul 2014;7(2):325–31.
57. Valiengo LC, Goulart AC, de Oliveira JF, et al. Transcranial direct current stimulation for the treatment of post-stroke depression: results from a randomised, sham-controlled, double-blinded trial. J Neurol Neurosurg Psychiatry 2017;88(2):170–5.
58. Vanderhasselt MA, De Raedt R, Namur V, et al. Transcranial electric stimulation and neurocognitive training in clinically depressed patients: a pilot study of the effects on rumination. Prog Neuropsychopharmacol Biol Psychiatry 2015;57:93–9.
59. Owen MJ, Sawa A, Mortensen PB. Schizophrenia. Lancet 2016;388(10039):86–97.
60. Conley RR. The burden of depressive symptoms in people with schizophrenia. Psychiatr Clin North Am 2009;32(4):853–61.
61. Shergill SS, Murray RM, McGuire PK. Auditory hallucinations: a review of psychological treatments. Schizophr Res 1998;32(3):137–50.
62. Kuo M-F, Paulus W, Nitsche MA. Therapeutic effects of non-invasive brain stimulation with direct currents (tDCS) in neuropsychiatric diseases. Neuroimage 2014;85:948–60.

63. Kubera KM, Barth A, Hirjak D, et al. Noninvasive brain stimulation for the treatment of auditory verbal hallucinations in schizophrenia: methods, effects and challenges. Front Syst Neurosci 2015;9:131.

64. Kapur S, Mamo D. Half a century of antipsychotics and still a central role for dopamine D 2 receptors. Prog Neuropsychopharmacol Biol Psychiatry 2003; 27(7):1081–90.

65. Silbersweig DA, Stern E, Frith C, et al. A functional neuroanatomy of hallucinations in schizophrenia. Nature 1995;378(6553):176.

66. Meyer-Lindenberg A. From maps to mechanisms through neuroimaging of schizophrenia. Nature 2010;468(7321):194–202.

67. Homan P, Kindler J, Hauf M, et al. Repeated measurements of cerebral blood flow in the left superior temporal gyrus reveal tonic hyperactivity in patients with auditory verbal hallucinations: a possible trait marker. Front Hum Neurosci 2013;7:304.

68. Brunelin J, Mondino M, Haesebaert F, et al. Efficacy and safety of bifocal tDCS as an interventional treatment for refractory schizophrenia. Brain Stimul 2012;5(3): 431–2.

69. Brunelin J, Mondino M, Gassab L, et al. Examining transcranial direct-current stimulation (tDCS) as a treatment for hallucinations in schizophrenia. Am J Psychiatry 2012;169(7):719–24.

70. Fitzgerald PB, McQueen S, Daskalakis ZJ, et al. A negative pilot study of daily bimodal transcranial direct current stimulation in schizophrenia. Brain Stimul 2014;7(6):813–6.

71. Mondino M, Haesebaert F, Poulet E, et al. Fronto-temporal transcranial direct current stimulation (tDCS) reduces source-monitoring deficits and auditory hallucinations in patients with schizophrenia. Schizophr Res 2015;161(2):515–6.

72. Bose A, Shivakumar V, Agarwal SM, et al. Efficacy of fronto-temporal transcranial direct current stimulation for refractory auditory verbal hallucinations in schizophrenia: a randomized, double-blind, sham-controlled study. Schizophr Res 2018;195:475–80.

73. Mondino M, Jardri R, Suaud-Chagny M-F, et al. Effects of fronto-temporal transcranial direct current stimulation on auditory verbal hallucinations and resting-state functional connectivity of the left temporo-parietal junction in patients with schizophrenia. Schizophr Bull 2015;42(2):318–26.

74. Smith RC, Boules S, Mattiuz S, et al. Effects of transcranial direct current stimulation (tDCS) on cognition, symptoms, and smoking in schizophrenia: a randomized controlled study. Schizophr Res 2015;168(1):260–6.

75. Fröhlich F, Burrello T, Mellin J, et al. Exploratory study of once-daily transcranial direct current stimulation (tDCS) as a treatment for auditory hallucinations in schizophrenia. Eur Psychiatry 2016;33:54–60.

76. Palm U, Keeser D, Hasan A, et al. Prefrontal transcranial direct current stimulation for treatment of schizophrenia with predominant negative symptoms: a double-blind, sham-controlled proof-of-concept study. Schizophr Bull 2016;42(5):1253–61.

77. Pondé PH, De Sena EP, Camprodon JA, et al. Use of transcranial direct current stimulation for the treatment of auditory hallucinations of schizophrenia–a systematic review. Neuropsychiatr Dis Treat 2017;13:347.

78. Gomes JS, Shiozawa P, Dias ÁM, et al. Left dorsolateral prefrontal cortex anodal tDCS effects on negative symptoms in schizophrenia. Brain Stimul 2015;8(5): 989–91.

79. Shiozawa P, Gomes JS, Ducos DV, et al. Effect of transcranial direct current stimulation (tDCS) over the prefrontal cortex combined with cognitive training for

treating schizophrenia: a sham-controlled randomized clinical trial. Trends Psychiatry Psychother 2016;38(3):175–7.

80. Weisman M, Bland R, Canino G, et al. The cross national epidemiology of obsessive-compulsive disorder. J Clin Psychiatry 1994;55(3 Suppl):5–10.

81. Stein DJ. Obsessive-compulsive disorder. Lancet 2002;360(9330):397–405.

82. Association AP. Diagnostic and statistical manual of mental disorders (DSM-5®). Arlington (VA): American Psychiatric Association; 2013.

83. Pallanti S, Hollander E, Bienstock C, et al. Treatment non-response in OCD: methodological issues and operational definitions. Int J Neuropsychopharmacol 2002; 5(2):181–91.

84. Milad MR, Rauch SL. Obsessive-compulsive disorder: beyond segregated cortico-striatal pathways. Trends Cogn Sci 2012;16(1):43–51.

85. de Wit S, Watson P, Harsay HA, et al. Corticostriatal connectivity underlies individual differences in the balance between habitual and goal-directed action control. J Neurosci 2012;32(35):12066–75.

86. Nauczyciel C, Le Jeune F, Naudet F, et al. Repetitive transcranial magnetic stimulation over the orbitofrontal cortex for obsessive-compulsive disorder: a double-blind, crossover study. Transl Psychiatry 2014;4(9):e436.

87. D'Urso G, Brunoni AR, Anastasia A, et al. Polarity-dependent effects of transcranial direct current stimulation in obsessive-compulsive disorder. Neurocase 2016; 22(1):60–4.

88. Volpato C, Piccione F, Cavinato M, et al. Modulation of affective symptoms and resting state activity by brain stimulation in a treatment-resistant case of obsessive–compulsive disorder. Neurocase 2013;19(4):360–70.

89. Narayanaswamy JC, Jose D, Chhabra H, et al. Successful application of add-on transcranial Direct Current Stimulation (tDCS) for treatment of SSRI resistant OCD. Brain Stimul 2015;8(3):655–7.

90. Hazari N, Narayanaswamy JC, Chhabra H, et al. Response to transcranial direct current stimulation in a case of episodic obsessive compulsive disorder. J ECT 2016;32(2):144–6.

91. D'Urso G, Brunoni AR, Mazzaferro MP, et al. Transcranial direct current stimulation for obsessive–compulsive disorder: a randomized, controlled, partial crossover trial. Depress Anxiety 2016;33(12):1132–40.

92. Mondino M, Haesebaert F, Poulet E, et al. Efficacy of cathodal transcranial direct current stimulation over the left orbitofrontal cortex in a patient with treatment-resistant obsessive-compulsive disorder. J ECT 2015;31(4):271–2.

93. Bation R, Poulet E, Haesebaert F, et al. Transcranial direct current stimulation in treatment-resistant obsessive–compulsive disorder: an open-label pilot study. Prog Neuropsychopharmacol Biol Psychiatry 2016;65:153–7.

94. Dinn WM, Aycicegi-Dinn A, Göral F, et al. Treatment-resistant obsessive-compulsive disorder: insights from an open trial of transcranial direct current stimulation (tDCS) to design a RCT. Neurol Psychiatry Brain Res 2016;22(3): 146–54.

Therapeutic Applications of Noninvasive Neuromodulation in Children and Adolescents

Deniz Doruk Camsari, MD[a], Melissa Kirkovski, PhD[b], Paul E. Croarkin, DO, MS[a],*

KEYWORDS

- Neuromodulation • Noninvasive brain stimulation
- Transcranial magnetic stimulation • TMS • Transcranial direct current stimulation
- tDCS • Adolescent depression • Autism spectrum disorder

KEY POINTS

- Neuromodulation is a rapidly developing field that will provide opportunities to develop new therapeutic modalities in child and adolescent psychiatry.
- Recent research has examined the feasibility and safety of transcranial direct current stimulation and transcranial magnetic stimulation in child and adolescent neuropsychiatric disorders.
- Enthusiasm for applying neuromodulatory tools in childhood and adolescent neuropsychiatric disorders must be moderated with systematic study, neurodevelopmental considerations, and rigorous ethical analyses.

INTRODUCTION

Noninvasive brain stimulation (NIBS) techniques have emerged as alternatives to invasive modalities given the ease of application, safety, tolerability, and reversibility. The

Financial Disclosures: Dr P.E. Croarkin has received research grant support from Pfizer (WS1926243), National Institute of Mental Health (K23MH10026 and R01MH113700), the Brain and Behavior Research Foundation (20883), and the Mayo Clinic Foundation. He has received equipment support from Neuronetics, Inc and receives supplies and genotyping services from Assurex Health, Inc for investigator-initiated studies. He is the primary investigator for a multicenter study of adolescent TMS funded by Neuronetics, Inc. Drs D.D. Camsari and M. Kirkovski have no financial disclosures.
^a Department of Psychiatry and Psychology, Mayo Clinic, 200 First Street Southwest, Rochester, MN 55905, USA; ^b Deakin Child Study Centre, School of Psychology, Deakin University, Geelong, VIC 3220, Australia
* Corresponding author.
E-mail address: croarkin.paul@mayo.edu

2 most well-studied forms of NIBS are transcranial magnetic stimulation (TMS) and transcranial electrical stimulation. Research protocols began applying brain stimulation techniques to children and adolescents in the early 1990s. Progress has been slow due to practical limitations and safety concerns.[1] As of 2017, there is no Food and Drug Administration–approved therapeutic use of NIBS techniques in children. Current evidence suggests potential use of NIBS techniques in children with depression, attention-deficit hyperactivity disorder (ADHD), epilepsy, autism, schizophrenia, dystonia, dyslexia, cerebral palsy, and Tourette syndrome (**Table 1**).[2–4]

TRANSCRANIAL MAGNETIC STIMULATION

The applications of TMS in children first started in the early 2000s and included both diagnostic and therapeutic approaches. Potential therapeutic applications of TMS in children include epilepsy, ADHD, autism spectrum disorder (ASD), depression, schizophrenia, and Tourette syndrome.[2] Single-pulse TMS is also used for presurgical mapping of the motor cortex and language areas.[5]

Safety and application guidelines for TMS were published in 2009 but focused on adults.[1]

In children and adolescents, recent systematic reviews suggest that both single-pulse and repetitive TMS have similar adverse effect profiles to adult populations.[3,6,7] The most commonly reported side effects are headache (11.5%), scalp discomfort (2.5%), twitching (1.2%), mood changes (1.2%), fatigue (0.9%), and tinnitus (0.6%).[3] The most serious side effect is seizure and to date there are 3 reported seizures in adolescents receiving TMS. These events occurred in the context of epileptogenic medication use,[8,9] alcohol consumption before the TMS session,[9] and application of deep TMS.[10] There are 2 reported instances of TMS-induced hypomania[8,11] and 2 reported cases of neurocardiogenic syncope, which were associated with preexisting circumstances.[12] No changes in cognitive functioning have been reported (**Fig. 1**).[13]

Major Depressive Disorder

Major depressive disorder is one of the most common psychiatric illnesses in children and adolescents. Suboptimal outcomes in the treatment of depression in children and adolescents have sparked interest focused on the study of novel, brain-based approaches such as TMS. Prior therapeutic TMS studies included 73 participants between the ages of 7 to 21 years in open trials, case studies, case series, and small sham-controlled trials. In a systematic review, Donaldson and colleagues[14] suggested that TMS may be an effective and well-tolerated treatment for treatment-resistant depression in adolescents. The most common TMS application was high-frequency TMS (10 Hz) over the left dorsolateral prefrontal cortex (L-DLPFC). TMS parameters varied in terms of number of sessions (10–30), session duration (10–37.5 min), and intensity (80%–120% of motor threshold [MT]). Among these studies, 2 open trials by Bloch and colleagues[11] (2008) and Wall and colleagues[15] (2011) showed statistically significant improvement in depressive symptoms measured by CDRS-R as well as the significant improvement in the Clinical Global Impression Severity of Illness Scales (CGI-S) with high-frequency TMS applied over the DLPFC. The study by Wall and colleagues differed from the study by Bloch and colleagues based on MT intensity (120% vs 80%), total number of pulses per session (3000 vs 400) and number of total TMS sessions (30 vs 14). A follow-up study by Bloch and colleagues[11] showed sustained improvement after 3 years.[13] Another open-label study by Wall and colleagues[16] in 2016 (n = 10) showed significant improvement (60% of participants) in depressive symptoms measured by CDRS-R, the Quick Inventory for Depressive

Table 1
Neuropsychiatric diseases included in neuromodulation trials in children and adolescents

	Depression	OCD	ADHD	Autism	Tourette Syndrome	Schizophrenia	Addiction	Dyslexia	Migraine	Cerebral Palsy	Dystonia	Epilepsy	Stroke	Headache
rTMS	X	—	X	X	X	X	—	—	—	X	—	X	X	—
TBS	—	—	—	X	X	—	—	—	—	—	—	—	—	—
tDCS	—	—	X	X	—	X	—	X	—	X	X	X	—	X
ECT	X	X	—	X	—	X	—	—	—	—	—	—	—	—
MST	X	—	—	—	—	—	—	—	—	—	—	—	—	—
eTNS	—	—	X	—	—	—	—	—	—	—	—	—	—	—

Abbreviations: ECT, electroconvulsive therapy; eTNS, external trigeminal nerve stimulation; MST, magnetic seizure therapy; OCD, obsessive-compulsive disorder; rTMS, repetitive transcranial magnetic stimulation; TBS, theta burst stimulation; tDCS, transcranial direct current stimulation.

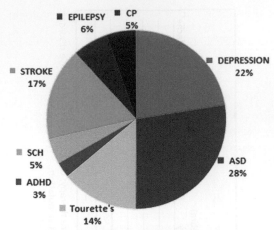

Fig. 1. Distribution of subjects in therapeutic TMS studies. SCH, schizophrenia; ASD, autism spectrum disorder; ADHD, attention-deficit hyperactivity disorder; CP, cerebral palsy.

Symptomatology Adolescent Seventeen-Item Self-Report (QIDS-A17-SR) and CGI-S after treatment and at 6-month follow-up. Initial studies suggest that high-frequency TMS treatments may modulate glutamatergic neurotransmission, and this presents an opportunity for precision medicine approaches to TMS.[17,18]

Autism Spectrum Disorder

ASD is diagnosed behaviorally by social impairments and the presence of restricted and repetitive patterns of behavior and interests. Early studies focused on ASD used conventional low-frequency (1 Hz) repetitive TMS applied to the prefrontal cortex daily over a period of time and demonstrated positive effects on behavioral and electrophysiological outcomes in children with ASD.[19,20] More recently, high-frequency theta-burst stimulation protocols applied to the motor cortex have also been investigated experimentally in this population.[21]

Tourette Disorder

TD is thought to involve hyperexcitability of the basal ganglia and motor cortex.[22,23] Among the few studies conducted in children with TD, low-frequency TMS (1 Hz, 110% MT, 10–20 sessions) applied over supplementary motor area has been shown to improve symptoms up to 6 months and was associated with increase in resting MT in children younger than 16 years.[24,25]

Attention-Deficit Hyperactivity Disorder

ADHD affects up to 12% of the population.[26] Initial treatment strategies include pharmacotherapy; yet, because of the unwanted side effects and risk for potential abuse, alternative treatments have emerged. In a study of 9 subjects (age 15–20 years), high-frequency TMS applied to the right prefrontal cortex (100% MT, 10 sessions) showed no difference between active and sham groups.[27]

Schizophrenia

Childhood onset schizophrenia is a rare disorder with an incidence less than 0.04%.[28] In adults, TMS inhibition of left temporoparietal region reduced auditory hallucinations in double-blind, randomized trials.[29,30] In children and young adults (age ≤18) limited studies showed improvement in positive and negative symptoms of schizophrenia with both high-frequency TMS delivered to the right frontal cortex (10 daily sessions of 20 Hz TMS) and low-frequency TMS applied to the left temporoparietal cortex (10 sessions of 1 Hz TMS).[31,32]

Neurologic Disorders

Inhibitory TMS (1 Hz for 20 minutes) applied over contralesional primary cortex showed improvement in hand functioning in patients aged 6 to 18 years with pediatric stroke,[33] especially when combined with constraint-induced movement therapy (CIMT) in a larger study.[34] In epilepsy, there are only a few case reports in children with intractable epilepsy that shows that low-frequency TMS (1 Hz) can lead to temporary reduction of epileptic activity.[35]

TRANSCRANIAL ELECTRICAL STIMULATION
Transcranial Direct Current Stimulation

In adults, tDCS has shown promise as an intervention for multiple neuropsychiatric disorders.[36] Experience in children and adolescents is limited to small randomized controlled trials (RCTs) and pilot studies,[4,37,38] but tDCS has potential as a tool to modulate cortical activity and promote neuroplasticity. It is appealing because it may prove more portable, safe, and accessible as compared with other techniques such as TMS **(Fig. 2)**.[39]

Electroconvulsive therapy (ECT) is safely used in adults with mood disorders with catatonia, psychotic features, and refractory to antidepressant therapy as well as in patients who refuse food and water intake or are acutely suicidal.[40] In children and adolescents it is often considered as a last resort likely due to factors such as stigma,

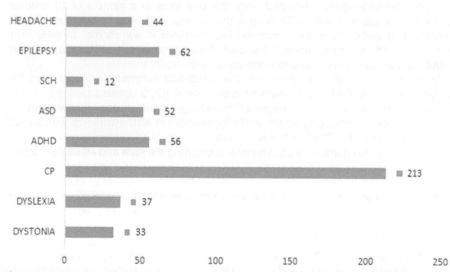

Fig. 2. Total number of subjects for each condition in TDCS studies. SCH, schizophrenia; ASD, autism spectrum disorder; ADHD, attention-deficit hyperactivity disorder; CP, cerebral palsy. (Data from Palm U, Segmiller FM, Epple AN, et al. Transcranial direct current stimulation in children and adolescents: a comprehensive review. J Neural Transm 2016;123(10):1219–34; and Muszkat D, Polanczyk GV, Dias TG, et al. Transcranial direct current stimulation in child and adolescent psychiatry. J Child Adolesc Psychopharmacol 2016;26(7):590–7.)

lack of clinical experience, concerns about long-term side effects, and legal restrictions.[41,42]

Major Depressive Disorder

In adults, prior studies demonstrate that depressed patients who underwent tDCS had greater response and remission rates,[43] but no prior studies have examined the effects of tDCS on depression in children and adolescents. Prior retrospective reviews suggest that electroconvulsive therapy can be effective in treating depression in children and adolescents with the rate of improvements up to 80% in unipolar depression and up to 90% in treatment-resistant depression.[41,42,44] Unfortunately, the dearth of RCTs and safety studies in children limits the use of ECT in younger patients.

Schizophrenia

In a double-blind sham-controlled trial, Mattai and colleagues[45] investigated the tolerability of bilateral anodal DLPFC (targeting cognitive difficulties) and bilateral cathodal and superior temporal (targeting auditory hallucinations) (2 mA for 20 min, 10 days) tDCS in 12 children with childhood-onset schizophrenia (age: 10–17 years). They found no difference between groups in terms of adverse effects or clinical measures suggesting that tDCS was well tolerated.

With regard to ECT trials, in a study with 13 participants with schizophrenia spectrum disorder (n = 13), Baeza and colleagues[46] showed that ECT lead to significant improvements in PANSS scores and CGI scores after acute phase of ECT and at 6 months. In a retrospective study of ECT, Puffer and colleagues[42] found significant improvement in CGI-I and CGI-S scores in 9 adolescents with psychotic disorder.

Autism Spectrum Disorders

Andrade and colleagues[47] targeted language problems in a sample of 14 children with 4 of the subjects with ASD. Across the sample, self-report measures indicate considerable variability in the perceived improvement in symptoms, ranging from "no change" to "very much better." One pilot study suggested that tDCS may improve syntax acquisition in children and adolescents with ASD.[48]

Other studies found improvement in the childhood autism rating scale and the Autism Treatment Evaluation Checklist with anodal tDCS applied over F3 (1 mA, 5 days).[49] Amatachaya and colleagues[50] found significant association between the electroencephalogram alpha activity and improvement in ASD symptoms with anodal tDCS applied over F3 (DLPFC) (2 mA, 20 min).

There are a small number of case reports supporting the safe and efficacious application of electroconvulsive therapy (ECT) to treat catatonia[51] and self-injurious behaviors[52] in children and adolescents with ASD. Moreover, ECT may also have had positive outcomes for some other characteristics of ASD in these cases, such as eye contact, verbal conversation,[53] and engagement in family activities.[52]

Attention-Deficit Hyperactivity Disorder

The neural basis of ADHD is thought to involve deficient inhibitory mechanisms that could be a potential target for tDCS.[54,55] In children, several studies showed improvement in inhibitory control with the stimulation of L-DLPFC.[56,57] For example, in a randomized crossover study (n = 20) anodal tDCS applied over the L-DLPFC improved the accuracy to responses in a Go-No-Go task, whereas cathodal tDCS improved No-Go accuracy suggesting improved inhibitory control.[57] Other studies looked at the effects of the slow oscillating tDCS on modulating cortical activity during non–

rapid eye movement sleep phase 2. Participants had improved reaction time and memory performance after slow oscillating tDCS.[58,59]

Epilepsy

Several case series with tDCS revealed reductions in epileptiform discharges in children with continuous spike and Wave during slow-wave sleep and Landau-Kleffner syndrome.[60] Initial pilot work in children suggested that tDCS reduced seizure frequency and severity in patients with generalized seizures due to cerebral palsy and other brain lesions,[61] Rasmussen encephalitis,[62] and focal cortical dysplasia.[63] In a randomized sham-controlled trial, Auvichayapat and colleagues[64] found a reduction in epileptiform discharges at 24 hours, 48 hours, and 4 weeks posttreatment following a single session of tDCS. In contrast, another study found no reduction in epileptiform activity.[65] Overall, tDCS has been well tolerated in patients with epilepsy except that a single case of seizure was reported during a course of tDCS.[66]

Cerebral Palsy/Dystonia

Dystonia is one of the most common movement disorders in children and does not always respond to classical pharmacologic interventions.[67] TDCS studies in dystonia have focused on combination of different therapeutic approaches with tDCS, including CIMT, visual reality, and treadmill. In a randomized clinical study of 20 patients with spastic cerebral palsy, anodal tDCS (1 mA, 20 min, 10 sessions total) applied over C3 combined with virtual reality mobility training improved velocity and cadence, mobility, and gross motor function.[68] Other studies showed similar results, including increase of body sway velocity,[69] decreased spasticity,[70] and improved static balance.[71] In contrast to aforementioned findings, Bhanpuri and colleagues[72] showed that anodal tDCS placed contralateral to the most affected limb worsened motor performance in patients with dystonia.

Dyslexia

Two studies explored the effects of tDCS in the treatment of dyslexia in children. In a sham-controlled study, Costanzo and colleagues[73] showed that anodal tDCS (1 mA, 20 min, 18 sessions) applied over the left parietotemporal region, with the cathode placed over the right homologue region, led to improved reading when combined with reading training. In a subsequent study, the investigators showed that cathodal tDCS applied over the left parietotemporal region increased the number of errors, whereas the anodal tDCS over the same region decreased the number of errors.[74]

FRONTIERS AND EMERGING TECHNOLOGIES
Trigeminal Nerve Stimulation and Magnetic Seizure Therapy

External stimulation of the trigeminal nerve (eTNS) and magnetic seizure therapy (MST) are emerging neuromodulatory techniques that have been shown to have therapeutic effects in adults. In an 8-week open-label pilot trial including 24 participants (between ages 7 and 14 years) with ADHD, eTNS administered at night time led to significant improvement in ADHD-IV Rating Scale and Conners Global Index.[75] There is a single case report in which the investigators reported full remission of depressive symptoms in an 18-year-old boy with refractory depression in the context of bipolar II disorder following 18 sessions of 100 Hz MST.[76]

DEVELOPMENTAL AND SAFETY CONSIDERATIONS

A recent systematic review that examined 48 studies with 513 children younger than 18 years supported the safety and feasibility of TMS and tDCS in children and adolescents.[3] Yet, in a recent commentary, Davis identified the potential gaps in translating brain stimulation techniques to children.[77] These include the unknown effects of stimulation in developing brains due to differences in anatomy and physiology, unknown side effects, limited translational data, and inherent ethical challenges in work with vulnerable populations.[77]

One of the most serious possible side effects of NIBS is seizure. MTs are typically higher in young children and reach adult levels by the age of 16 to 18 years.[78] As a result, higher stimulus intensities required in younger children might be associated with increased risk for adverse effects.[1] Moreover, infants and young children are thought to be especially prone to seizures due to increased glutamate sensitivity, reduced glutamate clearance, and incomplete GABA-mediated inhibition in the developing brain.[37] Therefore, further shift toward the excitatory activity induced by TMS could theoretically increase the seizure risk. Moreover, computational modeling studies suggest that typical intensities of tDCS results in higher densities and peak electrical fields in the cortex of children compared with that in adults.[79,80] Given the conductivity of the underlying biological tissues plays an important role in determining the maximum intensity and the distribution of the current that reaches to the cortex,[79] differences in skull size and composition can result in variability in the amount of the current delivered to the cortex, introducing not only safety concerns but also intersubject variability in dosing, making standardization more difficult. In addition, the relative size of the external auditory canal is smaller in young children resulting in higher resonance frequency,[81] which can increase the risk of acoustic injury during the delivery of TMS pulses.[1]

NEUROETHICS

Early guidelines regarding recruitment of children in TMS trials conclude that, unless there is compelling evidence for treatment of refractory cases, children should not be included in TMS trials due to concerns for interfering with normal neurodevelopment.[82]

Another important aspect to consider is potential applications of NIBS as a tool for neuroenhancement. It has been demonstrated that brain stimulation can enhance cognitive functions.[83] However, it is still unknown if improvement in one domain hinders the functioning of other domains.[84] Other concerns include emergence of unexpected effects such as unintentional behavioral responses or the discovery of incidental but clinically nonsignificant findings.[85]

In addition, tDCS or similar devices can be easily purchased online or constructed at home by simply watching online videos. Advertisement of these techniques without proper regulatory approvals could lead to inappropriate use of these techniques resulting in significant health issues.

SUMMARY

NIBS techniques have emerged as novel tools to promote plasticity and alleviate symptoms in neuropsychiatric disorders. Despite the intrinsic challenges in work with children and adolescents, the growing evidence suggests that brain stimulation will offer powerful and alternative tools to treat early onset neuropsychiatric disorders.

REFERENCES

1. Rossi S, Hallett M, Rossini PM, et al. Safety, ethical considerations, and application guidelines for the use of transcranial magnetic stimulation in clinical practice and research. Clin Neurophysiol 2009;120(12):2008–39.
2. Croarkin PE, Wall CA, Lee J. Applications of transcranial magnetic stimulation (TMS) in child and adolescent psychiatry. Intl Rev of Psyc 2011;23(5):445–53.
3. Krishnan C, Santos L, Peterson MD, et al. Safety of noninvasive brain stimulation in children and adolescents. Brain stimulation 2015;8(1):76–87.
4. Palm U, Segmiller FM, Epple AN, et al. Transcranial direct current stimulation in children and adolescents: a comprehensive review. J Neural Transm 2016; 123(10):1219–34.
5. Narayana S, Papanicolaou AC, McGregor A, et al. Clinical applications of transcranial magnetic stimulation in pediatric neurology. J Child Neurol 2015;30(9):1111–24.
6. Allen CH, Kluger BM, Buard I. Safety of transcranial magnetic stimulation in children: a systematic review of the literature. Pediatr Neurol 2017;68:3–17.
7. Hong YH, Wu SW, Pedapati EV, et al. Safety and tolerability of theta burst stimulation vs. single and paired pulse transcranial magnetic stimulation: a comparative study of 165 pediatric subjects. Front Hum Neurosci 2015;9:29.
8. Hu S-H, Wang S-S, Zhang M-M, et al. Repetitive transcranial magnetic stimulation-induced seizure of a patient with adolescent-onset depression: a case report and literature review. J Int Med Res 2011;39(5):2039–44.
9. Chiramberro M, Lindberg N, Isometsä E, et al. Repetitive transcranial magnetic stimulation induced seizures in an adolescent patient with major depression: a case report. Brain Stimul 2013;6(5):830–1.
10. Cullen KR, Jasberg S, Nelson B, et al. Seizure induced by deep transcranial magnetic stimulation in an adolescent with depression. J Child Adolesc Psychopharmacol 2016;26(7):637–41.
11. Bloch Y, Grisaru N, Harel EV, et al. Repetitive transcranial magnetic stimulation in the treatment of depression in adolescents: an open-label study. J ECT 2008; 24(2):156–9.
12. Kirton A, deVeber G, Gunraj C, et al. Neurocardiogenic syncope complicating pediatric transcranial magnetic stimulation. Pediatr Neurol 2008;39(3):196–7.
13. Mayer G, Aviram S, Walter G, et al. Long-term follow-up of adolescents with resistant depression treated with repetitive transcranial magnetic stimulation. J Ect 2012;28(2):84–6.
14. Donaldson AE, Gordon MS, Melvin GA, et al. Addressing the needs of adolescents with treatment resistant depressive disorders: a systematic review of rTMS. Brain Stimul 2014;7(1):7–12.
15. Wall CA, Croarkin PE, Sim LA, et al. Adjunctive use of repetitive transcranial magnetic stimulation in depressed adolescents: a prospective, open pilot study. J Clin Psychiatry 2011;72(9):1263–9.
16. Wall CA, Croarkin PE, Maroney-Smith MJ, et al. Magnetic resonance imaging-guided, open-label, high-frequency repetitive transcranial magnetic stimulation for adolescents with major depressive disorder. J Child Adolesc Psychopharmacol 2016;26(7):582–9.
17. Yang XR, Kirton A, Wilkes TC, et al. Glutamate alterations associated with transcranial magnetic stimulation in youth depression: a case series. J ECT 2014; 30(3):242–7.

18. Caetano SC, Fonseca M, Olvera RL, et al. Proton spectroscopy study of the left dorsolateral prefrontal cortex in pediatric depressed patients. Neurosci Lett 2005; 384(3):321–6.

19. Sokhadze EM, El-Baz AS, Sears LL, et al. rTMS neuromodulation improves electrocortical functional measures of information processing and behavioral responses in autism. Front Syst Neurosci 2014;8:134.

20. Sokhadze EM, El-Baz AS, Tasman A, et al. Neuromodulation integrating rTMS and neurofeedback for the treatment of autism spectrum disorder: an exploratory study. Appl Psychophysiol Biofeedback 2014;39(3–4):237–57.

21. Huang Y-Z, Rothwell JC. Theta burst stimulation. In: Marcolin MA, Padberg F, editors. Transcranial brain stimulation for treatment of psychiatric disorders. Basel (Switzerland): Karger; 2007. p. 187–203.

22. Gerard E, Peterson BS. Developmental processes and brain imaging studies in Tourette syndrome. J Psychosom Res 2003;55(1):13–22.

23. George MS, Sallee FR, Nahas Z, et al. Transcranial magnetic stimulation (TMS) as a research tool in Tourette syndrome and related disorders. Adv Neurol 2001;85: 225–35.

24. Kwon HJ, Lim WS, Lim MH, et al. 1-Hz low frequency repetitive transcranial magnetic stimulation in children with Tourette's syndrome. Neurosci Lett 2011;492(1):1–4.

25. Le K, Liu L, Sun M, et al. Transcranial magnetic stimulation at 1 Hertz improves clinical symptoms in children with Tourette syndrome for at least 6 months. J Clin Neurosci 2013;20(2):257–62.

26. Faraone SV, Sergeant J, Gillberg C, et al. The worldwide prevalence of ADHD: is it an American condition? World psychiatry 2003;2(2):104.

27. Weaver L, Rostain AL, Mace W, et al. Transcranial magnetic stimulation (TMS) in the treatment of attention-deficit/hyperactivity disorder in adolescents and young adults: a pilot study. J ECT 2012;28(2):98–103.

28. Driver DI, Gogtay N, Rapoport JL. Childhood onset schizophrenia and early onset schizophrenia spectrum disorders. Child Adolesc Psychiatr Clin N Am 2013; 22(4):539–55.

29. Hoffman RE, Boutros NN, Hu S, et al. Transcranial magnetic stimulation and auditory hallucinations in schizophrenia. Lancet 2000;355(9209):1073–5.

30. Hoffman RE, Hawkins KA, Gueorguieva R, et al. Transcranial magnetic stimulation of left temporoparietal cortex and medication-resistant auditory hallucinations. Arch Gen Psychiatry 2003;60(1):49–56.

31. Jardri R, Bubrovszky M, Demeulemeester M, et al. Repetitive transcranial magnetic stimulation to treat early-onset auditory hallucinations. J Am Acad Child Adolesc Psychiatry 2012;51(9):947–9.

32. Jardri R, Lucas B, Delevoye-Turrell Y, et al. An 11-year-old boy with drug-resistant schizophrenia treated with temporo-parietal rTMS. Mol Psychiatry 2007;12(4):320.

33. Kirton A, Chen R, Friefeld S, et al. Contralesional repetitive transcranial magnetic stimulation for chronic hemiparesis in subcortical paediatric stroke: a randomised trial. Lancet Neurol 2008;7(6):507–13.

34. Kirton A, Andersen J, Herrero M, et al. Brain stimulation and constraint for perinatal stroke hemiparesis The PLASTIC CHAMPS Trial. Neurology 2016;86(18): 1659–67.

35. Rotenberg A, Bae EH, Muller PA, et al. In-session seizures during low-frequency repetitive transcranial magnetic stimulation in patients with epilepsy. Epilepsy Behav 2009;16(2):353–5.

36. Szymkowicz SM, McLaren ME, Suryadevara U, et al. Transcranial direct current stimulation use in the treatment of neuropsychiatric disorders: a brief review. Psychiatr Ann 2016;46(11):642–6.
37. Hameed MQ, Dhamne SC, Gersner R, et al. Transcranial magnetic and direct current stimulation in children. Curr Neurol Neurosci Rep 2017;17(2):11.
38. Muszkat D, Polanczyk GV, Dias TGC, et al. Transcranial direct current stimulation in child and adolescent psychiatry. J child Adolesc Psychopharmacol 2016; 26(7):590–7.
39. Brunoni AR, Nitsche MA, Bolognini N, et al. Clinical research with transcranial direct current stimulation (tDCS): challenges and future directions. Brain stimulation 2012;5(3):175–95.
40. Fink M. Convulsive therapy: a review of the first 55 years. J Affect Disord 2001; 63(1):1–15.
41. Ghaziuddin N, Kutcher SP, Knapp P. Practice parameter for use of electroconvulsive therapy with adolescents. J Am Acad Child Adolesc Psychiatry 2004;43(12): 1521–39.
42. Puffer CC, Wall CA, Huxsahl JE, et al. A 20 year practice review of electroconvulsive therapy for adolescents. J child Adolesc Psychopharmacol 2016;26(7): 632–6.
43. Brunoni AR, Moffa AH, Fregni F, et al. Transcranial direct current stimulation for acute major depressive episodes: meta-analysis of individual patient data. Br J Psychiatry 2016;208(6):522–31.
44. Stein D, Weizman A, Bloch Y. Electroconvulsive therapy and transcranial magnetic stimulation: can they be considered valid modalities in the treatment of pediatric mood disorders? Child Adolesc Psychiatr Clin 2006;15(4):1035–56.
45. Mattai A, Miller R, Weisinger B, et al. Tolerability of transcranial direct current stimulation in childhood-onset schizophrenia. Brain stimulation 2011;4(4):275–80.
46. Baeza I, Flamarique I, Garrido JM, et al. Clinical experience using electroconvulsive therapy in adolescents with schizophrenia spectrum disorders. J child Adolesc Psychopharmacol 2010;20(3):205–9.
47. Andrade AC, Magnavita GM, Allegro JVBN, et al. Feasibility of transcranial direct current stimulation use in children aged 5 to 12 years. J Child Neurol 2014;29(10): 1360–5.
48. Schneider HD, Hopp JP. The use of the bilingual aphasia test for assessment and transcranial direct current stimulation to modulate language acquisition in minimally verbal children with autism. Clin Linguist Phon 2011;25(6–7):640–54.
49. Amatachaya A, Auvichayapat N, Patjanasoontorn N, et al. Effect of anodal transcranial direct current stimulation on autism: a randomized double-blind crossover trial. Behav Neurol 2014;2014:173073.
50. Amatachaya A, Jensen MP, Patjanasoontorn N, et al. The short-term effects of transcranial direct current stimulation on electroencephalography in children with autism: a randomized crossover controlled trial. Behav Neurol 2015;2015: 928631.
51. Wachtel LE, Griffin MM, Dhossche DM, et al. Brief report: Electroconvulsive therapy for malignant catatonia in an autistic adolescent. Autism 2010;14(4):349–58.
52. Wachtel LF, Contrucci-Kuhn SA, Griffin M, et al. ECT for self-injury in an autistic boy. Eur Child Adolesc Psychiatry 2009;18(7):458–63.
53. Wachtel LE, Kahng S, Dhossche DM, et al. ECT for catatonia in an autistic girl. Am J Psychiatry 2008;165(3):329–33.

54. Cosmo C, Baptista AF, de Araújo AN, et al. A randomized, double-blind, sham-controlled trial of transcranial direct current stimulation in attention-deficit/hyperactivity disorder. PLoS One 2015;10(8):e0135371.

55. Ditye T, Jacobson L, Walsh V, et al. Modulating behavioral inhibition by tDCS combined with cognitive training. Exp Brain Res 2012;219(3):363–8.

56. Bandeira ID, Guimarães RSQ, Jagersbacher JG, et al. Transcranial direct current stimulation in children and Adolescents with Attention-Deficit/Hyperactivity Disorder (ADHD) a pilot study. J child Neurol 2016;31(7):918–24.

57. Soltaninejad Z, Nejati V, Ekhtiari H. Effect of anodal and cathodal transcranial direct current stimulation on DLPFC on modulation of inhibitory control in ADHD. J Attent Disord 2015. 1087054715618792.

58. Munz MT, Prehn-Kristensen A, Thielking F, et al. Slow oscillating transcranial direct current stimulation during non-rapid eye movement sleep improves behavioral inhibition in attention-deficit/hyperactivity disorder. Front Cell Neurosci 2015; 9:307.

59. Prehn-Kristensen A, Munz M, Göder R, et al. Transcranial oscillatory direct current stimulation during sleep improves declarative memory consolidation in children with attention-deficit/hyperactivity disorder to a level comparable to healthy controls. Brain stimulation 2014;7(6):793–9.

60. Faria P, Fregni F, Sebastião F, et al. Feasibility of focal transcranial DC polarization with simultaneous EEG recording: preliminary assessment in healthy subjects and human epilepsy. Epilepsy Behav 2012;25(3):417–25.

61. Shelyakin AM, Preobrazhenskaya IG, Kassil' MV, et al. The effects of transcranial micropolarization on the severity of convulsive fits in children. Neurosci Behav Physiol 2001;31(5):555–60.

62. San-Juan D, Calcáneo Jde D, González-Aragón MF, et al. Transcranial direct current stimulation in adolescent and adult Rasmussen's encephalitis. Epilepsy Behav 2011;20(1):126–31.

63. Yook S-W, Park S-H, Seo J-H, et al. Suppression of seizure by cathodal transcranial direct current stimulation in an epileptic patient: a case report. Ann Rehabil Med 2011;35(4):579–82.

64. Auvichayapat N, Rotenberg A, Gersner R, et al. Transcranial direct current stimulation for treatment of refractory childhood focal epilepsy. Brain Stimulation 2013;6(4):696–700.

65. Varga ET, Terney D, Atkins MD, et al. Transcranial direct current stimulation in refractory continuous spikes and waves during slow sleep: a controlled study. Epilepsy Res 2011;97(1–2):142–5.

66. Ekici B. Transcranial direct current stimulation-induced seizure: analysis of a case. Clin EEG Neurosci 2015;46(2):169.

67. Mink JW. Special concerns in defining, studying, and treating dystonia in children. Mov Disord 2013;28(7):921–5.

68. Collange Grecco LA, de Almeida Carvalho Duarte N, Mendonça ME, et al. Effects of anodal transcranial direct current stimulation combined with virtual reality for improving gait in children with spastic diparetic cerebral palsy: a pilot, randomized, controlled, double-blind, clinical trial. Clin Rehabil 2015;29(12): 1212–23.

69. Lazzari RD, Politti F, Santos CA, et al. Effect of a single session of transcranial direct-current stimulation combined with virtual reality training on the balance of children with cerebral palsy: a randomized, controlled, double-blind trial. J Phys Ther Sci 2015;27(3):763–8.

70. Aree-uea B, Auvichayapat N, Janyacharoen T, et al. Reduction of spasticity in cerebral palsy by anodal transcranial direct current stimulation. J Med Assoc Thai 2014;97(9):954–62.
71. Grecco LA, Duarte NA, Zanon N, et al. Effect of a single session of transcranial direct-current stimulation on balance and spatiotemporal gait variables in children with cerebral palsy: A randomized sham-controlled study. Braz J Phys Ther 2014;18(5):419–27.
72. Bhanpuri NH, Bertucco M, Young SJ, et al. Multiday transcranial direct current stimulation causes clinically insignificant changes in childhood dystonia: a pilot study. J child Neurol 2015;30(12):1604–15.
73. Costanzo F, Varuzza C, Rossi S, et al. Evidence for reading improvement following tDCS treatment in children and adolescents with Dyslexia. Restor Neurol Neurosci 2016;34(2):215–26.
74. Costanzo F, Varuzza C, Rossi S, et al. Reading changes in children and adolescents with dyslexia after transcranial direct current stimulation. Neuroreport 2016;27(5):295–300.
75. McGough JJ, Loo SK, Sturm A, et al. An eight-week, open-trial, pilot feasibility study of trigeminal nerve stimulation in youth with attention-deficit/hyperactivity disorder. Brain stimulation 2015;8(2):299–304.
76. Noda Y, Daskalakis ZJ, Downar J, et al. Magnetic seizure therapy in an adolescent with refractory bipolar depression: a case report. Neuropsychiatr Dis Treat 2014;10:2049.
77. Davis NJ. Transcranial stimulation of the developing brain: a plea for extreme caution. Front Hum Neurosci 2014;8:600.
78. Eyre J. Development and plasticity of the corticospinal system in man. Neural Plast 2003;10(1–2):93–106.
79. Kessler SK, Minhas P, Woods AJ, et al. Dosage considerations for transcranial direct current stimulation in children: a computational modeling study. PLoS One 2013;8(9):e76112.
80. Minhas P, Bikson M, Woods AJ, et al. Transcranial direct current stimulation in pediatric brain: a computational modeling study. Paper presented at: Engineering in Medicine and Biology Society (EMBC), 2012 Annual International Conference of the IEEE2012. San Diego, CA, USA, August 28 - September 1, 2012.
81. Kruger B. An update on the external ear resonance in infants and young children. Ear and Hearing 1987;8(6):333–6.
82. George MS, Bohning DE, Loberbaum J, et al. Overview of transcranial magnetic stimulation. In: George MS, Belmaker RH, editors. Transcranial magnetic stimulation in clinical psychiatry. Washington, DC: American Psychiatric Publication; 2007. p. 1–38.
83. Snowball A, Tachtsidis I, Popescu T, et al. Long-term enhancement of brain function and cognition using cognitive training and brain stimulation. Curr Biol 2013;23(11):987–92.
84. Kadosh RC, Levy N, O'Shea J, et al. The neuroethics of non-invasive brain stimulation. Curr Biol 2012;22(4):R108–11.
85. Rajapakse T, Kirton A. Non-invasive brain stimulation in children: applications and future directions. Transl Neurosci 2013;4(2):217–33.

Therapeutic Applications of Invasive Neuromodulation in Children and Adolescents

Deniz Doruk Camsari, MD[a], Melissa Kirkovski, PhD[b],
Paul E. Croarkin, DO[a],*

KEYWORDS

- Neuromodulation • Invasive brain stimulation • Deep brain stimulation • DBS
- Vagal nerve stimulation • VNS • Children • Adolescents

KEY POINTS

- Vagal nerve stimulation has US Food and Drug Administration approval for intractable epilepsy in patients aged 4 and older.
- Deep brain stimulation has been used on a limited basis in youth with dystonia and intractable tic disorders.
- Further measured work with invasive neuromodulation for children and adolescents with debilitating neuropsychiatric disorders could provide new treatment options and expand current knowledge base of neurocircuitry across development.

INVASIVE NEUROMODULATION

Neuromodulation is a rapidly growing field that includes a variety of stimulation modalities. Although neuromodulation techniques have been used to treat medical conditions for thousands of years, contemporary neuromodulation began in the 1960s with the advent of deep brain stimulation (DBS). In adults, advances and growing evidence in the efficacy and safety of invasive neuromodulation techniques have already led to the study and in some cases US Food and Drug Administration (FDA) clearance for several indications. Parkinson disease, essential tremor, and

Financial Disclosures: Dr P.E. Croarkin has received research grant support from Pfizer, Inc (WS1976243), National Institute of Mental Health (K23MH10026 and R01MH113700), the Brain and Behavior Research Foundation (20883), and the Mayo Clinic Foundation. He has received equipment support from Neuronetics, Inc and receives supplies and genotyping services from Assurex Health, Inc for investigator-initiated studies. He is the primary investigator for a multicenter study of adolescent TMS funded by Neuronetics, Inc. Drs D.D. Camsari and M. Kirkovski have no financial disclosures.

[a] Department of Psychiatry and Psychology, Mayo Clinic, 200 First Street Southwest, Rochester, MN 55905, USA; [b] Deakin Child Study Centre, School of Psychology, Deakin University, Geelong, VIC 3220, Australia
* Corresponding author.
E-mail address: croarkin.paul@mayo.edu

Psychiatr Clin N Am 41 (2018) 479–483
https://doi.org/10.1016/j.psc.2018.04.008
0193-953X/18/© 2018 Elsevier Inc. All rights reserved.

epilepsy are the most widely studied conditions in adults.[1] As of 2017, FDA clearance in children is limited to use of vagal nerve stimulation (VNS) in drug-resistant epilepsy, and DBS in dystonia.

Vagal Nerve Stimulation

VNS is an invasive neuromodulatory technique that involves electrical stimulation of the 10th cranial nerve, the vagus nerve, via an implanted electrical stimulator. VNS is most commonly used to treat intractable epilepsy and treatment-resistant depression.[2] Common stimulation settings are 1 to 3 mA, 20 to 30 Hz, and 130 to 500 μs.[2] In 1997, the FDA approved the use of VNS in treatment of intractable epilepsy in adults and children aged 12 and older.[3] In 2017, another device was approved for partial-onset medication refractory epilepsy in patients as young as 4. A systematic review and meta-analysis of the efficacy of VNS in 326 children described a response rate of 38% (>50% reduction in seizure frequency). The study did note high variability and limited evidence.[4] In order to assess tolerability and side-effect profile, the investigators included additional case reports and retrospective studies, with a total of 1249 children included. Despite the high percentage of side effects (70%–80%), most of the patients tolerated these side effects well and continued treatment. Common side effects included procedure-related complications, including hoarseness (1%), dyspnea (<1%), fluid collection around the stimulator, and infection (3%). Other side effects were device-related complications, such as hardware failure (3%) and stimulus-related complications, such as aspiration (5%), due to vocal cord dysfunction during the stimulation period. Arrhythmias were noted as delayed complications. There were 5 sudden unexplained death in epilepsy patients and 4 unrelated deaths. The investigators also maintained that VNS may improve sleep quality, behavior, and mood and reduce treatment expense.[4]

Deep Brain Stimulation

DBS is one of the early brain stimulation techniques that emerged in 1960s and has since been used to treat multiple different neurologic and psychiatric conditions. DBS is an invasive procedure whereby the lead is placed in the targeted areas of the brain and is connected to the implanted pulse generator, which is extracranially placed. DBS is considered favorable as compared with surgical ablation procedures with regard to reversibility of the procedure and lower risk of complications.[5] The FDA cleared DBS for Parkinson disease tremor in 2001 and essential tremor in 1997. Other indications under FDA humanitarian device exemptions include dystonia in 2007, obsessive compulsive disorder in 2009, and closed loop stimulation for epilepsy.[6] Other areas of interest include major depressive disorder, Tourette syndrome, addictions, and obesity. In children, DBS use has been primarily limited to dystonia, but epilepsy, Tourette disorder (TD), and obsessive-compulsive disorder (OCD) have also been considered as potential targets.

Dystonia

When pharmacologic interventions fail to provide improvement, more invasive interventions such as pallidotomy and DBS are considered to treat symptoms and decrease disease burden in dsytonia.[7,8] The globus pallidus interna (GPi) has been the main target of DBS in treating dystonia in both adults[6] and children[9,10]; however, other regions, including the subthalamic nucleus and thalamic ventralis intermedius, have also been targeted. Bilateral stimulation of GPi with higher frequencies (100 Hz) has been reported to be the most common application of DBS in dystonia, yet lower frequencies have also been used.[8] Wider pulses were found to be poorly tolerated.[10] DBS has been shown to have superior efficacy especially in primary generalized dystonia.[11] Haridas and colleagues[9] demonstrated that in primary generalized dystonia patients (n = 22) under the age of 21, DBS is a safe method of treatment leading up to 94% improvement in Burke-Fahn-Marsden Dystonia Rating Scale motor scores at 3-year follow-up. Several factors have been identified as good prognostic factors,[8] including early intervention,[12,13] certain gene mutations,[12] and absence of other clinical features, such as contractures.[10] Other subgroups of dystonia were also explored in terms of DBS responsiveness, including dyskinetic cerebral palsy,[14] and pantothenate kinase associated neurodegeneration,[15] as well as other acquired dystonia due to prematurity and kern icterus, and neurodevelopmental and degenerative dystonia, but the evidence is limited.[8]

Tourette Disorder

In refractory cases of TD, DBS has been shown to be an effective treatment to reduce symptoms, but there are few studies in children and adolescents. An important limitation to use of DBS in children is the temporal decline in symptom severity by adulthood with almost 30% of the patients becoming symptom free, and 75% experiencing significant improvement in their symptoms over time.[16] Among the few case reports, Shahed and colleagues[17] showed that bilateral GPi-DBS in a 16-year-old patient with intractable Tourette syndrome was effective to reduce tic severity by 76% for motor and 68% for vocal tics leading to significant improvement in impairment, neurocognitive functions, and comorbid OCD symptoms. Similar improvements were reported in another study that included 2 patients under 18 years of age with the stimulation of centromedian parafascicular nucleus of thalamus.[18] Conversely, Dueck and colleagues[19] reported no improvement of symptoms with bilateral GPi-DB in a 16-year-old patient with TS and intellectual disability.

Obsessive-Compulsive Disorder

OCD is characterized by obsessions and compulsions, and its prevalence in children and adolescents is estimated to be 3%.[20] Neuroimaging studies have demonstrated disturbance of corticostriatothalamocortical circuits in OCD.[21,22] Initial treatment options include cognitive-behavioral therapy with exposure response prevention and pharmacotherapy; yet, approximately 50% of pediatric patients fail to respond to initial therapeutic approaches.[23] In certain circumstances, stereotactic ablation has been shown to be effective.[24] In adults, DBS was approved under humanitarian device exemption by the FDA in 2009 for the treatment of OCD. Common targets of DBS include the anterior capsule and the nucleus accumbens, leading up to 38% improvements and even remission. In children and adolescents, given the possibility of spontaneous remission into adulthood, invasive techniques remain a last resort. However, a 16-year-old patient with bilateral GPi-DBS had improvements in OCD symptoms.[25]

SUMMARY

Invasive brain stimulation techniques, such as DBS and VNS, have emerged as important therapeutic modalities for adults with Parkinson disease, essential tremor, treatment-resistant depression, OCD, and epilepsy. At present, systematic studies of DBS and VNS in children are lacking. As with noninvasive neuromodulation, future research and clinical practice with children receiving invasive forms of brain stimulation must involve careful consideration of ethical and neurodevelopmental concerns. In the future, noninvasive neuromodulation will likely present options for young patients with severe neuropsychiatric disorders and could inform developmental understandings of neurocircuitry.

REFERENCES

1. Youngerman BE, Chan AK, Mikell CB, et al. A decade of emerging indications: deep brain stimulation in the United States. J Neurosurg 2016;125(2):461–71.
2. Edwards CA, Kouzani A, Lee KH, et al. Neurostimulation devices for the treatment of neurologic disorders. Mayo Clin proc 2017;92(9):1427–44.
3. Schachter SC. Vagus nerve stimulation therapy summary five years after FDA approval. Neurology 2002;59(6 suppl 4):S15–29.
4. Klinkenberg S, Majoie H, Aalbers M, et al. Vagus nerve stimulation in children with epilepsy a review of literature on efficacy, secondary effects, and side-effects. VNS in children 2015;17.
5. Pahwa R, Lyons KE, Wilkinson SB, et al. Comparison of thalamotomy to deep brain stimulation of the thalamus in essential tremor. Mov Disord 2001;16(1): 140–3.
6. Tekriwal A, Baltuch G. Deep brain stimulation: expanding applications. Neurol Med Chir (Tokyo) 2015;55(12):861–77.
7. Mink JW. Special concerns in defining, studying, and treating dystonia in children. Mov Disord 2013;28(7):921–5.
8. Cif L, Coubes P. Historical developments in children's deep brain stimulation. Eur J Paediatr Neurol 2017;21(1):109–17.
9. Haridas A, Tagliati M, Osborn I, et al. Pallidal deep brain stimulation for primary dystonia in children. Neurosurgery 2011;68(3):738–43 [discussion: 743].
10. Marks WA, Honeycutt J, Acosta F, et al. Deep brain stimulation for pediatric movement disorders. Semin Pediatr Neurol 2009;16(2):90–8.
11. Coubes P, Roubertie A, Vayssiere N, et al. Treatment of DYT1-generalised dystonia by stimulation of the internal globus pallidus. Lancet 2000;355(9222):2220–1.
12. Vasques X, Cif L, Gonzalez V, et al. Factors predicting improvement in primary generalized dystonia treated by pallidal deep brain stimulation. Mov Disord 2009;24(6):846–53.
13. Isaias IU, Alterman RL, Tagliati M. Outcome predictors of pallidal stimulation in patients with primary dystonia: the role of disease duration. Brain 2008;131(7): 1895–902.
14. Koy A, Timmermann L. Deep brain stimulation in cerebral palsy: challenges and opportunities. Eur J Paediatr Neurol 2017;21(1):118–21.
15. Timmermann L, Pauls KAM, Wieland K, et al. Dystonia in neurodegeneration with brain iron accumulation: outcome of bilateral pallidal stimulation. Brain 2010; 133(3):701–12.
16. Bloch MH, Leckman JF. Clinical course of Tourette syndrome. J Psychosom Res 2009;67(6):497–501.
17. Shahed J, Poysky J, Kenney C, et al. GPi deep brain stimulation for Tourette syndrome improves tics and psychiatric comorbidities. Neurology 2007;68(2): 159–60.
18. Servello D, Porta M, Sassi M, et al. Deep brain stimulation in 18 patients with severe Gilles de la Tourette syndrome refractory to treatment: the surgery and stimulation. J Neurol Neurosurg Psychiatry 2008;79(2):136–42.
19. Dueck A, Wolters A, Wunsch K, et al. Deep brain stimulation of globus pallidus internus in a 16-year-old boy with severe Tourette syndrome and mental retardation. Neuropediatrics 2009;40(05):239–42.

20. Stewart S, Geller D, Jenike M, et al. Long-term outcome of pediatric obsessive–compulsive disorder: a meta-analysis and qualitative review of the literature. Acta Psychiatr Scand 2004;110(1):4–13.
21. Chiu C-H, Lo Y-C, Tang H-S, et al. White matter abnormalities of fronto-striato-thalamic circuitry in obsessive–compulsive disorder: a study using diffusion spectrum imaging tractography. Psychiatry Res Neuroimaging 2011;192(3): 176–82.
22. Sakai Y, Narumoto J, Nishida S, et al. Corticostriatal functional connectivity in non-medicated patients with obsessive-compulsive disorder. Eur Psychiatry 2011; 26(7):463–9.
23. Pediatric OCD Treatment Study (POTS) Team. Cognitive-behavior therapy, sertra-line, and their combination for children and adolescents with obsessive-compulsive disorder: the Pediatric OCD Treatment Study (POTS) randomized controlled trial. JAMA 2004;292(16):1969.
24. Liu K, Zhang H, Liu C, et al. Stereotactic treatment of refractory obsessive compulsive disorder by bilateral capsulotomy with 3 years follow-up. J Clin Neu-rosci 2008;15(6):622–9.
25. Sheppard DM, Bradshaw JL, Purcell R, et al. Tourette's and comorbid syndromes: obsessive compulsive and attention deficit hyperactivity disorder. A common etiology? Clin Psychol Rev 1999;19(5):531–52.

Clinical Usefulness of Therapeutic Neuromodulation for Major Depression
A Systematic Meta-Review of Recent Meta-Analyses

Alexander McGirr, MD, MSc, FRCPC[a],*, Marcelo T. Berlim, MD, MSc[b],*

KEYWORDS

- Major depression • Treatment-resistant depression • Neuromodulation
- Brain stimulation • Repetitive transcranial magnetic stimulation
- Transcranial direct current stimulation • Vagus nerve stimulation
- Deep brain stimulation

KEY POINTS

- Repetitive transcranial magnetic stimulation, transcranial direct current stimulation, vagus nerve stimulation, and deep brain stimulation are the most promising neuromodulation interventions for major depression.
- Repetitive transcranial magnetic stimulation is the most studied modality for major depression; its different active stimulation protocols have been generally associated with small to moderate effect sizes.
- Electroconvulsive therapy seems to be generally more effective than active repetitive transcranial magnetic stimulation for treating major depression.
- Although less studied than repetitive transcranial magnetic stimulation, active transcranial direct current stimulation has been associated with small to moderate effect sizes in major depression.
- Although research on vagus nerve stimulation and deep brain stimulation is challenging because of their invasiveness and the severity of the targeted pathology, they have demonstrated preliminary effectiveness.

Disclosure Statement: The authors report no potential conflicts of interest.
a Department of Psychiatry, Hotchkiss Brain Institute, Mathison Centre for Mental Health Research and Education, University of Calgary, TRW-4D68, 3280 Hospital Drive Northwest, Calgary, Alberta T2N 4Z6, Canada; b Neuromodulation Research Clinic, Depressive Disorders Program, Douglas Mental Health University Institute, McGill University, 6875 LaSalle Boulevard, Montréal, Québec H4H 1R3, Canada
* Corresponding authors.
E-mail addresses: alexander.mcgirr@ucalgary.ca (A.M.); nrc.douglas@me.com (M.T.B.)

Psychiatr Clin N Am 41 (2018) 485–503
https://doi.org/10.1016/j.psc.2018.04.009
0193-953X/18/© 2018 Elsevier Inc. All rights reserved.

psych.theclinics.com

Abbreviations	
CI	Confidence interval
cTBS	Continuous theta burst stimulation
DBS	Deep brain stimulation
DLPFC	Dorsolateral prefrontal cortex
HF-rTMS	High-frequency repetitive transcranial magnetic stimulation
iTBS	Intermittent theta burst stimulation
LF-rTMS	Low frequency repetitive transcranial magnetic stimulation
MD	Major depression
OR	Odds ratio
RD	Risk difference
SMD	Standardized mean difference
rTMS	Repetitive transcranial magnetic stimulation
TBS	Theta burst stimulation
tDCS	Transcranial direct current stimulation
VNS	Vagus nerve stimulation

INTRODUCTION

Major depression (MD) is characterized by the presence of depressed mood and/or anhedonia, as well as a number of somatic, vegetative, and psychological symptoms.[1] It is a debilitating condition that exacts enormous personal, social, and economic costs, including excessive mortality, disability, and secondary morbidity (eg, substance use disorders, suicidality).[2]

Although pharmacologic and psychosocial interventions remain the cornerstone of the management of MD, they are often unable to yield adequate clinical improvements in a large proportion of subjects.[3] Furthermore, medications, including antidepressants, are often associated with significant side effects such as, for example, metabolic abnormalities and sexual dysfunction.[1]

In recent years, a variety of novel therapeutic neuromodulation techniques targeting MD have become available. Among these, repetitive transcranial magnetic stimulation (rTMS), transcranial direct current stimulation (tDCS), vagus nerve stimulation (VNS), and deep brain stimulation (DBS) seem to be the most promising overall.[4] The body of primary empirical studies on their clinical usefulness in MD has been rapidly expanding, as have the meta-analyses aimed at quantitatively synthesizing this literature.[5] However, these studies have often produced inconsistent findings and, accordingly, have limited one's capacity to draw more definitive conclusions about the role of therapeutic neuromodulation for treating MD.

Consequently, we have carried out the present meta-review encompassing the past 10 years with the goal of critically appraising previously published meta-analyses. We hope that our findings will assist clinicians in optimizing their daily decision making, researchers in identifying where gaps exist in the current evidence base, and policy-makers in targeting resources more effectively.

METHODS

The protocol for this meta-review was registered with PROSPERO (CRD# 42017081833).

Search Strategy

We identified relevant systematic reviews with meta-analyses on the clinical usefulness of therapeutic neuromodulation for MD by searching 3 databases, namely, MEDLINE, EMBASE, and the Cochrane Database of Systematic Reviews, from January 1,

2007, to November 8, 2017. We also reviewed the reference lists of the included studies. The search results from each database were uploaded into a single library of Endnote X8 and all duplicates were electronically identified and then manually reviewed. The basic search procedures (including syntaxes, parameters, and results) are described in **Box 1**.

Study Selection

Meta-analyses were selected for inclusion using the following strategy: first, titles and abstracts were inspected; second, initially selected articles were read in full; third, articles fulfilling the a priori eligibility criteria were included in the meta-review.

Because there are disparate levels of evidence for each of the neuromodulation modalities considered in this meta-review, principally owing to the generally prohibitive nature of surgical randomized controlled trials (RCTs), we chose to apply different thresholds for metaanalysis inclusion. Specifically, meta-analyses on rTMS and tDCS were limited to those quantitatively synthesizing RCTs, whereas those on DBS and VNS were considered if they synthesized open-label trials in addition to RCTs.

Candidate studies had to satisfy the following criteria:

- Methodology: Systematic review with metaanalysis[6];
- Sample characteristics: Subjects aged 18 to 75 years with a diagnosis of MD (either unipolar or bipolar) according to criteria from the *Diagnostic and Statistical Manual of Mental Disorders, third edition*, or later[7] or the *International Classification of Diseases, 9th edition*, or later[8];
- Treatment characteristics: rTMS, tDCS, VNS or DBS used either as a monotherapy or as an augmentation strategy for MD; and
- Publication-related: Articles written in English and published in peer-reviewed journals.

Box 1
Electronic databases search

Date: January 1, 2007, to November 8, 2017

Syntaxes
  MEDLINE (PubMed)
    An advanced search was conducted on November 8, 2017, using the following search syntax: ("deep brain stimulation" OR "vagus nerve stimulation" OR "magnetic stimulation" OR "deep TMS" OR "direct current" OR "brain polarization") AND (meta-anal*[ti] OR metanal*[ti] OR "systematic review"[ti]) AND (depress*[ti] OR antidepress*[ti])
    This search retrieved 77 references.
  EMBASE (OVID interface)
    An advanced search was conducted on November 8, 2017, using the following search syntax: (deep brain stimulation or vagus nerve stimulation or magnetic stimulation or deep TMS or direct current or brain polarization).mp. and (meta-anal$ or metanal$ or systematic review).ti. and (depress$ or antidepress$).ti.
    This search retrieved 105 references after discarding duplicates.
  Cochrane Database of Systematic Reviews (CDSR)
    An advanced search was conducted on November 8, 2017, using the following syntax: ("deep brain stimulation" or "vagus nerve stimulation" or "magnetic stimulation" or "deep TMS" or "direct current" or "brain polarization") AND (meta-anal* OR metanal* OR "systematic review"):ti AND (depress* OR antidepress*):ti
    This search retrieved 27 references.

Studies were excluded if they enrolled subjects with "narrow" diagnoses (eg, post-partum MD) or secondary MD (eg, vascular depression).

Data Extraction and Synthesis

The following data were extracted from each included metaanalysis: publication year, treatment and control conditions (if applicable), number of primary studies, the pooled effect sizes and their 95% confidence intervals (CIs) for the main efficacy/effectiveness (ie, odds ratio [OR] for differential response and remission rates, and standardized mean difference [SMD] for pre–post depression scores), and acceptability (ie, ORs for differential dropout rates) analyses as well as the I^2 (an index for between-study heterogeneity). When the included meta-analyses reported other effect sizes (eg, Hedges's g, risk difference [RD], risk ratio, and event rate); these effects were converted, if applicable and whenever possible, to either an SMD or OR. Finally, we considered SMD with of values less than 0.2, 0.5 to 0.79, and greater than 0.8 to represent, respectively, small, moderate and large treatment effects.[9]

RESULTS
Literature Search

We retrieved 113 potential articles from MEDLINE, EMBASE, and the Cochrane Database of Systematic Reviews (see **Box 1**). Of these, 38 met our eligibility criteria.

Meta-analyses on repetitive transcranial magnetic stimulation for major depression

Of note, rTMS can either decrease or increase cortical excitability in relatively focal brain areas (reviewed further in Sarah L. Garnaat and colleagues' article, "Transcranial Magnetic Stimulation Therapy for Major Depressive Disorder," in this issue). Accordingly, frequencies of 1 Hz or less (ie, low-frequency rTMS [LF-rTMS]) are usually inhibitory, whereas frequencies of 5 Hz or greater (ie, high-frequency rTMS [HF-rTMS]) are usually excitatory.[10] In the context of MD, HF-rTMS and LF-rTMS have been applied, respectively, to the left and to the right dorsolateral prefrontal cortex (DLPFC).

In this meta-review, we included 29 meta-analyses on rTMS for MD; 3 studies were excluded because they either examined blinding integrity,[11] allowed open-label trials,[12] or only provided qualitative comparisons of rTMS interventions.[13]

Pooled repetitive transcranial magnetic stimulation protocols versus sham First, we examined 11 meta-analyses[10,14–22] that presented data pooling all active rTMS protocols compared with sham (**Table 1**, top panel).

SMDs for pre–post depression scores were reported by 7 meta-analyses, and ranged from 0.42 (95% CI, 0.18–0.66)[16] to 0.86 (95% CI, 0.57–1.15).[17] The 2 meta-analyses reporting the largest effect sizes had substantially smaller total sample sizes,[17,18] and their findings likely reflected immaturity of the literature at the time of data collection,[18] and possible unintentional errors in the application of eligibility criteria and/or bias in the search procedures.[17] With respect to response, 3 meta-analyses used RD as their effect size,[17,19,20] with 2 reporting similar results favoring active rTMS (ie, RD, 0.17 [95% CI, 0.10–0.23][19] and RD, 0.18 [95% CI, 0.06–0.30][20]), and the third, previously identified as having suffered from potential unintended biases,[17] reporting a substantially larger RD of 0.29 (95% CI, 0.15–0.44). Three meta-analyses originally reported ORs,[15,21,22] and although both reported higher response rates for active rTMS, their estimates differed somewhat (ie, ORs ranging from 2.49 [95% CI, 1.12–5.55][21] to 4.10 [95% CI, 2.85–5.90][15]), with the larger effect size possibly reflecting different study eligibility criteria.[15] Moreover, data relating to

Table 1
Meta-analyses examining the efficacy of active rTMS compared with sham for MD

Reference	Diagnosis	RCTs (n)	Patients (N)	SMD (95% CI)	SMD I² (%)	Response OR (95% CI)	Response I² (%)	Remission OR (95% CI)	Remission I² (%)	Dropout OR (95% CI)
Pooled rTMS protocols vs sham										
Gross et al,[18] 2007	BD + MDD	5	274	0.76 (0.51–1.01)	—	—	—	—	—	—
Lam et al,[19] 2008	BD + MDD	24	1092	0.48 (0.28–0.69)	>30	RD = 0.17 (0.10–0.23)[a]	>30	RD = 0.14 (0.06–0.21)[a]	>30	—
Slotema et al,[14] 2010	BD + MDD	34	1383	0.54 (NA)	54	—	—	—	—	—
Allan et al,[15] 2011	BD + MDD	31	—	0.64 (0.50–0.79)	43.5	4.10 (2.85–5.90)	41.7	—	—	—
Berlim et al,[11] 2013	BD + MDD	6	392	—	—	2.49 (1.12–5.55)	56.1	2.42 (1.27–4.60)	75.4	0.7 (0.35–1.41)
Gaynes et al,[22] 2014	BD + MDD	18	686	—	—	3.38 (2.24–5.10)	0	5.07 (2.50–10.30)	0	—
Kedzior et al,[16] 2014	BD + MDD	14	659	0.42 (0.18–0.66)	50	—	—	—	—	—
Liu et al,[17] 2014	BD + MDD	7	279	0.86 (0.57–1.15)	0	5.12 (2.11–12.45)[b]	17.7	—	—	RD = 0.01 (−0.04–0.07)[a]
Kedzior et al,[12] 2015	BD + MDD	16	495	0.48 (0.25–0.70)	—	—	—	—	—	—
Leggett et al,[35] 2015	BD + MDD	45	1335	—	27	3.53 (2.36–5.27)[b]	36.1	2.88 (1.79–4.64)	1.1	—
McGirr et al,[20] 2016	BD	19	181	—	—	2.39 (1.13–5.03)[b]	0	—	—	—
High-frequency rTMS vs sham										
Schutter,[24] 2009	BD + MDD	30	1164	0.39 (0.25–0.54)	—	—	—	—	—	—
Slotema et al,[14] 2010	BD + MDD	33	—	0.53 (NA)	—	—	—	—	—	—
Berlim et al,[23] 2014	BD + MDD	29	1371	—	—	3.30 (2.35–4.64)	2.97	3.28 (2.04–5.32)	0	0.96 (0.6–1.53)
Brunoni et al,[45] 2016	BD + MDD	43	—	—	—	3.28 (2.33–4.61)	34	—	—	1.04 (0.78–1.40)
Teng et al,[25] 2017	BD + MDD	30	1754	0.73 (0.47–1.00)	88	—	—	—	—	—

(continued on next page)

Table 1
(continued)

Reference	Diagnosis	RCTs (n)	Patients (N)	SMD (95% CI)	SMD I² (%)	Response OR (95% CI)	Response I² (%)	Remission OR (95% CI)	Remission I² (%)	Dropout OR (95% CI)
Low Frequency rTMS vs sham										
Schutter,[28] 2010	BD + MDD	9	252	0.63 (0.03–1.24)	—	—	—	—	—	—
Slotema et al,[14] 2010	BD + MDD	7	—	0.82 (NA)	—	—	—	—	—	—
Berlim et al,[27] 2013	BD + MDD	8	263	—	—	3.34 (1.39–8.01)	34.18	4.76 (2.13–10.64)	0	0.53 (0.19–1.45)
Brunoni et al,[45] 2016	BD + MDD	12	—	—	—	2.48 (1.22–5.05)	34	—	—	1.30 (0.72–2.34)
Bilateral rTMS vs sham										
Slotema et al,[14] 2010	BD + MDD	4	—	0.47 (NA)	—	—	—	—	—	—
Berlim et al,[29] 2013	BD + MDD	7	279	—	—	4.30 (1.94–9.52)	0	5.99 (1.65–21.76)	0	0.53 (0.20–1.36)
Zhang et al,[30] 2015	BD + MDD	7	278	—	—	4.05 (1.84–8.87)[b]	0	—	—	—
Brunoni et al,[45] 2016	BD + MDD	11	—	—	—	3.39 (1.91–6.02)	0	—	—	1.22 (0.38–3.53)
Theta burst stimulation vs sham										
Berlim et al,[33] 2017	BD + MDD	5	221	1.02 (0.34–1.7)	82	2.70 (1.4–2.8)	0	1.90 (0.9–4.5)	0.1	0.70 (0.25–1.98)

Abbreviations: BD, bipolar disorder; CI, confidence interval; MD, major depression; MDD, major depressive disorder; NA, not available; OR, odds ratio; RD, risk difference; RCT, randomized, controlled trial; rTMS, repetitive transcranial magnetic stimulation; SMD, standardized mean difference.
[a] Could not be recomputed as an OR because the raw data were not presented.
[b] Original estimate recomputed as an OR.

remission rates supported the overall higher efficacy of active rTMS, and the differences between the meta-analyses generally mirrored those observed for response. Finally, 2 meta-analyses[17,21] suggested similar acceptability between active rTMS protocols and sham.

High-frequency repetitive transcranial magnetic stimulation over the left dorsolateral prefrontal cortex versus sham Three meta-analyses[23–25] and 2 subgroup analyses[14,26] presented data on RCTs of active HF-rTMS compared with sham for MD (see **Table 1**, second panel).

SMDs for pre–post depressive symptoms were presented by 2 meta-analyses and 1 subgroup analysis and differed substantially from each other (ie, 0.39 [95% CI, 0.25–0.54],[24] 0.53 [95% CI, NA],[14] and 0.73 [95% CI, 0.47–1.00][25]), which might reflect varying search strategies and/or publication timeframes. In terms of response, 2 meta-analyses showed superiority for active HF-rTMS (ie, OR, 3.30 [95% CI, 2.35–4.64][23] and OR, 3.28 [95% CI, 2.33–4.61][26]), despite a large difference in the total number of included RCTs (ie, 29 and 43, respectively). Only 1 metaanalysis reported data on remission,[23] and it supported the higher efficacy of active HF-rTMS (ie, OR, 3.28 [95% CI, 2.04–5.32]). Finally, 2 meta-analyses[23,26] suggested similar acceptability between active HF-rTMS and sham.

Low-frequency repetitive transcranial magnetic stimulation over the right dorsolateral prefrontal cortex versus sham Two meta-analyses[27,28] and 2 subgroup analysis[14,26] synthesized RCTs examining LF-rTMS compared with sham for MD (see **Table 1**, third panel).

One metaanalysis[28] and 1 subgroup analysis[14] reported data on pre–post depressive symptoms and showed superior efficacy for active LF-rTMS (ie, SMD, 0.63 [95% CI, 0.03–1.24][28] and SMD, 0.82 [95% CI, NA][14]). With respect to response, 2 meta-analyses supported the efficacy of LF-rTMS (ie, ORs >2), although to marginally different degrees (ie, OR, 3.34 [95% CI, 1.39–8.01][27] and OR, 2.48 [95% CI, 1.22–5.05][26]). Aside from the different number of synthesized RCTs, there was no attributable source for the observed discrepancy. Only 1 metaanalysis examined remission, and it supported the superiority of active LF-rTMS (ie, OR, 4.76 [95% CI, 2.13–10.64][27]). Finally, 2 meta-analyses[26,27] suggested similar acceptability between active LF-rTMS and sham.

Bilateral repetitive transcranial magnetic stimulation over the dorsolateral prefrontal cortex versus sham One metaanalysis[29] and 3 subgroup analysis[14,26,30] synthesized RCTs examining bilateral rTMS compared with sham for MD (see **Table 1**, fourth panel).

One subgroup analysis[14] reported data on pre–post depressive symptoms and showed superior efficacy for active bilateral rTMS (ie, SMD, 0.47 [95% CI, NA]). With respect to response, the 3 meta-analyses supported the superiority of bilateral rTMS (ie, ORs >3), although to marginally different degrees (ie, ORs ranging from 3.39 [95% CI, 1.91–6.02][26] to 4.30 [95% CI, 1.94–9.52][29]). Aside from the different number of included RCTs, we could not identify a clear source for this discrepancy. The only metaanalysis examining remission reported a relatively large effect size favoring active bilateral rTMS (ie, OR, 5.99 [95% CI, 1.65–21.76]).[27] Finally, 2 meta-analyses[26,29] suggested similar acceptability between active bilateral rTMS and sham.

Theta burst stimulation over the dorsolateral prefrontal cortex versus sham Theta burst stimulation (TBS) is a novel rTMS protocol in which magnetic pulses are administered in bursts of 3 at high frequency (ie, 50 Hz), with an interburst interval of 200 ms or 5 Hz (ie, at the theta frequency).[31] Compared with standard rTMS, TBS usually requires less stimulation time as well as lower intensity[32] to produce longer lasting modulation of cortical excitability.[31] Three different TBS protocols have been used for MD: continuous TBS (cTBS) applied to the right DLPFC, intermittent TBS (iTBS) applied to the left DLPFC, and consecutive bilateral cTBS/iTBS to the DLPFC.[32]

To date there has been only a single metaanalysis[33] examining TBS compared with sham for MD (see **Table 1**, fifth panel) and it pooled iTBS, cTBS, and bilateral cTBS/iTBS protocols in its primary analyses.

Results on pre–post depressive symptoms demonstrated a relatively large effect size favoring active TBS (ie, SMD, 1.02 [95% CI, 0.34–1.7]), but substantial between-RCT heterogeneity (ie, I^2 = 82%). With respect to response, analysis supported the higher efficacy of TBS (ie, OR, 2.7 [95% CI, 1.4–2.8]); however, findings related to remission were nonsignificant. Finally, acceptability seemed to be similar between active TBS and sham.

High-frequency repetitive transcranial magnetic stimulation versus low-frequency repetitive transcranial magnetic stimulation One metaanalysis[34] and 2 subgroup analyses[26,35] examined the differential efficacy between HF-rTMS and LF-rTMS for MD (**Table 2**, first panel).

With respect to response, all meta-analyses failed to identify statistically significant differences between HF-rTMS and LF-rTMS. Moreover, only 1 metaanalysis examined remission, and found no differential efficacy between these 2 active rTMS protocols.[35] Finally, 2 meta-analyses suggested similar acceptability between HF-rTMS and LF-rTMS.[26,34]

Bilateral repetitive transcranial magnetic stimulation versus other repetitive transcranial magnetic stimulation protocols Two meta-analyses[30,36] examined the differential efficacy between active bilateral rTMS and other rTMS protocols for MD (see **Table 2**, second panel).

With respect to response and remission, neither metaanalysis found evidence of superiority for active bilateral rTMS compared with other rTMS protocols and there was substantial between-RCT heterogeneity (ie, I^2 ranging from 38% to 75%). Finally, 1 metaanalysis suggested similar acceptability between active bilateral rTMS and other rTMS protocols.[36]

Repetitive transcranial magnetic stimulation versus electroconvulsive therapy There have been 4 meta-analyses[37–40] and 1 subgroup analysis[14] on rTMS compared with ECT for MD (see **Table 2**, third panel).

One metaanalysis[37] and 1 subgroup analysis[14] reported data on pre–post depressive symptoms favoring ECT over rTMS (ie, SMD, −0.93 [95% CI, −1.61 to −0.26] and SMD, −0.47 [95% CI, NA], respectively). Three meta-analyses reported results on response,[38–40] with 1 finding no difference between ECT and rTMS,[38] and the other 2 reporting ECT to be significantly more effective (OR of 0.45 for both). Furthermore, 3 meta-analyses reported data on remission,[37,39,40] and found that ECT was superior to rTMS (with ORs ranging from 0.40 [95% CI, 0.23–0.68][39] to 0.46 [95% CI, 0.22–0.86][37]). Finally, 2 metaanalysis found similar acceptability between ECT and rTMS.[39,40]

Network meta-analyses of repetitive transcranial magnetic stimulation To date, there has been only 1 published network metaanalysis on rTMS for MD.[26] Briefly, in a network metaanalysis, multiple treatments are compared using both direct comparisons within RCTs and indirect "virtual" comparisons across RCTs based on a shared common comparator (eg, sham intervention).[41]

Table 2
Meta-analyses examining the differential efficacy of active rTMS protocols and of active rTMS compared with ECT for MD

Reference	Diagnosis	RCTs (n)	Patients (n)	SMD (95% CI)	SMD I² (%)	Response OR (95% CI)	Response I² (%)	Remission OR (95% CI)	Remission I² (%)	Dropout OR (95% CI)
High-frequency rTMS vs low-frequency rTMS										
Chen et al,[34] 2013	BD + MDD	7	221	—	—	1.15 (0.65–2.03)	0	—	—	2.71 (0.26–28.06)
Leggett et al,[35] 2015	BD + MDD	11	465	—	—	RR = 1.19 (0.97–1.46)[a]	0	RR = 1.29 (0.75–2.22)[a]	8.1	—
Brunoni et al,[45] 2016	BD + MDD	10	—	—	—	1.20 (0.70–2.04)	0	—	—	1.15 (0.38–3.53)
Bilateral rTMS vs other rTMS Protocols										
Chen et al,[36] 2014	BD + MDD	7	509	—	—	1.06 (0.58–1.91)	38	1.05 (0.52–2.11)	47	0.80 (0.25–2.50)
Zhang et al,[30] 2015	BD + MDD	10	634	—	—	1.95 (0.91–4.16)[b]	54	1.44 (0.37–5.63)[b]	75	—
rTMS vs ECT										
Slotema et al,[14] 2010	BD + MDD	6	215	−0.47 (NA)	28	—	—	—	—	—
Berlim et al,[37] 2013	BD + MDD	7	279	−0.93 (−1.61–0.26)	86.5	—	—	0.46 (0.22–0.96)	27.7	—
Xie et al,[40] 2013	BD + MDD	9	368	—	—	0.45 (0.13–0.89)	32	0.45 (0.13–0.89)	32	0.49 (0.29–0.85)
Ren et al,[39] 2014	BD + MDD	9	425	—	—	0.45 (0.21–0.97)[b]	49.8	0.40 (0.23–0.68)	13	1.07 (0.5–2.29)
Chen et al,[38] 2017	BD + MDD	7	509	—	—	0.64 (0.30–1.38)	—	—	—	—

Abbreviations: BD, bipolar disorder; CI, confidence interval; ECT, electroconvulsive therapy; MD, major depression; MDD, major depressive disorder; NA, not available; OR, odds ratio; RCT, randomized, controlled trial; RR, risk ratio; rTMS, repetitive transcranial magnetic stimulation; SMD, standardized mean difference.
[a] Could not be recomputed as an OR because the raw data were not presented.
[b] Original estimate recomputed as an OR.

With respect to response rates, the following active rTMS protocols were significantly more effective than sham: bilateral rTMS (OR, 3.96 [95% CI, 2.37–6.60]), HF-rTMS (OR, 3.07 [95% CI, 2.24–4.21]), LF-rTMS (OR, 2.37 [95% CI, 1.52–3.68]), TBS (OR, 2.54 [95% CI, 1.07–6.05]), and priming rTMS (OR, 4.66 [95% CI, 1.70–12.77]) (which involved a continuous, 15-minute train of LF-rTMS immediately preceded by twenty 5-second trains of 6 Hz HF-rTMS at low intensity[42]). The only rTMS intervention to separate from other active protocols in terms of higher response rates was bilateral rTMS compared with low-field synchronized rTMS (ie, OR, 3.65 [95% CI, 1.02–13.06]), a technique in which rotating magnets are used to deliver subthreshold sinusoidal waveform stimulation at the individual's alpha frequency.[43] Moreover, estimates relating to remission rates mirrored those observed for response (although they were more uncertain overall), with the exception of TBS, which was not found to be superior to sham. Also, priming rTMS was shown to be significantly more acceptable than sham, HF-rTMS, LF-rTMS, and synchronized rTMS.

Finally, there was evidence for large network heterogeneity for both response and remission, although there seemed to be little heterogeneity regarding dropout rates.

Meta-analyses on transcranial direct current stimulation for major depression

Five meta-analyses examining the efficacy of tDCS for MD were included in this meta-review[44–48] (Table 3), whereas 2 were excluded either because of a focus on tDCS-related affective switches[49] or the inclusion of open-label data.[50]

Transcranial direct current stimulation versus sham Five meta-analyses examined the efficacy of tDCS compared with sham for MD,[44–48] one of which considered individual patient-level data.[45]

In terms of pre–post depressive symptoms, 3 meta-analyses[45,47,48] reported significantly higher efficacy for active tDCS, with SMDs ranging from 0.30 (95% CI, 0.04–0.56)[47] to 0.37 (95% CI, 0.04–0.70),[48] whereas 1 failed to find support for the efficacy of tDCS[46] (however, the latter had the smallest pooled sample). With respect to response, 2 meta-analyses reported superior efficacy for active tDCS (OR, 1.63 [95% CI, 1.26–2.12][48] and OR, 2.44 [95% CI, 1.38–4.32][45]), and 2 reported negative results.[44,47] An examination of their methodologies suggests that Berlim and collaborators[44] only included RCTs published up until 2012 and, therefore, may have been statistically underpowered, and that Meron and colleagues[47] did not include a small RCT with very significant results[51] and also split the reporting for 1 RCT into 2 independent groups[52] (which may have influenced the final statistical weighting). Three meta-analyses examined remission,[44,45,48] and although the older one did not support the efficacy of tDCS,[44] the 2 more recent ones found superiority for active tDCS (ie, OR, 1.66 [95% CI, 1.32–2.10][48] and OR, 2.38 [95% CI, 1.22–4.64]). Finally, 2 meta-analyses[44,47] found similar acceptability between active tDCS and sham.

Meta-analyses on vagus nerve stimulation for major depression

Two meta-analyses[53,54] synthesized data on VNS for MD (Table 4). The first one[54] pooled 7 open-label trials (n = 399, mixed follow-up lengths), and reported a large effect size for change in depression scores from baseline (ie, SMD, 1.94 [95% CI, 1.36–2.52]), although with substantial between-study heterogeneity (ie, $I^2 = 83.86\%$). Moreover, it showed a heterogeneous response rate of 33.50% (95% CI, 23.9–44.8%; $I^2 = 69.82\%$).

The second metaanalysis,[53] using individual patient-level data, examined 6 clinical trials (with varied designs) and a total of 1460 patients with MD. The authors further investigated an independent sample of patients with treatment-resistant MD to bolster their "treatment as usual" comparison. Results at 96 weeks showed significantly

Table 3
Meta-analyses examining the efficacy of active tDCS compared with sham for MD

Reference	Diagnosis	RCTs (n)	Patients (n)	SMD (95% CI)	SMD I² (%)	Response OR (95% CI)	Response I² (%)	Remission OR (95% CI)	Remission I² (%)	Dropout OR (95% CI)
Kalu et al,[46] 2012	BD + MDD	6	176	0.74 (0.21–1.27)	61.4	—	—	—	—	—
Berlim et al,[44] 2013	BD + MDD	6	200	0.34 (0.12–0.57)	<2.5	1.97 (0.85–4.56)	7.5	2.13 (0.64–7.06)	0	0.89 (0.26–3.08)
Shiozawa et al,[48] 2014	BD + MDD	7	259	0.37 (0.04–0.70)	—	1.63 (1.26–2.12)	—	1.66 (1.32–2.10)	—	—
Meron et al,[47] 2015	BD + MDD	10	338	0.30 (0.04–0.57)	40	2.29 (0.69–7.58)[a]	0	—	—	1.12 (0.1–12.58)[a]
Brunoni et al,[45] 2016	BD + MDD	6	289	—	—	2.44 (1.38–4.32)	<2.5	2.38 (1.22–4.64)	<2.5	—

Abbreviations: BD, bipolar disorder; CI, confidence interval; MD, major depression; MDD, major depressive disorder; OR, odds ratio; RCT, randomized, controlled trial; SMD, standardized mean difference; tDCS, transcranial direct current stimulation.
[a] Original estimate recomputed as an OR.

Table 4
Meta-analyses examining the effectiveness of VNS for MD

Reference	Diagnosis	Studies (n)	Patients (n)	SMD (95% CI)	SMD I² (%)	Response ORª (95% CI)	Response I² (%)	Remission ORª (95% CI)	Remission I²
Martin & Martín-Sánchez,[54] 2012	BD + MDD	7	399	1.94 (1.36–2.52)	83.86	ER = 0.33 (0.24–0.45)	69.82	—	—
Berry et al,[53] 2013	BD + MDD	6	1576	—	—	3.19 (2.12–4.66)ᵇ	—	4.99 (2.93–7.76)ᵇ	—

Abbreviations: BD, bipolar disorder; CI, confidence interval; ER, event rate; MD, major depression; MDD, major depressive disorder; OR, odds ratio; SMD, standardized mean difference; VNS, vagus nerve stimulation.
ª Estimate calculated relative to "treatment as usual."
ᵇ At the 96-week follow-up.

higher rates of response and remission for depressed patients treated with VNS compared with "treatment as usual" (ie, OR, 3.19 [95% CI, 2.12–4.66] and OR, 4.99 [95% CI, 2.93–7.76], respectively).

Meta-analyses on deep brain stimulation for major depression

Two meta-analyses examined DBS for MD[55,56]; an additional study was excluded because it computed SMDs relative to simulated sham-treated patients.[57] Of the included metaanalysis, one restricted its scope to DBS of the subgenual/subcallosal cingulate,[55] whereas the other included several brain targets in addition to the latter (Table 5).[56]

Subgenual/subcallosal cingulate Both meta-analyses reported significant decreases in pre–post depressive symptoms at 12 months; however, their estimates varied substantially, and this was likely because Berlim and colleagues[55] restricted their analyses to trials with 12 or more months of prospective follow-up (and thus included a smaller total sample). Overall, the more restrictive metaanalysis[55] reported an SMD of 1.89 (95% CI, 1.15–2.64), whereas the more liberal one[56] reported an SMD of 3.02 (95% CI, 1.77–4.28). Finally, 1 metaanalysis reported rates of response and remission at 12 months of 39.90% (95% CI, 28.40%-52.80%) and 26.30% (95% CI, 13.00%-45.90%), respectively.[55]

Other brain targets Subgroup analyses[56] on different brain targets for DBS in MD reported the following significant SMDs for decreases in depressive symptoms compared with baseline: 1.19 (95% CI, 0.56–1.81) for the ventral capsule/ventral striatum (n = 55; mixed follow-up lengths), 1.40 (95% CI, 0.42–2.38) for the anterior limb of the internal capsule (n = 40; 12-month follow-up), 1.30 (95% CI, 0.44–2.16) for the nucleus accumbens (n = 14; mixed follow-up lengths), and 1.91 (95% CI, 0.81–3.01) for the medial forebrain bundle (n = 11; 12-month follow-up).

DISCUSSION

In the present meta-review, the authors summarized and critically appraised the meta-analytical literature on the use of therapeutic neuromodulation for MD published in the past decade. Overall, the majority of meta-analyses were dedicated to rTMS, followed by tDCS, and VNS/DBS. Although there were some differences with respect to estimates of clinical efficacy/effectiveness within each neuromodulation modality, there seems to be growing convergence as the respective fields gradually mature.

In terms of specific techniques, small to moderate effect sizes have been reported across active rTMS protocols. Moreover, analyses of response and remission rates suggest that the odds of improved outcomes are not only statistically but also clinically significant (ie, ORs >2). This literature has grown substantially over the past years, and analyses have become more refined and permitted comparison of different rTMS protocols both from pooled head-to-head RCTs as well as by network metaanalytical methods. Generally, few substantive differences between active rTMS protocols have been identified, though the network metaanalytical approach tentatively suggested that priming LF-rTMS (in comparison with sham, HF-rTMS, LF-rTMS, and synchronized rTMS) and bilateral rTMS (in comparison with synchronized rTMS) may be more acceptable and effective, respectively.[26] Moreover, the data comparing active rTMS with ECT demonstrated significant clinical superiority for the latter. Nevertheless, there remain substantial unanswered questions in this field that will hopefully be clarified as the primary literature expands. These questions include, for example, a more definitive determination of the usefulness of TBS protocols,[33] "accelerated"

Table 5
Meta-analyses examining the effectiveness of DBS for MD

Reference	Synthesized Time Point	Studies (n)	Patients (n)	SMD (95% CI)	SMD I² (%)	Response ER (95% CI)	Response I² (%)	Remission ER (95% CI)	Remission I² (%)	Dropout OR (95% CI)
Subgenual cingulate cortex										
Berlim et al,[55] 2014	12 mo	4	66	1.89 (1.15–2.64)	80.1	0.39 (0.28–0.52)	0.2	0.26 (0.13–0.45)	48.7	—
Zhou et al, in press	Mixed follow-up	6	77	3.02 (1.77–4.28)	83	—	—	—	—	—
Ventral capsule/ventral striatum										
Zhou et al, in press	Mixed follow-up	3	55	1.19 (0.56–1.81)	54	—	—	—	—	—
Anterior limb of the internal capsule										
Zhou et al, in press	12 mo	2	40	1.40 (0.42–2.38)	65	—	—	—	—	—
Nucleus accumbens										
Zhou et al, in press	Mixed follow-up	2	14	1.30 (0.44–2.16)	—	—	—	—	—	—
Medial forebrain bundle										
Zhou et al, in press	12 mo	2	11	1.91 (0.81–3.01)	0	—	—	—	—	—

Abbreviations: CI, confidence interval; DBS, deep brain stimulation; ER, event rate; MD, major depression; OR, odds ratio; SMD, standardized mean difference.

rTMS,[58] "deep" transcranial magnetic stimulation,[59] and the continuation/maintenance rTMS treatment.[60] Also, the stability of the medium-to long-term antidepressant effects of rTMS remains unclear, and this is especially relevant considering its labor-intensive and time-consuming nature.[4] Furthermore, the putative role of rTMS as a cognitive enhancer in MD[61] remains inadequately explored.

The field of tDCS for MD is rapidly growing and this is reflected in the number of currently available meta-analyses. Clearly, as more RCTs are published, the efficacy estimates will likely show a gradually more convincing separation between active tDCS and sham. As with rTMS, the effect sizes for tDCS seem to be in the small to moderate range, the odds of achieving response and remission straddle the threshold for clinical significance, and it seems to be an acceptable treatment overall. Future research on tDCS for MD should clarify, for example, whether differential efficacy exists between alternative protocols (eg, varying electrical currents and electrode placements) as well as the stability of its medium- to long-term antidepressant effects and its cognitive safety/benefits. Moreover, the usefulness of continuation/maintenance tDCS treatment should be further investigated.

Although psychosurgical interventions for MD have seen a resurgence in the last decade, they remain challenging to study owing to their invasiveness and the severity of the targeted pathology. Accordingly, the robustness of the scientific evidence associated with VNS and DBS for MD is inferior to that associated with noninvasive neuromodulation approaches. RCTs for psychosurgical interventions in MD are generally prohibitively expensive and their results have been often disappointing.[62–64] Yet, some brain targets have already passed this stringent test,[65] and interventions that have not demonstrated acute efficacy over sham have been tentatively shown, in longer term follow-up, to be associated with superior clinical outcomes when compared with "treatment as usual," although the interpretation of this finding remains complicated owing to issues inherent to psychosurgery. Clearly, substantial work is still needed to better clarify the neural network disturbances underlying MD as well as the putative ability of VNS and DBS to rectify them (particularly in patients for whom noninvasive neuromodulation has proved ineffective).

Limitations

This meta-review has a number of potential limitations. For example, the included meta-analyses often differed methodologically (eg, participant characteristics, treatment protocols, outcome assessments), and our findings are thus limited by their potential intrinsic shortcomings. Nevertheless, the reviewed studies are pioneering a nascent field and the associated variations in intervention can be difficult to capture with the metaanalytical method in these early stages of development. Also, because our literature search was limited to the last decade, meta-analyses published before 2007 were not directly assessed. Finally, as we limited our search to English-language articles, we may have missed studies published in other languages.

REFERENCES

1. Kupfer DJ, Frank E, Phillips ML. Major depressive disorder: new clinical, neurobiological, and treatment perspectives. Lancet 2012;379(9820):1045–55.
2. Sartorius N. The economic and social burden of depression. J Clin Psychiatry 2001;62(Suppl 15):8–11.
3. Rush AJ, Trivedi MH, Wisniewski SR, et al. Acute and longer-term outcomes in depressed outpatients requiring one or several treatment steps: a STAR*D report. Am J Psychiatry 2006;163(11):1905–17.

4. Schlaepfer TE, George MS, Mayberg H. WFSBP guidelines on brain stimulation treatments in psychiatry. World J Biol Psychiatry 2010;11(1):2–18.
5. Holtzheimer PE, Mayberg HS. Neuromodulation for treatment-resistant depression. F1000 Med Rep 2012;4:22.
6. Borenstein M, Hedges LV, Higgins JPT, et al. Introduction to meta-analysis. West Sussex (England): Wiley & Sons Ltd; 2009.
7. APA. Diagnostic and statistical manual of mental disorders (DSM-IV). 4th edition. Washington, DC: American Psychiatric Association; 1994.
8. WHO. The ICD-10 classification of mental and behavioural disorders: clinical descriptions and diagnostic guidelines. 10th edition. Geneva (Switzerland): World Health Organization; 1992.
9. Kraemer HC, Kupfer DJ. Size of treatment effects and their importance to clinical research and practice. Biol Psychiatry 2006;59(11):990–6.
10. Rosa MA, Lisanby SH. Somatic treatments for mood disorders. Neuropsychopharmacology 2012;37(1):102–16.
11. Berlim MT, Broadbent HJ, Van den Eynde F. Blinding integrity in randomized sham-controlled trials of repetitive transcranial magnetic stimulation for major depression: a systematic review and meta-analysis. Int J Neuropsychopharmacol 2013;16(5):1173–81.
12. Kedzior KK, Gellersen HM, Brachetti AK, et al. Deep transcranial magnetic stimulation (DTMS) in the treatment of major depression: an exploratory systematic review and meta-analysis. J Affect Disord 2015;187:73–83.
13. Micallef-Trigona B. Comparing the effects of repetitive transcranial magnetic stimulation and electroconvulsive therapy in the treatment of depression: a systematic review and meta-analysis. Depress Res Treat 2014;2014:135049.
14. Slotema CW, Blom JD, Hoek HW, et al. Should we expand the toolbox of psychiatric treatment methods to include Repetitive Transcranial Magnetic Stimulation (rTMS)? A meta-analysis of the efficacy of rTMS in psychiatric disorders. J Clin Psychiatry 2010;71(7):873–84.
15. Allan CL, Herrmann LL, Ebmeier KP. Transcranial magnetic stimulation in the management of mood disorders. Neuropsychobiology 2011;64(3):163–9.
16. Kedzior KK, Reitz SK. Short-term efficacy of repetitive transcranial magnetic stimulation (rTMS) in depression- reanalysis of data from meta-analyses up to 2010. BMC Psychol 2014;2(1):39.
17. Liu B, Zhang Y, Zhang L, et al. Repetitive transcranial magnetic stimulation as an augmentative strategy for treatment-resistant depression, a meta-analysis of randomized, double-blind and sham-controlled study. BMC Psychiatry 2014;14:342.
18. Gross M, Nakamura L, Pascual-Leone A, et al. Has repetitive transcranial magnetic stimulation (rTMS) treatment for depression improved? A systematic review and meta-analysis comparing the recent vs. the earlier rTMS studies. Acta Psychiatr Scand 2007;116(3):165–73.
19. Lam RW, Chan P, Wilkins-Ho M, et al. Repetitive transcranial magnetic stimulation for treatment-resistant depression: a systematic review and metaanalysis. Can J Psychiatry 2008;53(9):621–31.
20. McGirr A, Karmani S, Arsappa R, et al. Clinical efficacy and safety of repetitive transcranial magnetic stimulation in acute bipolar depression. World Psychiatry 2016;15(1):85–6.
21. Berlim MT, Van den Eynde F, Daskalakis ZJ. High-frequency repetitive transcranial magnetic stimulation accelerates and enhances the clinical response to antidepressants in major depression: a meta-analysis of randomized, double-blind, and sham-controlled trials. J Clin Psychiatry 2013;74(2):e122–9.

22. Gaynes BN, Lloyd SW, Lux L, et al. Repetitive transcranial magnetic stimulation for treatment-resistant depression: a systematic review and meta-analysis. J Clin Psychiatry 2014;75(5):477–89 [quiz: 489].

23. Berlim MT, van den Eynde F, Tovar-Perdomo S, et al. Response, remission and drop-out rates following high-frequency repetitive transcranial magnetic stimulation (rTMS) for treating major depression: a systematic review and meta-analysis of randomized, double-blind and sham-controlled trials. Psychol Med 2014;44(2):225–39.

24. Schutter DJ. Antidepressant efficacy of high-frequency transcranial magnetic stimulation over the left dorsolateral prefrontal cortex in double-blind sham-controlled designs: a meta-analysis. Psychol Med 2009;39(1):65–75.

25. Teng S, Guo Z, Peng H, et al. High-frequency repetitive transcranial magnetic stimulation over the left DLPFC for major depression: session-dependent efficacy: a meta-analysis. Eur Psychiatry 2017;41:75–84.

26. Brunoni AR, Chaimani A, Moffa AH, et al. Repetitive transcranial magnetic stimulation for the acute treatment of major depressive episodes: a systematic review with network meta-analysis. JAMA Psychiatry 2017;74(2):143–52.

27. Berlim MT, Van den Eynde F, Jeff Daskalakis Z. Clinically meaningful efficacy and acceptability of low-frequency repetitive transcranial magnetic stimulation (rTMS) for treating primary major depression: a meta-analysis of randomized, double-blind and sham-controlled trials. Neuropsychopharmacology 2013;38(4):543–51.

28. Schutter DJ. Quantitative review of the efficacy of slow-frequency magnetic brain stimulation in major depressive disorder. Psychol Med 2010;40(11):1789–95.

29. Berlim MT, Van den Eynde F, Daskalakis ZJ. A systematic review and meta-analysis on the efficacy and acceptability of bilateral repetitive transcranial magnetic stimulation (rTMS) for treating major depression. Psychol Med 2013;43(11):2245–54.

30. Zhang YQ, Zhu D, Zhou XY, et al. Bilateral repetitive transcranial magnetic stimulation for treatment-resistant depression: a systematic review and meta-analysis of randomized controlled trials. Braz J Med Biol Res 2015;48(3):198–206.

31. Huang Y-Z, Edwards MJ, Rounis E, et al. Theta burst stimulation of the human motor cortex. Neuron 2005;45:201–6.

32. Chung SW, Hoy KE, Fitzgerald PB. Theta-burst stimulation: a new form of TMS treatment for depression? Depress Anxiety 2015;32(3):182–92.

33. Berlim MT, McGirr A, Rodrigues Dos Santos N, et al. Efficacy of theta burst stimulation (TBS) for major depression: an exploratory meta-analysis of randomized and sham-controlled trials. J Psychiatr Res 2017;90:102–9.

34. Chen J, Zhou C, Wu B, et al. Left versus right repetitive transcranial magnetic stimulation in treating major depression: a meta-analysis of randomised controlled trials. Psychiatry Res 2013;210(3):1260–4.

35. Leggett LE, Soril LJ, Coward S, et al. Repetitive transcranial magnetic stimulation for treatment-resistant depression in adult and youth populations: a systematic literature review and meta-analysis. Prim Care Companion CNS Disord 2015;17(6).

36. Chen JJ, Liu Z, Zhu D, et al. Bilateral vs. unilateral repetitive transcranial magnetic stimulation in treating major depression: a meta-analysis of randomized controlled trials. Psychiatry Res 2014;219(1):51–7.

37. Berlim MT, Van den Eynde F, Daskalakis ZJ. Efficacy and acceptability of high frequency repetitive transcranial magnetic stimulation (rTMS) versus electroconvulsive therapy (ECT) for major depression: a systematic review and meta-analysis of randomized trials. Depress Anxiety 2013;30(7):614–23.

38. Chen JJ, Zhao LB, Liu YY, et al. Comparative efficacy and acceptability of elec-troconvulsive therapy versus repetitive transcranial magnetic stimulation for ma-jor depression: a systematic review and multiple-treatments meta-analysis. Behav Brain Res 2017;320:30–6.
39. Ren J, Li H, Palaniyappan L, et al. Repetitive transcranial magnetic stimulation versus electroconvulsive therapy for major depression: a systematic review and meta-analysis. Prog Neuropsychopharmacol Biol Psychiatry 2014;51:181–9.
40. Xie J, Chen J, Wei Q. Repetitive transcranial magnetic stimulation versus electro-convulsive therapy for major depression: a meta-analysis of stimulus parameter effects. Neurol Res 2013;35(10):1084–91.
41. Riley RD, Jackson D, Salanti G, et al. Multivariate and network meta-analysis of multiple outcomes and multiple treatments: rationale, concepts, and examples. BMJ 2017;358:j3932.
42. Fitzgerald PB, Hoy K, McQueen S, et al. Priming stimulation enhances the effec-tiveness of low-frequency right prefrontal cortex transcranial magnetic stimulation in major depression. J Clin Psychopharmacol 2008;28(1):52–8.
43. Leuchter AF, Cook IA, Jin Y, et al. The relationship between brain oscillatory ac-tivity and therapeutic effectiveness of transcranial magnetic stimulation in the treatment of major depressive disorder. Front Hum Neurosci 2013;7:37.
44. Berlim MT, Van den Eynde F, Daskalakis ZJ. Clinical utility of transcranial direct current stimulation (tDCS) for treating major depression: a systematic review and meta-analysis of randomized, double-blind and sham-controlled trials. J Psychiatr Res 2013;47(1):1–7.
45. Brunoni AR, Moffa AH, Fregni F, et al. Transcranial direct current stimulation for acute major depressive episodes: meta-analysis of individual patient data. Br J Psychiatry 2016;208(6):522–31.
46. Kalu UG, Sexton CE, Loo CK, et al. Transcranial direct current stimulation in the treatment of major depression: a meta-analysis. Psychol Med 2012;42(9):1791–800.
47. Meron D, Hedger N, Garner M, et al. Transcranial direct current stimulation (tDCS) in the treatment of depression: systematic review and meta-analysis of ef-ficacy and tolerability. Neurosci Biobehav Rev 2015;57:46–62.
48. Shiozawa P, Fregni F, Bensenor IM, et al. Transcranial direct current stimulation for major depression: an updated systematic review and meta-analysis. Int J Neuro-psychopharmacol 2014;17(9):1443–52.
49. Brunoni AR, Moffa AH, Sampaio-Junior B, et al. Treatment-emergent mania/hypo-mania during antidepressant treatment with transcranial direct current stimulation (tDCS): a systematic review and meta-analysis. Brain Stimul 2017;10(2):260–2.
50. Donde C, Amad A, Nieto I, et al. Transcranial direct-current stimulation (tDCS) for bipolar depression: a systematic review and meta-analysis. Prog Neuropsycho-pharmacol Biol Psychiatry 2017;78:123–31.
51. Fregni F, Boggio PS, Nitsche MA, et al. Treatment of major depression with trans-cranial direct current stimulation. Bipolar Disord 2006;8(2):203–4.
52. Brunoni AR, Valiengo L, Baccaro A, et al. The sertraline vs. electrical current ther-apy for treating depression clinical study: results from a factorial, randomized, controlled trial. JAMA Psychiatry 2013;70(4):383–91.
53. Berry SM, Broglio K, Bunker M, et al. A patient-level meta-analysis of studies eval-uating vagus nerve stimulation therapy for treatment-resistant depression. Med Devices (Auckl) 2013;6:17–35.
54. Martin JL, Martín-Sánchez E. Systematic review and meta-analysis of vagus nerve stimulation in the treatment of depression: variable results based on study designs. Eur Psychiatry 2012;27(3):147–55.

55. Berlim MT, McGirr A, Van den Eynde F, et al. Effectiveness and acceptability of deep brain stimulation (DBS) of the subgenual cingulate cortex for treatment-resistant depression: a systematic review and exploratory meta-analysis. J Affect Disord 2014;159:31–8.
56. Zhou C, Zhang H, Qin Y, et al. A systematic review and meta-analysis of deep brain stimulation in treatment-resistant depression. Prog Neuropsychopharmacol Biol Psychiatry 2018;82:224–32.
57. Smith DF. Exploratory meta-analysis on deep brain stimulation in treatment-resistant depression. Acta Neuropsychiatr 2014;26(6):382–4.
58. McGirr A, Van den Eynde F, Tovar-Perdomo S, et al. Effectiveness and acceptability of accelerated repetitive transcranial magnetic stimulation (rTMS) for treatment-resistant major depressive disorder: an open label trial. J Affect Disord 2015;173:216–20.
59. Levkovitz Y, Isserles M, Padberg F, et al. Efficacy and safety of deep transcranial magnetic stimulation for major depression: a prospective multicenter randomized controlled trial. World Psychiatry 2015;14(1):64–73.
60. Rachid F. Maintenance repetitive transcranial magnetic stimulation (rTMS) for relapse prevention in with depression: a review. Psychiatry Res 2018;262:363–72.
61. Martin DM, McClintock SM, Forster JJ, et al. Cognitive enhancing effects of rTMS administered to the prefrontal cortex in patients with depression: a systematic review and meta-analysis of individual task effects. Depress Anxiety 2017;34(11):1029–39.
62. Dougherty DD, Rezai AR, Carpenter LL, et al. A randomized sham-controlled trial of deep brain stimulation of the ventral capsule/ventral striatum for chronic treatment-resistant depression. Biol Psychiatry 2015;78(4):240–8.
63. Holtzheimer PE, Husain MM, Lisanby SH, et al. Subcallosal cingulate deep brain stimulation for treatment-resistant depression: a multisite, randomised, sham-controlled trial. Lancet Psychiatry 2017;4(11):839–49.
64. Rush AJ, Marangell LB, Sackeim HA, et al. Vagus nerve stimulation for treatment-resistant depression: a randomized, controlled acute phase trial. Biol Psychiatry 2005;58(5):347–54.
65. Bergfeld IO, Mantione M, Hoogendoorn ML, et al. Deep brain stimulation of the ventral anterior limb of the internal capsule for treatment-resistant depression: a randomized clinical trial. JAMA Psychiatry 2016;73(5):456–64.

Noninvasive Focused Ultrasound for Neuromodulation: A Review

Paul Bowary, MD[a],*, Benjamin D. Greenberg, MD, PhD[a,b,c]

KEYWORDS

• FUS • LIFU • Pulsation • Neuromodulation • Neurostimulation

KEY POINTS

• Low-intensity focused ultrasound (LIFU) can be used for intermittent (pulsation) or continuous brain stimulation for neuromodulation.

• LIFU is a potential alternative to other noninvasive neuromodulation techniques.

• LIFU offers potential ability to excite or inhibit neural activity, exquisite spatial resolution, and feasible use with simultaneous MRI.

• There remain substantial unanswered questions about the safety and efficacy of the technique at this early stage of its development.

INTRODUCTION

Focused ultrasound (FUS) has been of research and potential clinical interest as a neuromodulation method for over half a century.[1–5] However, over the past decade the interest in this technique has increased dramatically. High-intensity focused ultrasound (HIFU) is an approved technique for ablation of specific brain targets in the treatment of essential tremor[6,7] and chronic pain. Low-intensity focused ultrasound (LIFU) is unique among transcranial brain stimulation methods in combining exceptional spatial resolution (on the millimeter scale)[8–10] with the potential to target subcortical structures (deeper than 10 cm)[11] through the intact skull. It also has potential for inducing neuronal excitation or suppression without evidence of tissue damage.[12] Recent studies have shown neuromodulation effects—when LIFU is administered in pulsation mode[13]—translated onto behavioral outcomes,[14–16] electrophysiologic

Disclosure Statement: No disclosures.
[a] The Department of Psychiatry and Human Behavior, Alpert Medical School, Brown University, Providence, RI 02906, USA; [b] Butler Hospital, 345 Blackstone Boulevard, Providence, RI 02906, USA; [c] VA RR&D Center for Neurorestoration and Neurotechnology, Providence VA Medical Center, Providence, RI 02908, USA
* Corresponding author.
E-mail address: paul_bowary@brown.edu

Psychiatr Clin N Am 41 (2018) 505–514
https://doi.org/10.1016/j.psc.2018.04.010
0193-953X/18/© 2018 The Authors. Published by Elsevier Inc. This is an open access article under the CC BY-NC-ND license (http://creativecommons.org/licenses/by-nc-nd/4.0/).

recordings (electroencephalography [EEG]),[17–19] and functional MRI (fMRI).[20] Thus, LIFU may be useful in noninvasive neuromodulation. This article covers animal and human studies in this domain, including effects on tissue and blood-brain barrier (BBB) relevant to safety.

Ultrasound (US) waves are sound waves caused by cyclic mechanical vibrations occurring at frequencies higher than the upper audible human ear limit (>20 KHz). Although able to cause tissue heating at high intensities, US can be safe for human tissue when used at lower intensities, evidenced by its use for over the last several decades in clinical imaging. Whereas diagnostic ultrasonography uses frequencies in the megahertz range, transcranial ultrasound—and more specifically transcranial FUS —uses frequencies in the kilohertz range. This translates into more focused beams of US energy, targeting deeper brain structures and higher levels of precision compared with existing neuromodulatory approaches.

After a half-century hiatus, FUS is again center of vigorous research.[21–26] In the 1950s, Fry and colleagues[12] used FUS to produce a discrete lesion in the cat central nervous system while sparing nearby vasculature and tissue. They later demonstrated reversible suppression of evoked cortical potentials (visual cortex of cats) by FUS targeting the cat lateral geniculate nucleus. The same team showed that US close to the threshold for tissue damage caused reversible inhibition in animal's central nervous system, which they called "negative stimulation."[12] They were the first to consider the combination of high-intensity and high-frequency US and electrical fields for stimulation of neural structures—a theory that has not attracted research attention given significant high safety risks.[27] In 1990, Mihran and colleagues[28] were able to demonstrate significant alterations of nerve excitability in vitro using FUS pulsation.

It was not until 1995 that investigators pursued the use of nondestructive US to achieve lasting neuromodulation.[4] This line or research evaluated whether FUS could stimulate subcortical structures to induce different somatic outcomes and assist in the diagnosis of hearing disorders. In 1999, Hynynen and Sun[29] published an article describing the use of a helmet device in conjunction with real-time magnetic resonance (MR) and FUS for therapeutic practice. Since that time, the use of MR-guided FUS (MRgFUS) has been extensively explored in neurosurgery. MRgFUS is now approved by the US Food and Drug Administration (FDA) for thalamotomy-mediated treatment of essential tremor, as well as more than 26 publicly registered clinical trials targeting patients with brain tumors, Parkinson disease, Alzheimer disease, seizure disorders, and other neuropsychiatric disorders.[30–40]

In the mid 2000s, Hynynen, McDannold and colleagues[41–43] introduced the concept of disrupting the BBB using FUS coupled with the use of microbubbles (ie, <1 mm-diameter bubbles that oscillate on application of a sonic energy field and may thus reflect US wave trajectories). Since then, US-mediated opening of this barrier demonstrated potential for drastic improvement of the treatment of Alzheimer disease and may constitute a major turning point in neuro-oncology.[44]

Transcranial FUS can be divided into 2 major modalities: HIFU and LIFU[a]. In brief, HIFU is usually delivered to brain tissue as a continuous wave that has an acoustic intensity exceeding 200 W/cm^2. Its main mechanism is rapid heating of targeted tissue for ablation. In contrast, LIFU can stimulate intermittently (pulsation) or continuously

---

[a] In this article, the term LIFU will be used for low-intensity focused ultrasound delivered in pulsation mode, unless stated otherwise.

for nonheating–mediated neuromodulation. Delivery of US in a pulse mode is thought to further minimize chance of tissue heating. LIFU waves have an acoustic intensity that is less than 100 W/cm,[217,45] practically similar or even lower than the magnitude of diagnostic US intensities. This article focuses on the noninvasive and nonthermal effects (non–high-intensity ablative effects) of FUS and thus on the line of research that has been studying the potential of LIFU as a new amenity for transcranial stimulation.

OVERVIEW OF LOW-INTENSITY FOCUSED ULTRASOUND
Low-Intensity Focused Ultrasound: A Promising New Approach to Transcranial Stimulation

Today, brain stimulation has paved its way through research and clinical practice, whereas transcranial magnetic stimulation (TMS), transcranial current stimulation (TCS), and deep brain stimulation (DBS) are being broadly used or studied in neuropsychiatry. However, each of these approaches has known limitations, thus providing important areas of technical improvement. In particular, currently used brain stimulation techniques have low spatial resolution and thus lack specificity (TMS and TCS), are limited to superficial target points (TMS), or involve invasive procedures (DBS). LIFU, on the other hand, is able to focus an US beam through intact skull bone and thus precisely target small brain areas. FUS-induced changes were actually shown to be abolished when the US beam was centered 1 cm anterior or posterior to the region of interest, demonstrating spatial specificity that is superior to TMS and TCS.[17] Furthermore, unlike the technical difficulties of combining TMS and MRI,[11,46–49] simultaneous MR + FUS is already an FDA-approved intervention and thus ready for further investigation for neuropsychiatric use.

Low-Intensity Focused Ultrasound Neuromodulation: From Animal Studies to Human Trials

The neuromodulatory effects of FUS, more specifically LIFU, described earlier were demonstrated in a large number of animal studies over the past 20 years.[11,24,50,51] This article synthesizes this information and provides an integrated description of animal and human research outcomes.

Electroencephalography and bimodal modulatory effects

As mentioned earlier in this article, Fry and colleagues pioneered the studies of US effects on evoked EEG potentials in the 1950s. They specifically showed EEG suppression in a cat model, a phenomenon that was reproduced on rabbits[10] and rats[52,53] by different teams in 2011 to 2015 period. In 2011, Min and colleagues[18] were able to show that focused low-intensity pulsed sonication inhibited part of the seizure activity in a rat epilepsy model. The suppression was quantified by amount of epileptic EEG spikes. These spikes were shown to be mostly diminished—after sonication—in the frequency band that correlates with intensity of epilepsy. Human EEG studies were conducted in the same time period and were able to show similar transcranial FUS–induced suppression phenomenon. In 2014, Legon, Tyler, and colleagues demonstrated that amplitudes of S1-evoked potentials can be significantly attenuated (over different frequency bands than what is mentioned earlier) using LIFU. Those electrophysiologic outcomes were seen in conjunction with enhancement effects on sensory discrimination ability.[17,45] Thus, the results mentioned earlier showed similar LIFU-mediated EEG suppression effect in animals and humans, while targeting different subcortical or cortical areas, affecting multiple frequency bands, and leading to distinct neurologic and behavioral outcomes.

The number of US pulses delivered per second was shown to correlate with the described binary outcome. Sonication with a pulse repetition frequency (PRF) of 100 Hz was required to achieve *inhibition*, whereas increasing the PRF to 500 Hz would lead to almost an opposite effect, which is prolonged yet reversible "facilitation" of the evoked EEG response.[52,53] In fact, using MRgFUS—set at LIFU parameters—to sonicate S1 at a PRF of 500 Hz produced somatic and electrophysiologic outcomes identical to those induced by median nerve *stimulation*.

Behavioral and higher-level cognitive modulation using low-intensity focused ultrasound

In 2013, Deffieux and colleagues[15] demonstrated that LIFU can modulate visuomotor behavior in monkeys. Two awake macaque rhesus monkeys were trained to initiate a saccade in opposite direction to new visual targets. They were first required to fixate on a central target. Then, a red stimulus was introduced in the periphery while one of the monkeys was receiving a hemifield 320 kHZFUS stimulation. Anti-saccade (AS) latency was measured in both subjects and found to be temporarily delayed on the ipsilateral side of FUS frontal eye field stimulation. No similar effects were seen in sham stimulation or during control experiment (in this case, stimulation of premotor cortex). The main explanation of these outcomes is that FUS disrupted information processing across the frontal eye field, thus demonstrating FUS can modulate behavior. In the same year, Sanguinetti and colleagues[21] applied low-intensity/high-frequency (8 MHz) US for a total duration of 15 seconds over the posterior frontal cortex in humans and reported nonspecific improvement in mood and decreased pain sensation. This was followed by studies by Legon and colleagues[17,45] in 2014, where they showed evidence that FUS modulated the activity of S1 and enhanced discrimination ability.

Optimal Sonication Parameters

Ex-vivo/in-vitro studies conducted in 2008 and 2009 by 2 different researcher teams (Muratore and colleagues and Tyler and colleagues[54]) demonstrated that LIFU can cause time-locked action potentials, electrolyte imbalances, and signs of synaptic vesicle release.[55] Those 3 factors were considered as primary ingredients of neuromodulation. Then, multiple in-vivo animal studies that focused on these factors consistently showed that the stimulation parameters needed to elicit a response were stimulus duration of 10s to 100s of ms, high duty cycles (>50%), and lower rather than higher frequencies (250–350 KHzvs 500–650 KHz) to help minimize the concerns for acoustic beam refraction/absorption by the skull.[52,55–57]

These studies suggest that response ratio is closely related to intensity, duration, and duty cycle of the FUS stimulus. Kim and colleagues who have studied these parameters suggested the idea of a threshold, which they called "sweet spot." at which response peaks and above which it decreases. They suggested duty cycle of 50% and stimulus duration of 300 ms as the optimum "sweet spot" for their experiment on rats.[52] In this same study, LIFU pulsation was shown to require lower intensities than continuous LIFU to induce the same motor response, inviting researchers to use pulse-mode stimulation approach as a potentially safer technique for future clinical applications. This work was continued by Lee and colleagues, who used LIFU (pulsation) to target sheep brain and were able to develop the idea of "sweet spot" further. They demonstrated the presence of acoustic thresholds (sonication intensities) necessary to elicit both motor and visual evoked potentials. They also presented evidence of a graded response to FUS. Similar to findings in TMS studies, the magnitude of response in this study depended on the level of stimulation intensity.[58]

Role of Low-Intensity Focused Ultrasound in Neural and Functional Connectivity

Tufail and colleagues[55] sonicated primary motor cortex of mice using LIFU and were able to demonstrate direct movement of corresponding paws, whiskers, and tail. Min and colleagues[26] delivered FUS to the thalamus to modulate thalamocortical neurotransmitter levels. These, among other studies, demonstrated that LIFU can have its effects on both corticospinal and thalamocortical pathways—both important aspects of currently available treatments—indicating that LIFU can modulate clinically relevant targets.

In 2016, Lee and colleagues[59] sonicated the human primary visual cortex (V1) with LIFU. The introduction of fMRI in this study helped in showing that the sonication effects were not limited to the visual circuits but expanded to involve remote areas in the brain, mainly the attention networks in cognitive processing (fronto-temporoparietal areas and cerebellum) as well as the memory/navigation/recognition networks (parahippocampal gyrus and thalamus). Thus, LIFU targeting V1 increased neural activity at the level of stimulation as well as at the level of brain networks involved in higher-order visual and cognitive processing.[59]

In 2017, Sanguinetti and colleagues[23] reported possible changes in brain connectivity that may be associated with change in mood seen after FUS targeted the right inferior frontal gyrus (rIFG) in healthy volunteers. Specifically, using fMRI, they demonstrated increased connectivity in the dorsolateral prefrontal cortex, the medial prefrontal cortex, and rIFG (considered as cognitive control areas), whereas they also reported decreased connectivity between rIFG and parts of the limbic system.[23] This is the first time FUS, specifically LIFU, neuromodulation is demonstrated to affect neural network activity in humans.

Safety Concerns of Low-Intensity Focused Ultrasound

The acoustic energy of FUS can eventually be transformed into thermal or nonthermal energy. The latter can be categorized into mechanical force or cavitation (gas bubbles resulting from shockwave fluctuations).[60] Both thermal and sometimes cavitation effects of HIFU can be used in neurosurgery (eg, brain tumor ablation) or neurology (eg, ablation of epileptic foci). Although the possibility of tissue damage at this level of sonication is high, LIFU uses much lower levels of acoustic energy and seems to be safe. To this end, a review of multiple studies that involved histologic examination of tissue targeted with LIFU showed no signs of heat or cavitation.[11] Nevertheless, Lee and colleagues[58] who conducted the sheep study mentioned earlier recommended caution even in applying LIFU, because in their study microhemorrhages were seen on postsonication histology (V1 areas) of animals that received "highly repetitive" low-intensity sonication (which was quantified as every second for more than 500 times).

Table 1 depicts the main potential risks carried by FUS as well as details of how and when they are addressed. Following up on Hynynen, McDannold and colleagues'[41–43] studies related to temporary disruption of the BBB via FUS, few papers were published regarding safety of FUS-mediated BBB opening. Downs and colleagues[61] used FUS to open the BBB at the level of the caudate nucleus and the putamen of anesthetized primates and monitored safety through vital signs (VS)/physiologic changes checks, MRI analysis, and behavioral testing. No significant physiologic or

Table 1
Possible safety concerns associated with low-intensity focused ultrasound

	BBB Opening	Free Radicals	Overheating	Nonthermal Cavitation Effects	Hemorrhage
Risk	1. Prolonged BBB opening may promote unsafe brain entry of cells (eg, red blood cells, macrophages, viruses, bacteria, etc...) or proteins and peptides 2. Failure of the BBB to reclose	Sonication can form free radicals (short-lived yet very unstable)—possible inflammation and tissue damage	Typically generated at high acoustic intensity only (ideally not seen with LIFU)		
Recommendations	Cautious approach to controlling the degree of BBB opening may protect against some of these concerns[62]	Typically generated at high acoustic intensity only (ideally not seen with LIFU)			

major VS variations were reported. No evidence of hemorrhage was identified on MRI, whereas some edema in few subjects was fully reversible within 1 week.

Furthermore, continuous transcranial US stimulation has been used for decades in echoencephalography without safety concerns. Moreover, the FDA has determined and published the maximum allowed parameters of sonication for diagnostic purposes. These regulations cover the thermal index (level of heating), the mechanical index (level of mechanical effects), the spatial-peak temporal-average intensity (Ispta), and the spatial-peak pulse-average intensity (Isppa). Ispta and Isppa are in mW/cm^2 units (**Table 2**). Using these numbers as sonication limits when administering LIFU may be a safe approach toward determining specific LIFU safety parameters. Of note, in 2016, Lee and colleagues[59] stimulated V1 in humans without tissue damage using energy doses higher than the FDA limits described earlier, underscoring the safety of LIFU and also the importance of future research into more precise safety

Table 2
Food and Drug Administration limits of acoustic output level of diagnostic ultrasound

Acoustic Factor	Maximum Allowed Level
TI	6.0
MI	1.9
Ispta	720
Isppa	190

Abbreviations: Isppa, spatial-peak pulse-average intensity (unit is mW/cm2); Ispta, spatial-peak temporal-average intensity (unit is mW/cm2); MI, mechanical index; TI, thermal index.

parameters. However, as with any emerging technology, long-term follow-up safety studies are yet to be performed.

SUMMARY AND FUTURE DIRECTIONS

In this article, the authors described representative animal and human studies on ultrasonic neuromodulation. LIFU has significant potential for near-term implementation as a research and clinical tool. Reasons underscoring this potential include its ability to induce different patterns of neural activity, high spatial resolution, ease of application with fMRI, modest safety concerns, and early studies suggesting that LIFU might modulate neural networks involved in psychiatric disorders. These advantages being stated, there remains important work regarding parameter estimation and ideal use of LIFU in neuropsychiatric disorders and careful testing in controlled trials before LIFU will be clinically available.

REFERENCES

1. Lynn JG, Putnam TJ. Histology of cerebral lesions produced by focused ultrasound. Am J Pathol 1944;20(3):637–49.
2. Fry WJ, Barnard JW, Fry EJ, et al. Ultrasonic lesions in the mammalian central nervous system. Science 1955;122(3168):517–8.
3. Rinaldi PC, Jones JP, Reines F, et al. Modification by focused ultrasound pulses of electrically evoked responses from an in vitro hippocampal preparation. Brain Res 1991;558(1):36–42.
4. Gavrilov LR, Tsirulnikov EM, Davies IA. Application of focused ultrasound for the stimulation of neural structures. Ultrasound Med Biol 1996;22(2): 179–92.
5. Ballantine HT Jr, Bell E, Manlapaz J. Progress and problems in the neurological applications of focused ultrasound. J Neurosurg 1960;17(5):858–76.
6. Lipsman N, Schwartz ML, Huang Y, et al. MR guided focused ultrasound thalamotomy for essential tremor: a proof-of-concept study. Lancet Neurol 2013; 12(5):462–8.
7. Martin E, Jeanmonod D, Morel A, et al. High-intensity focused ultrasound for noninvasive functional neurosurgery. Ann Neurol 2009;66(6):858–61.
8. Mehić E, Xu JM, Caler CJ, et al. Increased anatomical specificity of neuromodulation via modulated focused ultrasound. PLoS One 2014;9(2):e86939.
9. Robertson JLB, Cox BT, Jaros J, et al. Accurate simulation of transcranial ultrasound propagation for ultrasonic neuromodulation and stimulation. J AcoustSoc Am 2017;141(3):1726.
10. Yoo S-S, Bystritsky A, Lee J-H, et al. Focused ultrasound modulates region-specific brain activity. Neuroimage 2011;56(3):1267–75.
11. Rezayat E, Toostani IG. A review on brain stimulation using low intensity focused ultrasound. BasicClinNeurosci 2016;7(3):187–94.
12. Fry FJ, Ades HW, Fry WJ. Production of reversible changes in the central nervous system by ultrasound. Science 1958;127(3289):83–4.
13. Fini M, Tyler WJ. Transcranial focused ultrasound: a new tool for non-invasive neuromodulation. Int Rev Psychiatry 2017;29(2):168–77.
14. Lee W, Kim H, Lee S, et al. Creation of various skin sensations using pulsed focused ultrasound: evidence for functional neuromodulation. Int J ImagSyst Tech 2014;24(2):167–74.
15. Deffieux T, Younan Y, Wattiez N, et al. Low-intensity focused ultrasound modulates monkey visuomotor behavior. CurrBiol 2013;23(23):2430–3.

16. Kim H, Lee SD, Chiu A, et al. Estimation of the spatial profile of neuromodulation and the temporal latency in motor responses induced by focused ultrasound brain stimulation. Neuroreport 2014;25(7):475–9.

17. Mueller J, Legon W, Opitz A, et al. Transcranial focused ultrasound modulates intrinsic and evoked EEG dynamics. Brain Stimul 2014;7(6):900–8.

18. Min B-K, Bystritsky A, Jung K-I, et al. Focused ultrasound-mediated suppression of chemically-induced acute epileptic EEG activity. BMCNeurosci 2011;12:23.

19. Yu K, Sohrabpour A, He B. Electrophysiological source imaging of brain networks perturbed by low-intensity transcranial focused ultrasound. IEEE Trans Biomed Eng 2016;63(9):1787–94.

20. Leo AI, Mueller JK, Grant A, et al. Transcranialfocused ultrasound for BOLD fMRI signal modulation in humans. ConfProcIEEEEng Med BiolSoc 2016;2016: 1758–61.

21. Sanguinetti JL, Smith EE, Tyler WJ, et al. Transcranial ultrasound (Tus) brain stimulation affects mood in healthy human volunteers with a prototype ultrasound device. Psychophysiology 2014;51:S42.

22. Meng Y, Suppiah S, Mithani K, et al. Current and emerging brain applications of MR-guided focused ultrasound. J TherUltrasound 2017;5:26.

23. Sanguinetti J, Allen JJB. Transcranial ultrasound improves mood and affects resting state functional connectivity in healthy volunteers. Brain Stimulation: Basic, Translational, and Clinical Research in Neuromodulation 2017;10(2):426.

24. Baek H, Pahk KJ, Kim H. A review of low-intensity focused ultrasound for neuromodulation. Biomed EngLett 2017;7(2):135–42.

25. Gavrilov LR, Tsirulnikov EM. Focused ultrasound as a tool to input sensory information to humans [review]. AcoustPhys 2012;58(1):1–21.

26. Min BK, Yang PS, Bohlke M, et al. Focused ultrasound modulates the level of cortical neurotransmitters: potential as a new functional brain mapping technique. Int J ImagSyst Tech 2011;21(2):232–40.

27. Fry WJ. Electrical stimulation of brain localized without probes–theoretical analysis of a proposed method. J AcoustSoc Am 1968;44(4):919–31.

28. Mihran RT, Barnes FS, Wachtel H. Temporally-specific modification of myelinated axon excitability in vitro following a single ultrasound pulse. Ultrasound Med Biol 1990;163:297–309.

29. Hynynen K, Sun J. Trans-skull ultrasound therapy: the feasibility of using image-derived skull thickness information to correct the phase distortion. IEEE Trans UltrasonFerroelectrFreqControl 1999;46(3):752–5.

30. Ram Z, Cohen ZR, Harnof S, et al. Magnetic resonance imaging-guided, high-intensity focused ultrasound for brain tumor therapy. Neurosurgery 2006;59(5): 949–55.

31. McDannold N, Clement GT, Black P, et al. Transcranial magnetic resonance imaging-guided focused ultrasound surgery of brain tumors: initial findings in 3 patients. Neurosurgery 2010;66(2):323–32.

32. Bauer R, Martin E, Haegele-Link S, et al. Noninvasive functional neurosurgery using transcranialMR imaging-guided focused ultrasound. ParkinsonismRelatDisord 2014;20(Suppl 1):S197–9.

33. Na YC, Chang WS, Jung HH, et al. Unilateral magnetic resonance-guided focused ultrasound pallidotomy for Parkinson disease. Neurology 2015;85(6): 549–51.

34. Tsai S-J. Therapeutic potential of transcranial focused ultrasound for Rett syndrome. Med SciMonit 2016;22:4026–9.

35. Mueller JK, Ai L, Bansal P, et al. Numerical evaluation of the skull for human neuromodulation with transcranial focused ultrasound. J Neural Eng 2017;14(6): 066012.
36. Elias WJ, Khaled M, Hilliard JD, et al. A magnetic resonance imaging, histological, and dose modeling comparison of focused ultrasound, radiofrequency, and gamma knife radiosurgery lesions in swine thalamus. J Neurosurg 2013;119(2): 307–17.
37. McDannold N, Livingstone M, Top CB, et al. Preclinical evaluation of a low-frequency transcranial MRI-guided focused ultrasound system in a primate model. Phys Med Biol 2016;61(21):7664–87.
38. Hameroff S, Trakas M, Duffield C, et al. Transcranial ultrasound (TUS) effects on mental states: a pilot study. Brain Stimul 2013,6(3).409–15.
39. Piper RJ, Hughes MA, Moran CM, et al. Focused ultrasound as a non-invasive intervention for neurological disease: a review. Br J Neurosurg 2016;30(3): 286–93.
40. Krishna V, Sammartino F, Rezai A. A review of the current therapies, challenges, and future directions of transcranial focused ultrasound technology: advances in diagnosis and treatment. JAMA Neurol 2018;75(2):246–54.
41. Hynynen K, McDannold N, Vykhodtseva N, et al. Noninvasive MR imaging-guided focal opening of the blood-brain barrier in rabbits. Radiology 2001; 220(3):640–6.
42. McDannold N, Vykhodtseva N, Raymond S, et al. MRI-guided targeted blood-brain barrier disruption with focused ultrasound: histological findings in rabbits. Ultrasound Med Biol 2005;31(11):1527–37.
43. McDannold N, Vykhodtseva N, Hynynen K. Use of ultrasound pulses combined with Definity® for targeted blood-brain barrier disruption: a feasibility study. Ultrasound Med Biol 2007;33(4):584–90.
44. Chu PC, Liu HL, Lai HY, et al. Neuromodulation accompanying focused ultrasound-induced blood-brain barrier opening. SciRep 2015;5:15477.
45. Legon W, Sato TF, Opitz A, et al. Transcranial focused ultrasound modulates the activity of primary somatosensory cortex in humans. Nat Neurosci 2014;17(2): 322–9.
46. Ulmer S, Jansen O. Combining transcranial magnetic stimulation with (f) MRI. Berlin: Spriner Heidelberg; 2013. p. 283–97, fMRI.
47. Peterchev AV, Wagner TA, Miranda PC, et al. Fundamentals of transcranial electric and magnetic stimulation dose: definition, selection, and reporting practices. Brain Stimulation 2012;5(4):435–53.
48. Mueller JK, Legon W, Tyler WJ. Analysis of transcranial focused ultrasound beam profile sensitivity for neuromodulation of the human brain. arXiv:150302019 [q-bio]. 2015.
49. Lee W, Chung Y-A, Jung Y, et al. Simultaneous acoustic stimulation of human primary and secondary somatosensory cortices using transcranial focused ultrasound. BMCNeurosci 2016;17(1):68.
50. Naor O, Krupa S, Shoham S. Ultrasonic neuromodulation. J NeuralEng 2016; 13(3):031003.
51. Bystritsky A, Korb AS, Douglas PK, et al. A review of low-intensity focused ultrasound pulsation. Brain Stimulation 2011;4(3):125–36.
52. Kim H, Chiu A, Lee SD, et al. Focused ultrasound-mediated non-invasive brain stimulation: examination of sonication parameters. Brain Stimul 2014;7(5):748–56.
53. Lee W, Kim H, Jung Y, et al. Image-guided transcranial focused ultrasound stimulates human primary somatosensory cortex. Sci Rep 2015;5:8743.

54. Tyler WJ, Tufail Y, Finsterwald M, et al. Remote excitation of neuronal circuits using low intensity, low-frequency ultrasound. PLoS One 2008;3(10):e3511.
55. Tufail Y, Matyushov A, Baldwin N, et al. Transcranial pulsed ultrasound stimulates intact brain circuits. Neuron 2010;66(5):681–94.
56. King RL, Brown JR, Newsome WT, et al. Effective parameters for ultrasound-induced in vivo neurostimulation. Ultrasound Med Biol 2013;39(2):312–31.
57. King RL, Brown JR, Pauly KB. Localization of ultrasound-induced in vivo neurostimulation in the mouse model. Ultrasound Med Biol 2014;40(7):1512–22.
58. Lee W, Lee SD, Park MY, et al. Image-guided focused ultrasound-mediated regional brain stimulation in sheep. Ultrasound Med Biol 2016;42(2):459–70.
59. Lee W, Kim H-C, Jung Y, et al. Transcranial focused ultrasound stimulation of human primary visual cortex. Scientific Rep 2016;6:34026.
60. O'Brien WD. Ultrasound-biophysics mechanisms. ProgBiophysMolBiol 2007; 93(1–3):212–55.
61. Downs ME, Buch A, Sierra C, et al. Long-term safety of repeated blood-brain barrier opening via focused ultrasound with microbubbles in non-human primates performing a cognitive task. PLoSOne 2015;10(5):e0125911.
62. Bystritsky A, Korb AS. A review of low-intensity transcranial focused ultrasound for clinical applications. CurrBehavNeurosci Rep 2015;2:60–6.

The Future of Brain Stimulation Treatments

Kevin A. Caulfield, MS[a,b,*], Mark S. George, MD[a,b]

KEYWORDS

- tDCS • LIFUP • Focused ultrasound • tACS • Speed of onset • Durability • Circuit

KEY POINTS

- Over the past 80 years, several trends emerged in the field of brain stimulation that are likely to continue into the future, including being less invasive, more focal, better integrated with behavior, and using less energy.
- There are also several exciting new methods that may be disruptive in the field, including pulsed ultrasound stimulation and temporally interfering fields.
- The future growth of brain stimulation is promising. The focal nature of the stimulation produces minimal systemic side effects.
- Technology continues to advance to create even better stimulation methods. And we better understand the neuroplasticity methods by which to change the brain.

INTRODUCTION

Since Cerletti's first use of electroconvulsive therapy (ECT) in 1938, several themes have emerged in the field of brain stimulation. These include, with new technologies and even within existing technologies, gradual decreases in stimulation intensity, greater focality of treatment, increased specificity of brain stimulation targets, and greater public acceptance of therapeutic neuromodulation.

Remember that modern neuromodulation arose on a foundation of psychopharmacologic advancements in the 1920s and 1930s. Manfred Sankel and Ladislaus von Meduna recognized that overdoses of insulin and pentylenetetrazol (metrazol) that caused seizures improved schizophrenic symptoms.[1–3] Drawing on these clinical observations, Ugo Cerletti, an Italian epileptologist, developed ECT in 1938 as a means of producing seizures to remediate psychoses and, later, depression.[4] Cerletti's ECT 80 years ago was an epoch-shifting invention. For the first time, researchers and clinicians could reliably stimulate the human brain and the field of brain stimulation (or neuromodulation) was born. The next paradigm-shifting neuromodulation

[a] Brain Stimulation Laboratory, Medical University of South Carolina, 67 President Street, 502 North, Charleston, SC 29425, USA; [b] Ralph H. Johnson VA Medical Center, 109 Bee Street, Charleston, SC 29401, USA
* Corresponding author. 67 President Street, 502 North, Charleston, SC 29425.
E-mail address: caulfiel@musc.edu

Psychiatr Clin N Am 41 (2018) 515–533
https://doi.org/10.1016/j.psc.2018.05.004
0193-953X/18/© 2018 Elsevier Inc. All rights reserved.

invention, transcranial magnetic stimulation (TMS), grew out of creative thinking in response to a tricky problem and highlights how the field has historically moved toward using less invasive, lower energy stimulation. In 1980 at Queen Square in London, UK, Patrick Merton and Bert Morton found that transcranial electrical stimulation, applied at around 60 to 100 mA of electrical current through the scalp, could effectively cause muscle twitches and phosphenes (flashes of light) yet was too uncomfortable and even painful to tolerate.[5–7] Ingeniously reasoning that briefly pulsing electrical current through a loop of metal wire would create an electromagnetic field (Faraday's law), which in turn could cause neuronal discharge at the cortex without direct electrical stimulation through the skull, Tony Barker, working in Sheffield, UK, took aim at creating the first modern TMS device. Over several years and many failed machines (and some big explosions!), Barker was able to create a TMS machine and coil that could stimulate the cortex without significant pain. Now there was a method of focal and relatively pain-free brain stimulation of the superficial cortex in an awake and alert human! The subsequent neuroimaging revolution of the 1980s and 1990s was the key that unlocked the therapeutic potential of TMS and continues to be the background for evaluating and using neuromodulation. New neuroimaging methods, such as PET and MRI, allowed scientists to observe, for the first time, the structural and functional status of the brain, in health and pathology, and in real time (ie, before death). Armed with this information, neuroscientists now had maps of where potentially to apply transcranial brain stimulation in different diseases. In 1994, psychiatrists began to use TMS in medication-resistant depression (as defined by inadequate clinical response to ≥2 pharmacologic therapies).[8] Several multisite, double-blind controlled clinical trials, including the industry-independent OPT-TMS trial published in 2010,[9] firmly established its efficacy in acutely treating depression. In 2008, the US Food and Drug Administration (FDA) first cleared a TMS device, and now 6 TMS devices are FDA cleared for the acute treatment of depression. Herein, we highlight the key considerations and trends of neuromodulation and discuss and digest the use of several new preclinical and clinical brain stimulation technologies.

CONSIDERATION 1: NEUROMODULATION HAS BECOME LESS INVASIVE

A hallmark feature of neuromodulation over the past 80 years is the decreasing invasiveness of stimulation. By less invasive, we refer to the trend of subsequently developed forms of noninvasive brain stimulation using less strength of electrical or electromagnetic current over time (**Fig. 1**). To understand this, it is best to compare the amount of electricity that each brain stimulation method actually delivers. Many of us do not have a working knowledge of a milliamp, like we do an inch or a pound (or kilogram). We can, however, understand energy as how long it takes to power a light bulb (because this gets reflected in a utility bill we pay each month!). Using this scale ECT, which uses the greatest amount of energy in a single treatment session, only applies enough voltage and current to power a 60W light bulb for a mere 10 seconds. (Much to the surprise of even our laboratory's brilliant biomedical engineer, whose off-the-cuff guess was orders of magnitude longer). A single treatment session of the subsequent forms of neuromodulation would power the same light bulb for even less time: all less than 4 seconds!.

Another way to grasp this is to compare the summed amount of exogenous energy applied over a treatment session or treatment course to the amount of endogenous energy used by the brain in the same amount of time (**Fig. 2**). Because the human brain operates at 20 W, it produces enough energy constantly to power the 60 W light bulb one-third of the amount of time of the course of stimulation. For the 4 weeks a typical

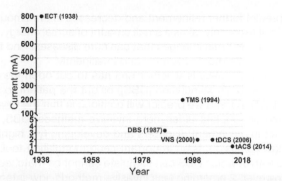

Fig. 1. The amount of delivered electrical current (mA) in brain stimulation techniques has decreased over time. Year indicates first clinical use of each stimulation method; current refers to current delivered in a single pulse (deep brain stimulation [DBS], electroconvulsive therapy [ECT], transcranial magnetic stimulation [TMS], vagal nerve stimulation [VNS]) or steady electrical current (transcranial alternating current stimulation [tACS], transcranial direct current stimulation [tDCS]).

ECT course of 8 to 12 sessions takes, the background brain activity uses enough energy to power a 60 W light bulb for 806,400 seconds. This background brain energy creation and use is more than 80,000 times greater than the extrinsic energy that ECT delivers! That is, during a course of ECT, doctors deliver only 1/80,000 of the energy the brain uses over that time. A small addition indeed. All the brain stimulation methods use relatively amazingly small amounts of energy compared with the idling energy use of the background organ, the brain. Given the trend toward decreasing amounts of stimulation, the difference between the energy applied relative to the brain use is even more pronounced for TMS (TMS delivers 1/1,000,000 [millionth] the amount of energy the brain uses over 6 weeks). As the field of neuromodulation

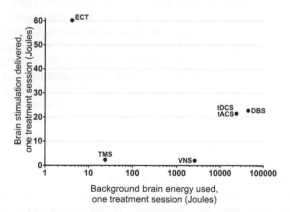

Fig. 2. The amount of background brain energy used during the course of one treatment session dwarfs the amount of brain stimulation energy delivered, electroconvulsive therapy being the sole exception. We calculated the total brain stimulation energy from the actual duration of current delivery (taking into account frequency, number of pulses, phase, and pulse width). DBS, deep brain stimulation; ECT, electroconvulsive therapy; tACS, transcranial alternating current stimulation; tDCS, transcranial direct current stimulation; TMS, transcranial magnetic stimulation; VNS, vagal nerve stimulation.

progresses, we predict further refinement and decreases in the amount of energy we deliver to the brain. It likely only takes a small amount of actual energy, precisely delivered and timed, to create brain changes that can cure diseases. And the field is using even these small amounts more efficiently and intelligently.

Another form of invasiveness is whether one has to cut open the skull and insert something (as in deep brain stimulation [DBS]) or put the patient to sleep to deliver the charge (as in ECT). A trend we predict will continue is that the newer, noninvasive techniques replace or supplant older more invasive methods. DBS, which has had high clinical impact in movement disorders and developing (yet highly debated) evidence for treating depression, is an important neuromodulation tool. The specificity and subcortical depth at which DBS can stimulate cannot be matched with other current methods. However, 2 emerging less invasive methods, low-intensity focused ultrasound pulsations (LIFUP) and temporally interfering (TI) electric fields (EFs), have the potential to noninvasively stimulate focal locations deep in the brain (without surgery). We describe each of these and show how they may become disruptive brain stimulation methods in the near future.

Low-Intensity Focused Ultrasound Pulsation

LIFUP uses multiple ultrasound transducers in a cap placed on the scalp to produce high-frequency (100 Hz) sonications for 30 seconds at a time for 10 trains of pulses. Unlike traditional ultrasound, which constantly transmits ultrasound and listens to the echo to form an image, LIFUP delivers the ultrasound in packets or pulses. For reasons that are not clear, pulsed ultrasound causes neurons to depolarize and fire. Bones typically block ultrasound waves. Cleverly, however, one can deliver the ultrasound from multiple sources and use the skull as a lens, to actually shape and focus the convergent beam deeper in the brain. The clinical use of LIFUP thus uses MRI scans taken before stimulation to position and calculate how multiple ultrasonic pulsations will converge at a location in the brain (taking into account the bone dispersion of the beam from the skull). Because each transducer cannot individually cause neuronal discharge, neuronal firing can be focused both deep (2–12 cm under the cap; for comparison, traditional TMS can stimulate 1–3.4 cm^2 deep[10,11]) and focally (as small as 0.5 mm in diameter, and up to 1000 mm; the focality of a standard, commercially available 70-mm figure-of-8 TMS coil is roughly 50 mm^2[10,11]). Interestingly, the pulse width of the carrying frequency of LIFUP (0.5 ms) is strikingly similar to that used in all other pulsed neuromodulation therapies (DBS, 0.6 ms; ECT, 0.5 ms; TMS, 0.2 ms; vagal nerve stimulation [VNS], 0.5 ms), suggesting that this timeframe is mechanistically meaningful. This is a good example of the common background science of brain stimulation that transcends the individual methods.

Researchers have examined the effects of LIFUP in preclinical and clinical settings, confirming its ability to safely stimulate neural tissue,[12–15] proposing cellular mechanisms for its efficacy,[14–21] and now starting to use LIFUP in human patients. Monti and colleagues[22] (2016) described a case study in which they used LIFUP to stimulate a comatose patient's thalamus. Two pre-LIFUP assessments rated the patient as being in minimally conscious state. After sonication, the patient recovered motor and oromotor functions the next day, advancing to full language comprehension and communication by nodding and shaking his head. At 5 days post-LIFUP, the patient attempted to walk. Although this study was neither blinded nor sham controlled, the first application of therapeutic LIFUP in a human patient was encouraging and we expect more therapeutic applications of LIFUP and potential clinical trials in the future. If LIFUP continues to show clinical usefulness, it has the potential to supplant the role of DBS without the need for surgery. The key barrier to LIFUP replacing DBS for clinical applications is that, by and large, DBS is used in a manner where the device is inserted and turned constantly on without attempting to fundamentally change circuit dynamics or behavior so that you could remove the device. Obviously, patients cannot permanently wear a LIFUP helmet. However, to the degree that we learn how to stimulate in ways that permanently change circuit behavior (long-term depression or long-term potentiation) without ablation, we may be able to substitute several sessions of LIFUP that can train and rewire the brain instead of permanently implanting hardware. LIFUP can certainly stimulate deep and focal and noninvasively and, thus, may be a key next step in brain stimulation.

Temporally Interfering Electric Fields

Another potentially disruptive tool deserves mention in this discussion of future directions. Boyden and colleagues (2017) recently pioneered another brain stimulation approach that can noninvasively stimulate deep in the brain (at least of mice). This method, called TI EFs or temporal interference,[23] is similar to LIFUP in that it applies brain stimulation deep in the brain by using converging noninvasive sources of stimulation. However, the mechanism differs. Whereas LIFUP uses ultrasound sonications, TI uses very high-frequency ($\geq$1000 Hz) oscillating EFs applied at multiple locations on the scalp. Because all neurons (even in nonprimates) seem to apply a low-pass filter to electrical signals from the neural membrane (ie, neurons do not discharge from very high-frequency stimulation),[24] very-high frequency stimulation will not directly cause neuronal firing. Creatively drawing on this principle, Boyden's team applied 2 TI EFs to each side of a transgenic mouse's head, with each EF differing by only 10 Hz (sinusoidal currents at 2010 and 2000 Hz). They found that, where the EFs intersected, the effective stimulation frequency was the difference between the 2 higher frequencies (10 Hz). They demonstrated that this method could noninvasively stimulate deep brain regions in the mouse like the hippocampus. Like LIFUP, TI has the potential to treat brain disorders where stimulation of a deep pathologic locus might matter. Although no studies to date have investigated the use of TI in humans or animal disease models, barring some unexpected safety issue, TI may have translational applications in the near future. (Some researchers, however, are questioning whether this approach will actually work in a much larger human brain, with the increased volume of tissue. The intensity of current applied may need to be very high, perhaps similar to ECT. If this is true, one would likely have to perform TI under anesthesia, limiting to some degree the potential applications.) Nevertheless, the possibility of noninvasive focal stimulation without surgery is exciting.

Transcutaneous Auricular Nerve Stimulation

There is a developing noninvasive approach to targeting the vagus nerve called transcutaneous vagus nerve stimulation (also transcutaneous auricular nerve stimulation [taVNS] and for transcutaneous cervical nerve stimulation). As is the case with LIFUP and TI, taVNS obviates the need for surgical implantation of a brain stimulation (VNS) device. (Remember that cervical VNS largely involves surgery for implanting the electrode around the vagus and implanting the generator in the chest wall.) Reasoning that the auricular branch of the vagus nerve runs close to the middle third and lower third surface of the auricle, researchers have successfully stimulated the vagus nerve using ear clips. For a control site, they have stimulated nearby over the earlobe (which is not innervated by the vagal nerve).[25] taVNS increases blood flow to vagal afferent pathways[26,27] and can change resting state functional connectivity in depressed patients.[28,29] One sham-controlled study found taVNS-induced changes in cerebral blood flow to limbic and temporal brain structures (decreased activation in the amygdala, hippocampus, parahippocampal gyrus, and the middle and superior temporal gyrus; increased activation in the insula, precentral gyrus, and the thalamus) with concurrent mood improvements (as measured by the Adjective Mood Scale).[27] Finally, preliminary clinical evidence for taVNS in depression has been promising. To date, there have been 2 randomized, sham-controlled studies in taVNS for depression. One study enrolled 37 patients for 10 daily stimulation sessions, finding a 48% decrease in Beck Depression Inventory scores from pretreatment to posttreatment in the taVNS condition with no significant difference in the sham condition.[30] The other study enrolled 160 patients who underwent 4 to 12 weeks of daily, showing that 27% of taVNS patients were responders after 4 weeks, with no responders after 4 weeks in the sham condition.[31] One notable difference between the taVNS studies in depression and the much larger body of literature with implanted cervical VNS is that to date, researchers have only tested taVNS in "garden variety" depression (ie, not treatment-resistant depression). Moreover, cervical VNS seems to have slow onset of response but is markedly durable. No one has studied taVNS for more than 6 weeks.

In sum, taVNS holds potential as a noninvasive therapeutic neuromodulatory tool, with researchers continuing to explore further applications of this approach. Animal and now human studies have shown that pairing a behavior with vagus stimulation improves plasticity changes in the brain. Thus, researchers are now pairing cervical or auricular VNS with tones (to treat tinnitus) or speech rehabilitation (for aphasia).

Transcranial Direct Current Stimulation and Transcranial Alternating Current Stimulation

Last, there is a class of noninvasive neuromodulation methods that use a different strategy than all other forms of transcranial stimulation. Although ECT, TMS, LIFUP, and TI focus on directly causing neurons to fire, transcranial direct current stimulation (tDCS) passes low amounts of subthreshold electrical stimulation (typically 1-2 mA, but up to 4 mA of current) from an anode to a cathode on the scalp to increase the neuronal resting potential in brain regions near the electrode, making neurons more likely to fire. Because these forms of neuromodulation do not cause neuronal discharge, researchers often pair tDCS with a behavioral task, such as using cognitive–behavioral therapy with anodal left dorsolateral prefrontal cortex (DLPFC) stimulation for the treatment of depression.[32]

To date, tDCS has had mixed (and sometimes hotly contested) behavioral and therapeutic results in humans. Some tDCS reviews, such as one evaluating the effects of double-blind, sham-controlled studies using tDCS for major depression,[33] have suggested that tDCS has roughly the same effect size as TMS for depression. A recent metaanalysis for tDCS in depression, including only randomized, sham-controlled, double-blind studies lasting between 5 and 15 sessions, found significantly higher response (34% vs 19%) and remission (23.1% vs 12.7%) rates in active versus sham tDCS.[34] However, a recent international clinical trial found tDCS has only weak antidepressant effects.[35] In contrast, a series of tDCS reviews by Horvath and associates[36–39] in 2015 contend that tDCS has no cognitive or clinical benefit aside from changing TMS motor threshold Adding fuel to the controversy, a recent cadaver study using more than 200 implanted electrodes initially found that 1 to 2 mA of tDCS does not reach the cortex. Subsequent analyses in rat and human cadavers and patients suggest that 4 to 6 mA of current are necessary for 25% of the current to reach the cortex.[40,41] Disappointingly, much of the tDCS work to date may have been massively underdosed. Despite the varied literature, tDCS remains popular in experimental and potential neurotherapeutic use owing to its low cost (tDCS devices can be purchased for as little as $30) and favorable side effect profile (to date, tDCS has never caused a seizure[42]).

One potential explanation for the wide variance of tDCS findings is that, unlike every FDA-cleared therapeutic brain stimulation method, tDCS uniquely does not have a behavioral method for determining the needed dose within an individual. In contrast, we can calculate the seizure threshold for ECT,[43] motor threshold for TMS,[44–47] tremor suppression or dose titration for DBS,[48,49] and voice changes or sensation for VNS.[50] In the future, we expect that neuroscientists will evaluate how different measures, such as TMS motor threshold, can be used to determine and individualize tDCS dose for each patient. tDCS modeling, especially those based on each patient's MRI scan and taking into account the electrode sizes and location, could also help to inform stimulation parameters and individualized tDCS dosing.[51,52] Until we can determine for each subject whether tDCS is having a behavioral change, we predict it will struggle as a treatment modality despite its simplicity and low cost.

An even more recent development is a related form of low current electrical stimulation called transcranial alternating current stimulation (tACS). tACS passes sinusoidal, oscillating currents of 0.5 to 200 Hz and around 1 mA between 2 electrodes placed on the scalp and holds clinical promise, particularly in neurologic or psychiatric states in which there is a known oscillatory abnormality (eg, alpha frequency).[53] Frohlich and McCormick's[54] (2010) rigorous testing of oscillatory currents on different in vivo and in vitro ferret brain preparations highlighted certain stimulation parameters that seem to be crucial for efficacious tACS. Among these is the concept that weak exogenous oscillatory EFs can only entrain slow oscillations close to their intrinsic frequencies (a concept referred to as Arnold's tongue[55]). In the coming years, we expect more experiments to use tACS and further refine its potential therapeutic applications.

CONSIDERATION 2: HOW SMALL OR PRECISE SHOULD THE STIMULATION BE?

When using prefrontal TMS to treat depression, we do not yet have a method for precisely locating the best spot for treatment. In the absence of this, one company, Brainsway, has developed larger broader coils that stimulate bigger areas of cortex. It is unclear now whether there are differences in efficacy or side effects between the traditional figure-of-8 coils and the broader and deeper coils, but this difference highlights the issues involved in evermore focal or broad stimulation.

A broad, less precise stimulation method risks not only stimulating the desired region, but also other regions and circuits. These collateral circuits may produce unwanted side effects. Early work on this topic by Cohen Kadosh in 2013 suggests that tDCS to the left DLPFC that enhanced performance on a math task could come at the cognitive expense of another, symbol learning task.[56] This consideration that Cohen Kadosh raises in the realm of cognitive enhancement may never become truly germane to clinical conditions in which the potential benefit of the treatment (eg, remediating depression) will likely easily outweigh most possible side effects from the neuromodulation approach. However, we would not be surprised to see greater consideration of the side effects of neuromodulation, perhaps especially when neuropsychiatrists apply broader and deeper stimulation such as with the H-coil, in the future.

Will We Have Robots Delivering Brain Stimulation in the Future?

To our knowledge, no studies to date have examined the effects of TMS pulse precision versus dispersion and how this may affect clinical response in TMS for depression. Do you lose efficacy if the coil moves slightly within a session or from day to day? Highlighting the degree to which neuroscientists have considered this variable, they have already developed the technology for robotically delivered brain stimulation. Researchers are beginning to assess the use of robot-guided neuronavigated TMS, which can hold the coil position constant within 2 mm, even adjusting to the patient's head movements.[57] One clinical study investigated the use of robot-guided, neuronavigated 20-Hz TMS for the treatment of neuropathic pain, demonstrating a modest effect of treatment (77.5% of patients had a mean pain relief of 41% that lasted an average of 15.6 days). However, without a sham stimulation condition and with no comparison between robot-guided TMS and hand or coil arm-held TMS, it is difficult to assess how the 2 approaches differ, if at all. Another experiment thoroughly evaluated the EF induced in the brain in a 2 (coil holder vs robotized TMS that followed the head) × 3 (avoiding head motion, using a head rest, and moving the head freely) design.[58] Although the induced EF was greatly reduced for coil holder conditions (19.7%–32%), indicating less consistency between brain stimulation target from the start to end of the session, the robotized TMS only had reduced EFs of 1.4% to 4.9%. Furthermore, the orientation of the induced EF changed by 5.5° to 7.6° for the coil holder and only 0.2° to 0.4°, again demonstrating that a robotic coil holder results in greater consistency within a stimulation session. Whether this extra precision matters in clinical applications remains to be shown.

Other researchers looking at robot-guided neuronavigated TMS have suggested that the best utility in using this technology is assisting inexperienced users to accurately and reproducibly position the TMS coil.[59,60] We are intrigued by the prospect of automating TMS as well as other forms of brain stimulation.

CONSIDERATION 3: WILL USING CLOSED-LOOP STIMULATION WITH INDIVIDUAL TAILORING OF DOSE ALLOW WIDER ACCESSIBILITY TO QUALITY TREATMENTS AND MORE CONSISTENT OUTCOMES?

Another potential consideration in automating clinical TMS for depression or other conditions is whether closed-loop motor threshold finding would help to consistently dose treatment. The term closed loop implies a fully automated system that modifies the parameters or location of stimulation based on a biomarker, without any action by a human. To date, 1 study by Meincke and colleagues[61] (2016) examined the use of robotic coil positioning with a closed loop target search in a 7 × 7 grid around each participant's motor cortex. The robot moved a figure-of-8 coil around the grid in a randomized fashion, with a computer program recording the motor-evoked potential (MEP) from each stimulation location. Once an MEP-positive location was found (as defined by having ≥50 μV MEPs), the robot targeted adjacent targets in the grid. Once the robot stimulated each position in the grid, it delivered 15 pulses per MEP-positive location and estimated the motor threshold at each spot using an algorithm.[62]

One drawback to this study from Meincke and colleagues is the amount of time it took to locate the best possible motor hotspot. Although it may take trained TMS technicians less than 5 minutes, this closed-loop, robotized method took an average of 66 minutes. In the future, we are curious to see the effects of handheld, closed-loop motor threshold finding that requires fewer pulses per location to find the optimal motor hotspot in a timelier fashion and without the need for MRI scans or a TMS-delivering robot.

Closed loop systems are now being used with DBS for epilepsy (Neuropace, FDA approved), and Parkinson's disease. Many other closed loop DBS methods are being investigated, where stimulation is triggered by a biomarker from the patient (typically electroencephalography) and then the stimulation is also progressively modified to improve clinical outcomes. The same is being done with closed-loop tACS during sleep.[63]

CONSIDERATION 4: DISCOVERING THE BEST PATTERNS OF STIMULATION THAT CAN PRODUCE LONG-TERM AND LASTING THERAPEUTIC CHANGES (THE HOLY GRAIL)

As researchers increased the armamentarium of the neuromodulation toolbox, the field began to observe stark variance in the timing and durability of response between different types of stimulation. One of the authors of this article (MSG) previously wrote on this topic in 2010, positing that the time of onset response for a brain stimulation method and disease often correlates with the time of relapse if the method is stopped (ie, faster response, faster relapse).[64] Sackeim's rule, as some have called this, is an interesting hypothesis. If it is true, it reflects the underlying translational mechanisms of the brain stimulation therapy, and whether they are promoting and creating true durable plasticity and changes in the brain (axonal growth or neurogenesis), or rather creating quick, and likely temporary modifications of brain function. Herein we compare and contrast the timing of response and relapse for DBS, ECT, TMS (10 Hz and intermittent theta burst stimulation [iTBS]), and VNS, and discuss the methods researchers are using to delay or prevent relapse. In the future, we expect neuroscientists to study these relationships and adjust stimulation protocols to effect longer lasting neurologic and psychiatric change.

Deep Brain Stimulation

High-frequency DBS (>100 Hz) of the subthalamic nucleus has been a revelatory treatment for Parkinson's disease, with near immediate cessation of tremor in Parkinson's disease.[65,66] As long as the DBS device is in the brain and turned on (with adequate stimulation parameters), the tremor will be treated for many years. However, if a lead breaks or the battery depletes, the tremor returns almost immediately (starting within a few seconds and reaching maximum amplitude after just 2 minutes), in accordance with Sackeim's rule. That is, in general, using the common methods today, there is no durability of the therapeutic effect of DBS for tremor in Parkinson's disease beyond the instant of stimulation.

In contrast, the same technology, DBS, applied in much the same manner to treat dystonia, has a markedly slower onset of action over weeks to months, and the therapeutic effects do not always immediately return if the device malfunctions. Instead, the dystonic symptoms can take weeks to months to reemerge.[67,68] Even within 1 neuromodulation technique, GPi DBS (globus pallidus interna), for 2 different disorders, Sackeim's rule seems to hold true.

For depression, the DBS literature is more varied,[69,70] perhaps owing to multiple stimulation targets[71] (subgenual cingulate, ventral capsule, medial forebrain bundle, and nucleus accumbens). Although there may not be enough clinical studies to conclude much about the relationship between time of response and time of relapse, the seminal DBS study in depression by Mayberg and colleagues[72] (2005) included an interesting manipulation for one patient. After 6 months of subgenual cingulate DBS, the researchers turned the stimulation off for 4 weeks in a patient who had remitted, without telling the patient (Hamilton Depression Rating Scale [HAMD] score from 29 at baseline to 4 after 6 months of DBS). After 2 weeks of DBS off, the patient's HAMD was 9, and after 4 weeks, the HAMD was 10. After Mayberg and colleagues turned the DBS back on, the patient resumed stimulation and once again remitted.

Electroconvulsive Therapy

Considered to be the gold standard of neuromodulation for depression, ECT has a very high remission rate (around 70%) in even highly treatment-resistant patients.[73] ECT patients also respond to treatment quickly, with 54% of patients having a 50%

or greater decrease in their HAMD score after just 3 treatments.[74] However, in line with Sackeim's observation, this fast response tends to come with a quick relapse if nothing else is done, with more than 50% of patients relapsing within 6 months.[75,76] Researchers have investigated different ways to mitigate this steep drop-off in HAMD score, with continuation (maintenance) ECT treatments once every few weeks as a promising possibility,[77–81] with a consensus paper published in 2018 recommending maintenance ECT and pharmacology to prevent or delay relapse.[82] The use of maintenance brain stimulation that attempts to retain the effects of treatment after the induction course is over is a common trend (as discussed in the 10-Hz TMS section elsewhere in this article), and we expect to see further investigation and refinement in this area.

Ten-Hertz Transcranial Magnetic Stimulation

If DBS and ECT are paragons of fast response-fast relapse neuromodulation, high-frequency (10 Hz) TMS for depression seems to have a more moderate timing of response and relapse, particularly when clinics use maintenance TMS.

A large, multisite, retrospective, naturalistic study by Carpenter and colleagues[83] (2012) used standard high frequency (10-Hz) prefrontal TMS for depression found that after 30 sessions (6 weeks), 58.0% of the 307 patients treated met the criteria for response. Another study by Cohen and colleagues[84] (2009) tracked depression patients throughout their treatment course and through 6 months after treatment. Of greatest interest to Fregni's group was monitoring the durability of remission to TMS for depression in 204 of the 474 patients treated for depression. Of the patients who remitted (HAMD score of <8), the improvement in mood lasted an average of 119.3 days, with 75.3% at 2 months, 60.0% at 3 months, 42.7% at 4 months, and 22.6% at 6 months retaining the effect.

One important consideration with 10-Hz TMS, as with ECT, is whether maintenance TMS treatments can prevent or delay relapse.[85,86] One study by Janicak and colleagues[86] (2010), offered TMS patients maintenance treatment when patients met criteria for symptom worsening and followed their outcomes up to 24 weeks after acute TMS treatment. With maintenance treatment, only 10 of 99 patients (10.1%) relapsed. Although there was no sham control or statistical comparison to nonmaintenance durability of TMS treatments, the evidence was compelling enough for maintenance TMS to become fairly commonplace among TMS clinics worldwide.

Intermittent Theta Burst Stimulation

There may not be a more enticing new neuromodulation stimulation method on the potential verge of large-scale clinical trials than iTBS. TBS, first developed by Huang and colleagues[87] (2005), mimics endogenous hippocampal neuronal firing by using 50 bursts per second of 3 pulses each, delivered at the theta frequency of 5 Hz.[88] Theta burst exists in 2 varieties: intermittent or iTBS, which delivers theta bursts for 2 seconds each with 8 seconds in between trains (eg, 20 trains of iTBS given over 200 seconds), and continuous TBS (cTBS), which delivers theta bursts all at once (eg, 40 seconds of cTBS for 600 pulses). Based on how iTBS and cTBS, respectively, enhanced and suppressed the size of the MEPs from the motor cortex, iTBS is viewed as long-term potentiation like and cTBS is considered to be long-term depression like, although the evidence from varying stimulation parameters (eg, comparing 600 vs 1200 pulses of iTBS and cTBS) seem to be less consistent.[89]

Clinically, iTBS over the left DLPFC has shown potential for treating depression.[90] Although the inferences we can draw from most of these initial studies are limited by their lack of double-blind and sham-controlled experimental designs, there are several compelling themes to note.

First, iTBS seems to have similar clinical TMS effects as 10-Hz TMS with far fewer pulses. One study by Bakker and colleagues[91] (2015) retrospectively compared the response and timing of response in 185 major depression patients who had received once daily clinical 10 Hz TMS (n = 98; 6000 pulses per day) or iTBS (n = 87; 1200 pulses per day) treatments over the prefrontal cortex over several weeks and showed nearly indistinguishable rates of response between the 2 conditions (50.6% response for 10 Hz; 48.5% response for iTBS), which improved almost identically by week and from the end of treatment (4 weeks) to posttreatment (taken 8 weeks after treatment cessation). At 8 weeks posttreatment, the durability of the antidepressant effects of 10 Hz TMS and iTBS were indistinguishable (both groups retained antidepressant effects). In sum, iTBS intriguingly had roughly the same clinical effect, at least initially, with far fewer pulses (20% of the amount of pulses in the 10-Hz TMS condition). A more recent randomized but still not double-blind study shows no clinical difference between theta burst TMS (600 pulses, 5 minutes for each session) and conventional TMS (3000 pulses, 20 minutes).[92]

Second, within iTBS, the timing of response and relapse both seem to follow Sackeim's rule but can change based on how often stimulation occurs (ie, once daily treatments vs multisession/day treatments).

Williams and colleagues[93] (2018) recently published a study that tested the effects of neuronavigated, high-dose iTBS for depression (1800 pulses per session at 90% of resting motor threshold, for 10 sessions per day and 5 days for 90,000 total pulses). Six patients with highly treatment-resistant depression (each patient had undergone at least 1 course of ECT and 1 course of 10-Hz TMS, with an average duration of illness of 32 years, and failure to respond to conventional psychotherapy and pharmacology) underwent treatment with remarkable effects. Five of 6 patients met criterion for response (mean HAMD scores for all patients decreasing from 28.8 to 7.0), and 4 met the criterion for remission (HAMD scores <7). However, of the 5 patients who responded to the treatment, only one retained a 50% improvement in HAMD score for 2 weeks after treatment, and no patients met criterion for remission (lowest HAMD, 14; mean HAMD, 19.3).

With no sham control, it is not possible to definitively affirm Sackeim's rule in this case because the initial response and remission could have been due to a placebo effect. However, these preliminary data are a compelling addition to the fast response, fast relapse mantra and are particularly interesting because the method of application within a single form of neuromodulation (iTBS) seems to determine the durability of response. We expect future studies to investigate how to optimize iTBS treatment for depression and whether it is possible to mitigate the tradeoff between timing of response and relapse (perhaps through maintenance iTBS treatments).

Vagus Nerve Stimulation

Building on pioneering animal work in the mid-1980s demonstrating the anticonvulsive utility of VNS in animals,[94–96] multiple research groups demonstrated the therapeutic antiepileptic[97–99] utility of VNS for humans. Anecdotal mood improvements secondary to anticonvulsive activity and PET imaging studies[100] hinted at its potential therapeutic value for depression.[101–103] On the Sackeim's rule continuum, VNS for depression falls on the deep end of slow response, slow relapse. The therapeutic effects take several months to occur but seems to be quite durable over several years with continued treatment.[104–107] One study by Aaronson and colleagues[108] (2017), followed VNS patient outcomes (based on percentage of patients meeting response or remission criteria on the Montgomery-Asberg Depression Rating Scale) in 3-month intervals for 5 years after VNS implantation. Notably, it took 12 months for roughly 50% of VNS patients to reach response criteria (slow response), but patients continued to improve between each 3-month interval over a treatment-as-usual control condition, with nearly 70% of patients reaching response criteria at 5 years after VNS implantation (slow relapse rate and high durability of antidepressant effects).

CONSIDERATION 5: COMBINING BRAIN STIMULATION WITH SPECIFIC BRAIN ACTIVITY TO MOST EFFECTIVELY ENGAGE CIRCUITS AND MODIFY BEHAVIOR

This is a relatively simple and obvious concept, and many studies now confirm that coupling behavioral activation with stimulation produces better clinical effects than either alone. Hebb was correct.

CONSIDERATION 6: ARE THERE IMPORTANT BIOMARKERS OR OTHER VARIABLES THAT PREDICT THERAPEUTIC RESPONSE TO NEUROMODULATION? HOW CAN WE USE THESE FACTORS TO INDIVIDUALIZE TREATMENT?

Because not every patient responds to neuromodulation treatment, neuroscientists aim to identify if there are biomarkers or other predictors of response. There are many enticing possibilities that may assist the selection of treatment targets and which patients may be most suited to receive TMS or other neurotherapeutics, and we discuss two of the factors herein.

Neuroscientists have almost exclusively used functional neuroimaging, such as PET and functional MRI, for retrospective descriptive and observational purposes. However, there is a growing body of work focusing on how intrinsic functional connectivity (ie, how different regions of the brain tend to correlate or anticorrelate in activity) can be used to prospectively determine TMS targets. Fox and colleagues[109] (2012) were among the first investigators to test how the TMS target for clinically treated depression patients using the 5-cm rule, and its functional connectivity to the subgenual cingulate, differed between responders and nonresponders. His research group found that the more effective stimulation site was significantly more anticorrelated with the subgenual cingulate, suggesting that these results could be applied prospectively to determine the best possible stimulation target. Prospective applications of these findings have confirmed that greater anticorrelation between the DLPFC and subgenual cingulate correlate with better response to TMS for depression and that TMS changes the connectivity between the default mode and frontoparietal central execute networks.[110] In the future, we expect more research in the area of how neuroimaging can prospectively influence TMS targets as the field of neuromodulation trends toward more refinement and higher individualization of treatment. It will be interesting to see if neuropsychiatrists someday base stimulation targets on each individual's intrinsic functional connectivity. Although this is theoretically feasible, our laboratory's neuroimaging experts estimate that, with the current technology, there would be a serious cost–benefit ratio to weigh, with the prerequisite time experimenters need to assess for an individual's functional connectivity to reveal itself being around 90 minutes in the scanner.

Building on what Fox and others have found, Drysdale and colleagues[111] (2017) set out to identify different biotypes (neurophysiologic subtypes based on different patterns of dysfunctional connectivity in limbic and frontostriatal networks) in depression. To do this, the authors applied a machine learning algorithm that clustered patients into distinct groups based on whole-brain patterns of abnormal functional connectivity. This identified 2 groups of network patterns that either involved frontal/orbitofrontal areas or the limbic system (amygdala, subgenual cingulate, lateral prefrontal cortex, ventral hippocampus, and ventral striatum). On top of core depressive symptoms, the researchers identified which connectivity features correlated with different items on the HAMD inventory and further delineated the depressive subtypes into 4 biotypes.

Of the top core clinical features of depression that the 4 biotypes shared (eg, low mood, anhedonia, fatigue, and lack of energy that are associated with the insula, orbitofrontal cortex, ventromedial prefrontal cortex, and various subcortical areas), they differed on other clinical symptoms. Notably, types 1 and 4 had increased anxiety, types 3 and 4 had greater anhedonia and psychomotor slowing, and types 1 and 2 had lower energy and more fatigue, which all significantly correlated with brain activity in affiliated regions. Most intriguing to the field of neuromodulation, the authors identified which biotypes responded best to 10-Hz clinical rTMS, which greatly differed among groups. Although the majority of biotype 1 (82.5%) and biotype 3 (61.0%) patients had a 25% or greater decrease in HAMD score from TMS, only 25.0% and 29.6% in biotypes 2 and 4 had similar improvements. Moving forward, we expect that the push toward greater individualization of treatment will continue. If it is not currently feasible to have each patient get an MRI scan before treatment, perhaps biotyping based on HAMD responses could assist in identifying which patients will respond. Notably, clinical symptoms did not track well with the imaging-defined biotypes.

SUMMARY

Brain stimulation methods use the brain's currency (electricity) to precisely change neuronal firing. Because of the focal nature of the intervention, there are no drug–drug interactions. The amount of energy these approaches use is rather modest, and often thousands (even millions) of times less than what the brain is using in the same amount of time as a treatment. New methods are surfacing each year and surely more technologies and treatment strategies are on the way.

REFERENCES

1. Sakel M. A new treatment of schizophrenia. Am J Psychiatry 1937;93(4):829–41.
2. Fink M, Ladislas J. Meduna, M.D. 1896–1964. Am J Psychiatry 1999;156(11): 1807.
3. Gazdag G, Bitter I, Ungvari GS, et al. Laszlo Meduna's pilot studies with camphor inductions of seizures: the first 11 patients. J ECT 2009;25(1):3–11.
4. Endler NS. The origins of electroconvulsive therapy (ECT). Convuls Ther 1988; 4(1):5–23.
5. Merton PA, Morton HB. Stimulation of the cerebral cortex in the intact human subject. Nature 1980;285:227.
6. Merton PA, Morton HB. Electrical stimulation of human motor and visual cortex through the scalp. Proc Aust Physiol Pharmacol Soc 1980;305:9–10.
7. Merton PA, Hill DK, Morton HB, et al. Scope of a technique for electrical stimulation of human brain, spinal cord, and muscle. Lancet 1982;2(8298):597–600.
8. George MS, Wassermann EM, Williams WA, et al. Daily repetitive Transcranial Magnetic Stimulation (rTMS) improves mood in depression. Neuroreport 1995; 6:1853–6.
9. George MS, Lisanby SH, Avery D, et al. Daily left prefrontal transcranial magnetic stimulation therapy for major depressive disorder: a sham-controlled randomized trial. Arch Gen Psychiatry 2010;67(5):507–16.

10. Hanlon C. Blunt or precise? A note about the relative precision of figure-of-eight rTMS coils. Brain Stimul 2017;10(2):338–9.

11. Deng ZD, Lisanby SH, Peterchev AV. Electric field depth-focality tradeoff in transcranial magnetic stimulation: simulation comparison of 50 coil designs. Brain Stimul 2013;6(1):1–13.

12. Tufail Y, Matyushov A, Baldwin N, et al. Transcranial pulsed ultrasound stimulates intact brain circuits. Neuron 2010;66(5):681–94.

13. Yoo S-S, Bystritsky A, Lee J-H, et al. Focused ultrasound modulates region-specific brain activity. Neuroimage 2011;56(3):1267–75.

14. Min BK, Yang PS, Bohlke M, et al. Focused ultrasound modulates the level of cortical neurotransmitters: potential as a new functional brain mapping technique. Int J Imaging Syst Technol 2011;21(2):232–40.

15. Tyler WJ, Tufail Y, Finsterwald M, et al. Remote excitation of neuronal circuits using low-intensity, low-frequency ultrasound. PLoS One 2008;3(10):e3511.

16. Yang PS, Kim H, Lee W, et al. Transcranial focused ultrasound to the thalamus is associated with reduced extracellular GABA levels in rats. Neuropsychobiology 2012;65(3):153–60.

17. Choi JB, Lim SH, Cho KW, et al. The effect of focused ultrasonic stimulation on the activity of hippocampal neurons in multi-channel electrode. Paper presented at: Neural Engineering (NER), 2013 6th International IEEE/EMBS Conference on, Osaka, Japan, July 3–7, 2013.

18. Wahab RA, Choi M, Liu Y, et al. Mechanical bioeffects of pulsed high intensity focused ultrasound on a simple neural model. Med Phys 2012;39(7Part1): 4274–83.

19. Krasovitski B, Frenkel V, Shoham S, et al. Intramembrane cavitation as a unifying mechanism for ultrasound-induced bioeffects. Proc Natl Acad Sci U S A 2011; 108(8):3258–63.

20. Plaksin M, Shoham S, Kimmel E. Intramembrane cavitation as a predictive bio-piezoelectric mechanism for ultrasonic brain stimulation. Phys Rev X 2014;4(1): 011004.

21. Schiff ND, Giacino JT, Kalmar K, et al. Behavioural improvements with thalamic stimulation after severe traumatic brain injury. Nature 2007; 448(7153):600.

22. Monti MM, Schnakers C, Korb AS, et al. Non-invasive ultrasonic thalamic stimulation in disorders of consciousness after severe brain injury: a first-in-man report. Brain Stimul 2016;9(6):940–1.

23. Grossman N, Bono D, Dedic N, et al. Noninvasive deep brain stimulation via temporally interfering electric fields. Cell 2017;169(6):1029–41.e16.

24. Hutcheon B, Yarom Y. Resonance, oscillation and the intrinsic frequency preferences of neurons. Trends Neurosci 2000;23(5):216–22.

25. Fallgatter A, Neuhauser B, Herrmann M, et al. Far field potentials from the brain stem after transcutaneous vagus nerve stimulation. J Neural Transm 2003; 110(12):1437–43.

26. Dietrich S, Smith J, Scherzinger C, et al. A novel transcutaneous vagus nerve stimulation leads to brainstem and cerebral activations measured by functional MRI/Funktionelle Magnetresonanztomographie zeigt Aktivierungen des Hirnstamms und weiterer zerebraler Strukturen unter transkutaner Vagusnervstimulation. Biomed Tech (Berl) 2008;53(3):104–11.

27. Kraus T, Hösl K, Kiess O, et al. BOLD fMRI deactivation of limbic and temporal brain structures and mood enhancing effect by transcutaneous vagus nerve stimulation. J Neural Transm 2007;114(11):1485–93.

28. Fang J, Rong P, Hong Y, et al. Transcutaneous vagus nerve stimulation modulates default mode network in major depressive disorder. Biol Psychiatry 2016;79(4):266–73.
29. Liu J, Fang J, Wang Z, et al. Transcutaneous vagus nerve stimulation modulates amygdala functional connectivity in patients with depression. J Affect Disord 2016;205:319–26.
30. Hein E, Nowak M, Kiess O, et al. Auricular transcutaneous electrical nerve stimulation in depressed patients: a randomized controlled pilot study. J Neural Transm 2013;120(5):821–7.
31. Rong P, Liu J, Wang L, et al. Effect of transcutaneous auricular vagus nerve stimulation on major depressive disorder: a nonrandomized controlled pilot study. J Affect Disord 2016;195:172–9.
32. D'Urso G, Mantovani A, Micillo M, et al. Transcranial direct current stimulation and cognitive-behavioral therapy: evidence of a synergistic effect in treatment-resistant depression. Brain Stimul 2013;6(3):465–7.
33. Shiozawa P, Fregni F, Benseñor IM, et al. Transcranial direct current stimulation for major depression: an updated systematic review and meta-analysis. Int J Neuropsychopharmacol 2014;17(9):1443–52.
34. Brunoni AR, Moffa AH, Fregni F, et al. Transcranial direct current stimulation for acute major depressive episodes: meta-analysis of individual patient data. Br J Psychiatry 2016;208(6):522–31.
35. Brunoni AR, Moffa AH, Sampaio-Junior B, et al. Trial of electrical direct-current therapy versus escitalopram for depression. N Engl J Med 2017;376(26):2523–33.
36. Horvath JC. New quantitative analyses following Price & Hamilton's critique do not change original findings of Horvath et al. Brain Stimul 2015;8(3):665–6.
37. Horvath JC. Are current blinding methods for transcranial direct current stimulation (tDCS) effective in healthy populations? Clin Neurophysiol 2015;126(11):2045–6.
38. Horvath JC, Forte JD, Carter O. Quantitative review finds no evidence of cognitive effects in healthy populations from single-session transcranial direct current stimulation (tDCS). Brain Stimul 2015;8(3):535–50.
39. Horvath JC, Forte JD, Carter O. Evidence that transcranial direct current stimulation (tDCS) generates little-to-no reliable neurophysiologic effect beyond MEP amplitude modulation in healthy human subjects: a systematic review. Neuropsychologia 2015;66:213–36.
40. Vöröslakos M, Takeuchi Y, Brinyiczki K, et al. Direct effects of transcranial electric stimulation on brain circuits in rats and humans. Nat Commun 2018;9(1):483.
41. Chhatbar PY, Kautz SA, Takacs I, et al. Evidence of transcranial direct current stimulation-generated electric fields at subthalamic level in human brain in vivo. Brain Stimul 2018. [Epub ahead of print].
42. Bikson M, Grossman P, Thomas C, et al. Safety of transcranial direct current stimulation: evidence based update 2016. Brain Stimul 2017;10(5):983–5.
43. van Waarde JA, van Oudheusden LJ, Tonino BA, et al. MRI characteristics predicting seizure threshold in patients undergoing electroconvulsive therapy: a prospective study. Brain Stimul 2013;6(4):607–14.
44. Herbsman T, Forster L, Molnar C, et al. Motor threshold in transcranial magnetic stimulation: the impact of white matter fiber orientation and skull-to-cortex distance. Hum Brain Mapp 2009;30(7):2044 55.
45. Anderson BS, George MS. A review of studies comparing methods for determining transcranial magnetic stimulation motor threshold: observation of

movement or electromyography assisted. J Am Psychiatr Nurses Assoc 2009; 15(5):304–13.

46. Mishory A, Molnar C, Koola J, et al. The maximum-likelihood strategy for determining transcranial magnetic stimulation motor threshold, using parameter estimation by sequential testing is faster than conventional methods with similar precision. J ECT 2004;20(3):160–5.

47. Kozel FA, Nahas Z, DeBrux C, et al. How the distance from coil to cortex relates to age, motor threshold and possibly the antidepressant response to repetitive transcranial magnetic stimulation. J Neuropsychiatry Clin Neurosci 2000;12: 376–84.

48. Lozano AM. Deep brain stimulation therapy. BMJ 2012;344:e1100.

49. Schwalb JM, Hamani C. The history and future of deep brain stimulation. Neurotherapeutics 2008;5(1):3–13.

50. George MS, Sackeim HA, Rush AJ, et al. Vagus nerve stimulation: a new tool for brain research and therapy. Biol Psychiatry 2000;47:287–95.

51. Truong DQ, Hüber M, Xie X, et al. Clinician accessible tools for GUI computational models of transcranial electrical stimulation: BONSAI and SPHERES. Brain Stimul 2014;7(4):521–4.

52. Huang Y, Datta A, Bikson M, et al. Realistic vOlumetric-Approach to Simulate Transcranial Electric Stimulation–ROAST–a fully automated open-source pipeline. [Epub ahead of print].

53. Herrmann CS, Rach S, Neuling T, et al. Transcranial alternating current stimulation: a review of the underlying mechanisms and modulation of cognitive processes. Front Hum Neurosci 2013;7:279.

54. Frohlich F, McCormick DA. Endogenous electric fields may guide neocortical network activity. Neuron 2010;67(1):129–43.

55. Frohlich F. Tuning out the blues–thalamo-cortical rhythms as a successful target for treating depression. Brain Stimul 2015;8(6):1007–9.

56. Iuculano T, Kadosh RC. The mental cost of cognitive enhancement. J Neurosci 2013;33(10):4482–6.

57. Lancaster JL, Narayana S, Wenzel D, et al. Evaluation of an image-guided, robotically positioned transcranial magnetic stimulation system. Hum Brain Mapp 2004;22(4):329–40.

58. Richter L, Trillenberg P, Schweikard A, et al. Stimulus intensity for hand held and robotic transcranial magnetic stimulation. Brain Stimulation: Basic Translational, Clin Res Neuromodulation 2013;6(3):315–21.

59. Richter L, Bruder R, Schweikard A. Hand-assisted positioning and contact pressure control for motion compensated robotized transcranial magnetic stimulation. Int J Comput Assist Radiol Surg 2012;7(6):845–52.

60. Ginhoux R, Renaud P, Zorn L, et al. A custom robot for transcranial magnetic stimulation: first assessment on healthy subjects. Paper presented at: Engineering in Medicine and Biology Society (EMBC), 2013 35th Annual International Conference of the IEEE, 2013.

61. Meincke J, Hewitt M, Batsikadze G, et al. Automated TMS hotspot-hunting using a closed loop threshold-based algorithm. NeuroImage 2016;124: 509–17.

62. Awiszus F. TMS and threshold hunting. Supplements to clinical neurophysiology, vol. 56. Amsterdam (The Netherlands): Elsevier; 2003. p. 13–23.

63. Lustenberger C, Boyle MR, Alagapan S, et al. Feedback-controlled transcranial alternating current stimulation reveals a functional role of sleep spindles in motor memory consolidation. Curr Biol 2016;26(16):2127–36.

64. George MS. Time course of therapeutic response, and durability, of the different brain stimulation methods–from the Editor-in Chief's desk. Brain Stimul 2010; 3(4):185–6.
65. Blahak C, Bazner H, Capelle HH, et al. Rapid response of parkinsonian tremor to STN-DBS changes: direct modulation of oscillatory basal ganglia activity? Mov Disord 2009;24(8):1221–5.
66. Cooper SE, Kuncel AM, Wolgamuth BR, et al. A model predicting optimal parameters for deep brain stimulation in essential tremor. J Clin Neurophysiol 2008;25(5):265–73.
67. Pretto TE, Dalvi A, Kang UJ, et al. A prospective blinded evaluation of deep brain stimulation for the treatment of secondary dystonia and primary torticollis syndromes. J Neurosurg 2008;109(3):405–9.
68. Isaias IU, Alterman RL, Tagliati M. Deep brain stimulation for primary generalized dystonia: long-term outcomes. Arch Neurol 2009;66(4):465–70.
69. Kennedy SH, Giacobbe P, Rizvi SJ, et al. Deep brain stimulation for treatment-resistant depression: follow-up after 3 to 6 years. Am J Psychiatry 2011;168(5): 502–10.
70. Dougherty DD, Rezai AR, Carpenter LL, et al. A randomized sham-controlled trial of deep brain stimulation of the ventral capsule/ventral striatum for chronic treatment-resistant depression. Biol Psychiatry 2015;78(4):240–8.
71. Zhou C, Zhang H, Qin Y, et al. A systematic review and meta-analysis of deep brain stimulation in treatment-resistant depression. Prog Neuropsychopharmacol Biol Psychiatry 2018;82:224–32.
72. Mayberg HS, Lozano AM, Voon V, et al. Deep brain stimulation for treatment-resistant depression. Neuron 2005;45(5):651–60.
73. Petrides G, Fink M, Husain MM, et al. ECT remission rates in psychotic versus nonpsychotic depressed patients: a report from CORE. J ECT 2001;17(4): 244–53.
74. Husain MM, Rush AJ, Fink M, et al. Speed of response and remission in major depressive disorder with acute electroconvulsive therapy (ECT): a Consortium for Research in ECT (CORE) report. J Clin Psychiatry 2004;65(4): 485–91.
75. Sackeim HA, Haskett RF, Mulsant BH, et al. Continuation pharmacotherapy in the prevention of relapse following electroconvulsive therapy: a randomized controlled trial. JAMA 2002;285:1299–307.
76. Tew JD Jr, Mulsant BH, Haskett RF, et al. Relapse during continuation pharmacotherapy after acute response to ECT: a comparison of usual care versus protocolized treatment. Ann Clin Psychiatry 2007;19(1):1–4.
77. Elias A, Phutane VH, Clarke S, et al. Electroconvulsive therapy in the continuation and maintenance treatment of depression: systematic review and meta-analyses. Aust N Z J Psychiatry 2018;52(5):415–24.
78. Brown ED, Lee H, Scott D, et al. Efficacy of continuation/maintenance electroconvulsive therapy for the prevention of recurrence of a major depressive episode in adults with unipolar depression: a systematic review. J ECT 2014; 30(3):195–202.
79. Rodriguez-Jimenez R, Bagney A, Torio I, et al. Clinical usefulness and economic implications of continuation/maintenance electroconvulsive therapy in a Spanish National Health System public hospital: a case series. Rev Psiquiatr Salud Ment 2015;8(2).75–82.
80. McCall WV. Finally, evidence for continuation electroconvulsive therapy in major depressive disorder. J ECT 2016;32(4):221.

81. Jelovac A, Kolshus E, McLoughlin DM. Relapse following successful electrocon-vulsive therapy for major depression: a meta-analysis. Neuropsychopharmacol-ogy 2013;38(12):2467.

82. Gill SP, Kellner CH. Clinical practice recommendations for continuation and maintenance electroconvulsive therapy for depression: outcomes from a review of the evidence and a consensus workshop held in Australia in May 2017. J ECT 2018. [Epub ahead of print].

83. Carpenter LL, Janicak PG, Aaronson ST, et al. Transcranial Magnetic Stimulation (TMS) for major depression: a multisite, naturalistic, observational study of acute treatment outcomes in clinical practice. Depress Anxiety 2012;29(7):587–96.

84. Cohen RB, Boggio PS, Fregni F. Risk factors for relapse after remission with re-petitive transcranial magnetic stimulation for the treatment of depression. Depress Anxiety 2009;26(7):682–8.

85. Li X, Nahas Z, Anderson B, et al. Can left prefrontal rTMS be used as a mainte-nance treatment for bipolar depression? Depress Anxiety 2004;20(2):98–100.

86. Janicak PG, Nahas Z, Lisanby SH, et al. Durability of clinical benefit with trans-cranial magnetic stimulation (TMS) in the treatment of pharmacoresistant major depression: assessment of relapse during a 6-month, multisite, open-label study. Brain Stimul 2010;3(4):187–99.

87. Larson J, Lynch G. Induction of synaptic potentiation in hippocampus by patterned stimulation involves two events. Science 1986;232(4753):985–8.

88. Huang Y-Z, Edwards MJ, Rounis E, et al. Theta burst stimulation of the human motor cortex. Neuron 2005;45(2):201–6.

89. Gamboa OL, Antal A, Moliadze V, et al. Simply longer is not better: reversal of theta burst after-effect with prolonged stimulation. Exp Brain Res 2010;204(2):181–7.

90. Li C-T, Chen M-H, Juan C-H, et al. Efficacy of prefrontal theta-burst stimulation in refractory depression: a randomized sham-controlled study. Brain 2014;137(7):2088–98.

91. Bakker N, Shahab S, Giacobbe P, et al. rTMS of the dorsomedial prefrontal cor-tex for major depression: safety, tolerability, effectiveness, and outcome predic-tors for 10 Hz versus intermittent theta-burst stimulation. Brain Stimul 2015;8(2):208–15.

92. Blumberger DM, Vila-Rodriguez F, Thorpe KE, et al. Effectiveness of theta burst versus high-frequency repetitive transcranial magnetic stimulation in patients with depression (THREE-D): a randomised non-inferiority trial. Lancet 2018;391(10131):1683–92.

93. Williams NR, Sudheimer KD, Bentzley BS, et al. High-dose spaced theta-burst TMS as a rapid-acting antidepressant in highly refractory depression. Brain 2018;141(3):e18.

94. Zabara J. Peripheral control of hypersynchronous discharges in epilepsy. Elec-troencephalogr Clin Neurophysiol 1985;61:5162.

95. Zabara J. Time course of seizure control to brief, repetitive stimuli. Epilepsia 1985;26:518.

96. Zabara J. Inhibition of experimental seizures in canines by repetitive vagal stim-ulation. Epilepsia 1992;33(6):1005–12.

97. Penry JK, Dean JC. Prevention of intractable partial seizures by intermittent vagal stimulation in humans: preliminary results. Epilepsia 1990;31(s2):S40–3.

98. Ben-Menachem E, Mañon-Espaillat R, Ristanovic R, et al. Vagus nerve stimula-tion for treatment of partial seizures: 1. A controlled study of effect on seizures. Epilepsia 1994;35(3):616–26.

99. Handforth A, DeGiorgio C, Schachter S, et al. Vagus nerve stimulation therapy for partial-onset seizures A randomized active-control trial. Neurology 1998; 51(1):48–55.

100. Henry TR, Bakay RA, Votaw JR, et al. Brain blood flow alterations induced by therapeutic vagus nerve stimulation in partial epilepsy: I. Acute effects at high and low levels of stimulation. Epilepsia 1998;39(9):983–90.

101. Rush AJ, George MS, Sackeim HA, et al. Vagus nerve stimulation (VNS) for treatment-resistant depressions: a multicenter study. Biol Psychiatry 2000; 47(4):276–86.

102. Sackeim HA, Rush AJ, George MS, et al. Vagus nerve stimulation (VNS™) for treatment-resistant depression: efficacy, side effects, and predictors of outcome. Neuropsychopharmacology 2001;25(5):713–28.

103. George MS, Rush AJ, Marangell LB, et al. A one-year comparison of vagus nerve stimulation with treatment as usual for treatment-resistant depression. Biol Psychiatry 2005;58(5):364–73.

104. Sackeim HA, Brannan SK, Rush AJ, et al. Durability of antidepressant response to vagus nerve stimulation (VNS). Int J Neuropsychopharmacol 2007;10(6): 817–26.

105. Rush AJ, Sackeim HA, Marangell LB, et al. Effects of 12 months of vagus nerve stimulation in treatment-resistant depression: a naturalistic study. Biol Psychiatry 2005;58(5):355–63.

106. Rush AJ, Marangell LB, Sackeim HA, et al. Vagus nerve stimulation for treatment-resistant depression: a randomized, controlled acute phase trial. Biol Psychiatry 2005;58(5):347–54.

107. Nahas Z, Marangell LB, Husain MM, et al. Two-year outcome of vagus nerve stimulation (VNS) for treatment of major depressive episodes. J Clin Psychiatry 2005;66(9):1097–104.

108. Aaronson ST, Sears P, Ruvuna F, et al. A 5-year observational study of patients with treatment-resistant depression treated with vagus nerve stimulation or treatment as usual: comparison of response, remission, and suicidality. Am J Psychiatry 2017;174(7):640–8.

109. Fox MD, Buckner RL, White MP, et al. Efficacy of transcranial magnetic stimulation targets for depression is related to intrinsic functional connectivity with the subgenual cingulate. Biol Psychiatry 2012;72(7):595–603.

110. Liston C, Chen AC, Zebley BD, et al. Default mode network mechanisms of transcranial magnetic stimulation in depression. Biol Psychiatry 2014;76(7): 517–26.

111. Drysdale AT, Grosenick L, Downar J, et al. Resting-state connectivity biomarkers define neurophysiological subtypes of depression. Nat Med 2017;23(1):28.

Moving?

Make sure your subscription moves with you!

To notify us of your new address, find your **Clinics Account Number** (located on your mailing label above your name), and contact customer service at:

Email: journalscustomerservice-usa@elsevier.com

800-654-2452 (subscribers in the U.S. & Canada)
314-447-8871 (subscribers outside of the U.S. & Canada)

Fax number: 314-447-8029

**Elsevier Health Sciences Division
Subscription Customer Service
3251 Riverport Lane
Maryland Heights, MO 63043**

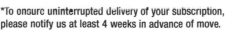

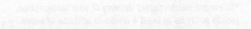